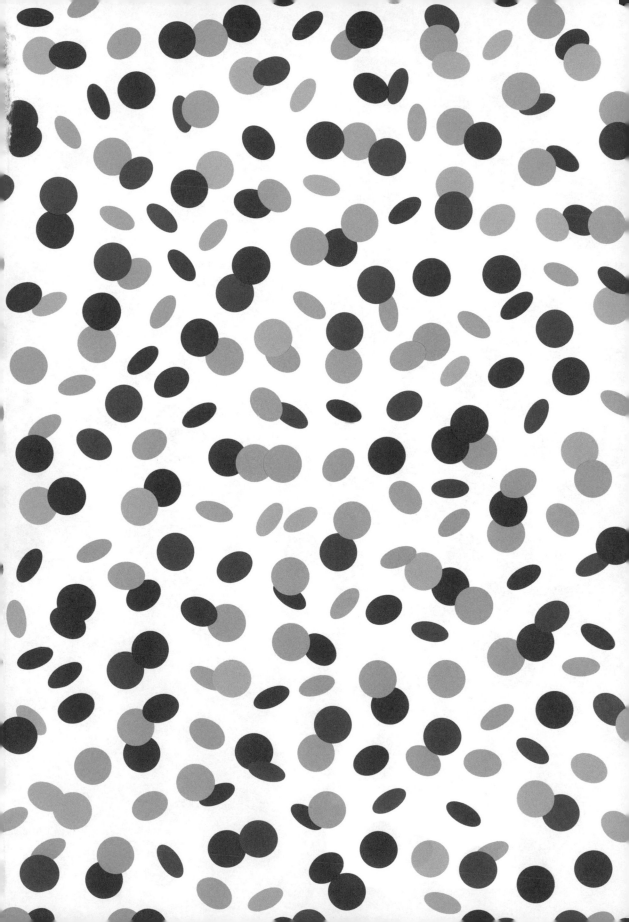

Making Sense of
Medicine

Global Health Humanities

Series Editors: Susan Hogan and Anna Greenwood

This new book series looks at the global health humanities from a number of perspectives, incorporating:

- medical humanities
- health humanities (broadly defined)
- history of medicine
- arts and health.

A wide range of critical studies interrogating the epistemology of knowledge production will be considered. Forms of health knowledge production will be questioned. This series is attentive to the mutually constitutive nature of gender, sexual identity, cultural identity, disability, age and other categories of difference that shape social practices and individual lives. This sensitivity to cultural perspectives forms a critical, and distinctive, lens for the series. Topics of interest include, but not restricted to, global health inequalities and the health humanities; critical reflections on global health humanities; conceptualisations of health; global health in health humanities scholarship; global maternal health; critical analysis of representations of health and illness across cultures; gender inequality; gender issues in the arts and health.

Global Health Humanities is targeted to appeal to health humanities scholars, clinicians and carers, and arts and humanities practitioners, as well as the learned general public.

Titles:

Making Sense of Medicine: Material Culture and the Reproduction of Medical Knowledge (2022)
Edited by John Nott and Anna Harris

Making Sense of Medicine

Material Culture and the Reproduction of Medical Knowledge

EDITED BY
John Nott and Anna Harris,
with special contributions by Rachel Vaden Allison,
Harro van Lente, Candida F. Sánchez Burmester,
Andrea Wójcik and Sally Wyatt

⬤ **intellect**
Bristol, UK / Chicago, USA

First published in the UK in 2022 by Intellect, The Mill, Parnall Road,
Fishponds, Bristol, BS16 3JG, UK

First published in the USA in 2022 by Intellect, The University of Chicago
Press, 1427 E. 60th Street, Chicago, IL 60637, USA

A catalogue record for this book is available from the British Library.

Copy editor: MPS Limited
Cover and layout designer: Aleksandra Szumlas
Cover photo: Models used to practice physical examination skills at
Maastricht University's Skillslab. Image courtesy of Anna Harris.
Production manager: Sophia Munyengeterwa
Typesetter: Aleksandra Szumlas

Paperback ISBN 978-1-78938-577-9
ePDF ISBN 978-1-78938-578-6
ePUB ISBN 978-1-78938-579-3

Part of the Global Health Humanities series
Print ISSN 2752-8545 / Online ISSN 2752-8553

Printed and bound by Gomer

To find out about all our publications, please visit our website.
There you can subscribe to our e-newsletter, browse or download our current
catalogue, and buy any titles that are in print.

www.intellectbooks.com

This is a peer-reviewed publication.

CONTENTS

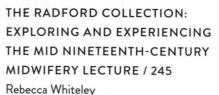

INTRODUCTION

WHAT MATTERS IN MEDICAL EDUCATION?

John Nott and Anna Harris

Medical knowledge manifests in materials, and materials are integral to the reproduction of medical knowledge. From the novice student to the expert practitioner, those who study and work in and around medicine rely on material guidance in their everyday practice and as they seek to further their craft. Students, just as experts, pore over textbooks, photographs and films. They put up and copy down chalkboard illustrations, manipulate plastic models and inspect organic specimens fixed in formalin. They pass through grand university libraries and try not to contaminate anything in cramped surgical theatres. Students, just as experts, learn within an expansive material culture of medicine, they learn from explicitly educative materials, from the workaday tools used for diagnosis and in treatment, they learn in everyday spaces and as part of sprawling infrastructures. While the specific constellation of material varies across time and space, many materials have remained constant, key actors in the spread of medical practices and in the steady, global expansion of biomedical frameworks of health and disease. This collection focuses on the materials, objects, tools and technologies, which facilitate the reproduction of medical knowledge and often reify understandings of medical science.

Medical materials are usually considered, in the humanities and social sciences at least, with a mind to their content – in terms of the information they convey or their particular representation of the body or of disease (see, for instance, Kemp and Wallace 2000; Sappol 2017). Far less attention has been paid to their materiality, their origins and their individual object trajectories. Where materials are produced, where they have travelled and ended up, how they are used and by whom, their affective and sensory qualities, and what materials they are used in conjunction with are just some of ways that materials bear express relevance to their epistemic effects. These questions have, in recent years, been the concern of a growing number of historians (Hallam 2008; Wils et al. 2017), anthropologists (Saunders 2008; Prentice 2013; Rice 2013; Taylor 2011), sociologists (Underman 2020; Pasveer 2006), medical educators (Fenwick 2013) and practicing physicians (Kneebone 2020), some of whom have contributed to this collection.

To date, historical reflections on the material culture of medical knowledge have tended to focus on the circulation of scientific materials as drivers of curiosity, as the empirical foundation of medicine, and as the basis for further investigation (Dupré and Lüthy 2011; MacGregor 2007). Where research has considered the material culture of medical knowledge, its focus has often concerned a small collection of artistically and culturally influential artefacts. Despite what is often a rather narrow focus, historians have, however, begun to pay greater attention to the material and practical history of knowledge in general (Smith et al. 2014), and to the material transmission of medical knowledge in particular (Hendriksen 2014; Margócsy et al. 2018). Despite this, there has been limited historicisation of educative technologies in the more immediate past and historical studies have been slow to engage with the rich seam of philosophical and social science research regarding scientific materialities (Clever and Ruberg 2014; Schouwenburg 2015; Guerrini 2016).

For some time now, philosophers have sought to bring matter to life, emphasising the 'vibrant material that runs alongside and inside humans' (Bennett 2010: viii) in order to provide a radical challenge to the anthropocentric focus of traditional ontology. Materials are, instead, seen as actants – to take the terminology of Science and Technology Studies (STS) (Latour 2007) – sources of action which, just as humans, are capable of doing things, making a difference and effecting events. These ideas have been applied to, adapted in or entirely reconsidered by various fields of social science research. In anthropology, Tim Ingold takes that artefacts are 'the crystallization of activity within a relational field' (Ingold 2002: 345). The unstable material, social, intellectual, emotional and economic contexts which constitute the 'relational field' contributes to the processual and relational nature of objects. To describe these properties means telling their stories (Ingold 2007).

Anthropologist Daniel Miller also focuses on materials, but from a different, archaeologically inspired ethnographic tradition, which has considered material culture in a dramatic range of sites across the world (Miller 2010, 2013), or in the homes of an otherwise unremarkable south London street (Miller 2008). Telling the stories of the things which surround us, by choice or by chance, offers subtle insight into intangible aspects of the human condition. Archaeologists continue to highlight the timelessness of these conclusions and seek to bring social science and philosophical insights back to the object-centred field of archaeology. Ian Hodder (2012), for example, drawing in part from research on Neolithic sites in southern Turkey, emphasises that interdependent relationships between people and things have always been a defining aspect of human culture. These dependencies are the cause of endless 'entanglements' between people and things. This collective cultural reliance on objects has made room for the suggestion that embodied interactions with material culture are integral in the development of human cognition (Malafouris 2013). This collection is inspired by and engages with these various traditions in philosophy, STS, anthropology and archaeology. Across the collection, chapters and essays consider matter as vibrant, as acting, affective and relating, as entangled with medical traditions and knowledge. They are all stories of the material assemblages which effect medical learning, exploring the ways such matter interacts, overlaps, competes, surpasses, becomes obsolete and offers something different from each other.

Materials and technologies are – across a wide range of academic disciplines – increasingly understood as both silent witnesses and agential actors in the development of biomedical practices the world over. Building in no small part from Bruno Latour's (Latour and Woolgar 1979; Latour 2000) contribution to this literature, material analyses have been foundational for social constructionist understandings of science and technology. This collection both draws from and contributes to these ideas, questioning, in particular, the relationship between biomedical fact and the contested epistemologies which are built into the materials of modern medicine. In this respect, many of these chapters contribute to Karen Barad's view that culture may be shaped by the material world just as readily as matter is shaped by culture, and that matter is 'not a thing, but a doing, a congealing of agency' (Barad 2003: 822). Similar conclusions have been extended to considerations of bodily materialities. Annemarie Mol's praxiographic philosophy of disease, for example, takes that bodies, biologies and pathologies are enacted through sociomaterial practices and, as such, depend upon 'everything and everyone that is active while [they are] being practiced' (Mol 2002: 32–33).

The tangled nature of materials and practices in medicine speaks to a tradition in the social sciences and humanities which explores embodied, sensory engagements. These ideas have been used to develop empirical work on the visceral, felt and enlivened bodily experiences of medical practitioners and their engagement with materials in the pursuit of medical knowledge (Prentice 2013; Rice 2013; Maslen 2015; Harris 2016; Hammer 2018). Throughout the volume, readers will find frequent mention of foundational texts on these topics, such as Rachel Prentice's (2013) ethnography of surgical education, Charles Goodwin's (1994) influential account of professional vision, and Lorraine Daston and Peter Galison's work on trained judgement (2010). Prentice's work has stretched the bounds of ethnographic study of objects in medical education, using an STS approach, in order to include the designers of medical materials. Goodwin paved the way for a more thoroughly materialist analysis of a historically constituted architecture for perception, using legal video footage and dirt colour charts as examples. Daston and Galison have been at the vanguard of an emergent historical interrogation of embodied knowledge and its representation.

In history, the material turn has come about in conversation with more experimental researchers. In the history of science, research on embodied or 'gestural' knowledge is studied through re-enactment, hands-on experimentation (Sibum 1995; Heering 2008; Fickers and van den Oever 2011; Krebs 2017) and, more recently, film (Craddock, this volume). Academic interest in embodied knowledge often goes hand in hand with attention to the sensory ways of knowing, both as a topic and method of study. As such, this collection also builds on a tradition of sensuous scholarship in anthropology and history (Classen 1993; Stoller 1997; Howes and Classen 2014). More recently, scholars such as Jennifer Gabrys (2019) and others in STS (Helmreich 2019) have been decentring the human in sensing practices, in order to show the ways in which objects also have sensory capacities. Attuning to the sensory nature of materials in the reproduction of medicine opens up questions of how knowledge may and may not travel and why materials matter in medical epistemology. Indeed, if we embrace epistemology as something which is always also sensorial and embodied, it becomes impossible to divorce the reproduction of medicine from the materials through which it is reproduced.

Notes on ordering: Instructions for the reader

Across 26 chapters, each of which offers insight into the various material constellations of biomedical reproduction, this collection contributes to ongoing attempts to bring order to medicine. We consider ordering as a set of practices that shapes the world (Law and Lynch 1988) and are, as such, highly reflexive of the ways in which this collection has itself been ordered. There is, in fact, not one mode of ordering in this book but many. The most obvious, and in some ways the least analytical, is the alphabetical list of objects and materials around which each chapter centres. In arranging this book alphabetically, we contribute to a long history of ordering in medicine, one which is characterised by alphabetical classifications of, for instance, disease, the International Classification of Diseases (ICD) being the most well-known. The ICD is also used as the central example in Geoffrey Bowker and Susan Leigh Star's (2000) study of 'classification and its consequences'. As the history of the ICD makes plain, attempts at ordering and classification have rarely reflected the deepening of scientific consensus but are, instead, usually the result of conflict and compromise amongst an international cast of actors. This collection is both a homage to and departure from practices of ordering contained within these epistemic technologies.

As with other playful reflections on the objects and subjects of science (Daston 2004; Geissler et al. 2017), we engage with experimental approaches and various modes of ordering as a means to push against the traditional form of edited collections. Short ruminations sit alongside longer academic essays; visual material is elevated beyond illustration and taken to be material, sensorial evidence; various presentations of research blur the line between data and data analysis. Multiple methodologies are also pursued, not only traditional social scientific and historical methods, like ethnography and archival research, but also artistic investigation (Koski and Ostherr, this volume), re-enactment on film (Craddock, this volume) or the embroidered observations of artists in surgical residencies (Kneebone and Oakes, this volume). Notes have been made from artist's notebooks (Kneebone and Oakes, this volume) and as fieldnotes (Wojcik et al., this volume), scrapbooks considered as resources (Dandona, this volume), and the work involved in the upkeep of historical artefacts is not hidden but is developed as part of the analysis (Saward, this volume). Theoretical insights are drawn from film theory (Bonah and Danet, this volume), art history (Dandona, this volume) and semiotics (Aland et al., this volume). Stories are told in the collection as instructions (Allison, this volume), scripts (Guarrasi, this volume), or in footnotes (Kumoji and Nott, this volume). The form of this collection ultimately reflects its primary argument – that the material construction of epistemic objects is relevant to, and intimately involved in, the reproduction of medical knowledge.

Universalism and standardisation

Making sense of medicine has always required a degree of order and standardisation, but the chapters in this collection resist the image of biomedicine as a monolithic, singular entity, as in an older tradition of medical sociology. By attending to the minutiae of material culture in medicine, these chapters instead contribute to a more recent body of literature which takes that biomedicine exists as a shifting tangle of frameworks, paradigms and practices that are hybrid, plural, multiple and readily contaminated by localised norms and alternative epistemologies (see, for instance, Mol 2002). This practical instability contradicts the assumptions of universalism which underlie biomedical practices (Lock and Nguyen 2010) and which are often reproduced in epistemic materials claiming to present an objective, fixed understanding of human biology (Daston and Galison 2010). Many of the materials detailed in this collection exist within this enduring tradition. Anne Katrine Kleberg Hansen (this volume), for instance, explains how typographies of fatness were, in the mid-twentieth century, reified and reproduced through the medium of photography. Other chapters suggest that the local production of teaching materials offers intimately local forms of medicine (e.g Langwick and Mosha; Kumoji and Nott, both in this volume). This is not simply a disciplinary effort, in the Foucaldian sense, but, as Drew Danielle Belsky (this volume) explains with reference to the contemporary manufacture of medical illustration, also provides an often overlooked form of medical care.

Threads and traces

With this in mind, materiality is broadly defined throughout this collection. Understood not just as 'object[s], but as a relational material configuration' (Elliott with Hall, this volume: 381), material assemblages – interactions which are especially apparent in the case of Ivana Guarrasi's simulated heart (this volume) – leave palpable 'traces' through the world (Aland et al., this volume). This approach allows for ornate medical school buildings, as in Annmarie Adam's (this volume) architectural history of McGill University's Pathology Institute to sit alongside Paul Craddock's (this volume) research into the pedagogic value of a modest cigarette paper. Architectural change at McGill invites questions, for example, of how medical disciplines are defined. While Craddock's cigarette paper, a sheer and fragile little sheet, offers a hidden history of skill in medical practice, Fleur Oakes' *Textile Body*, a beautifully threaded and tactile rendering of her surgical observations, encapsulates a long history of surgical practice that her co-author, collaborator and surgeon Roger Kneebone, is part of. In this respect, each of these chapters helps to unpick the socio-material foundations of science along lines pioneered in the Marxist-feminist philosophy of Donna Haraway. 'Any interesting being in technoscience', Haraway wrote in 1997, 'like a textbook, molecule, equation, mouse, pipette, bomb, fungus, technician, agitator, or scientist can – and often should – be teased open to show the sticky economic, technical, political, organic, historical, mythic, and textual threads that make up its tissues' (68; see also Dumit 2014). As we have argued elsewhere (Nott and Harris 2020), within the deconstructed material sitings of modern medicine are 'sticky threads' which bear relevance to contemporary practice; this collection presents a further attempt at unravelling and cataloguing these tangled relationships. We believe that what the chapters highlight, when taken together, is that the objects of medical reproduction resist stable classifications, that they are in fact never one thing, but mean different things at different times, in different places. As Claire Wendland writes, in her chapter in this volume, they constantly move 'through social worlds' (384).

Sensory, embodied and affective knowing

This integration of materials allows for reflection on embodied, sensorial experiences of knowing and learning in medicine. Christian Bonah and Joël Danet (this volume), for instance, question the prevailing assumption that media and film is mostly visual. As in Rachel Vaden Allison's consideration of chalk and chalkboards (this volume), other chapters refer explicitly to the multisensorality of a teaching practice. Christine den Harder and Anna Harris (this volume) use the example of a half-filled water balloon as an improvised medical simulator in order to explain the sensory-material affordances which are often overlooked in the commercial manufacture of teaching tools, while Kelly Underman's chapter (this volume) examines the sensoriality of gloves in training gynaecological examinations. Andrea Wojcik (this volume) concerns herself with the sensory limitations of a simulated wound in medical school assessment, while Peter Winter (this volume) and Denielle Elliott alongside Dominic Hall (this volume) consider the sensorial differences that teaching objects afford. Kaisu Koski and Kirsten Ostherr (this volume) similarly illustrate how bodily interactions with everyday objects facilitate medical students' breaking of bad news, practices which are usually considered as an exercise in language alone.

The affective, sensory influence of material culture is apparent also in the objects found in clinical spaces. David Theodore's history of the Nurseserver (this volume), a piece of postwar hospital furniture designed in pursuit of efficiency, emphasises the haptic knowledge which is necessary for the provision of care. As Theodore's chapter shows, medicine – in a practical sense – is learned in conjunction with materials which are largely abstracted from cognitive forms of knowledge. These objects promote the practical skills that contribute to the craft of medicine and that are also invaluable in its reproduction. This is, in part, what Harriet Palfreyman (this volume) notes in her history of surgical illustration in mid-century Manchester. The skill necessary for the artistic reproduction of the body mediates the haptic and visual expertise of the surgeon. This is, in fact, common of all of the materials considered here, whether analogue or digital (see, for instance, chapters by Winter; Lehne; Saward; Aland et al.; Elliott with Hall, all this volume).

Centres and peripheries

In considering both the history and the geography of medical knowledge, this collection traces the spread of biomedical practices out of Enlightenment Europe. As the image on the cover of this collection suggests, it is the Euro-North American experience which has dominated the history of biomedical epistemology, and White bodies still tend to dominate material representations of the biomedical body in educative settings.

While some chapters reiterate this narrative, others provide means to resist it. Stacey Langwick and Mary Mosha (this volume) proffer the garden as a site for postcolonial resistance through a more holistic approach to biomedicine, while Craddock (this volume) gives space to disciplinary differences, offering up embroidery as a practical, embodied way of knowing the body. Readers might, then, consider reading along geographic or temporal lines. A significant amount of the collection focuses on historical centres of biomedical epistemology, on sites in Europe and North America. Rebecca Whiteley's (this volume) focus on medical illustrations in the nineteenth-century Manchester speaks, for instance, to the closeness of the library, museum and lecture theatre in Europe at the time – the material-spatial constellations which supported a particular tradition of medical knowledge reproduction, even into in the age of clinical medicine. This material focus is updated and mechanised in contributions by Angela Saward, Jakob Lehne and Peter Winter (all this volume). Their respective focus on the development of medical film for professional development in the United Kingdom; on early networks of ultrasound machines and their operators; and on radiography education in contemporary British settings offers insight into the cutting-edge material networks which bind medical advancement with technological change.

Other chapters, however, probe the geographical limits of biomedical hegemony, and move into spaces where biomedicine has had lively competition from rival understandings of health and disease. Lan Li (this volume), for example, addresses the tensions arising from conflicting approaches to modernisation in twentieth-century China. In doing so, they explains how contested ideas present themselves in scientific and epistemic materials. Langwick and Mosha (this volume) mobilise Swahili medical concepts and materialities in their Tanzanian hospital garden in order to cultivate pedagogic innovations and a notion of therapeutic sovereignty *within* a biomedical framework. These are often also areas in which colonisation has played some role, spaces where biomedicine has been utilised as an arm of European empire. Focusing on both Malawian and North American medical schools, Wendland (this volume) describes the stethoscope – that imperious symbol of medical insight – as a powerful materialisation of esoteric knowledge, and as an arbiter of professional status. However Robert Kumoji and John Nott (this volume) suggest that the localised production of teaching materials - in this case in Ghana's oldest and largest pathology museum - offers a means to resist historical centres of knowledge production.

Pasts and presents

In recording the quiet manufacture of its material culture, the collection can also be read with a mind to the history of medicine. Many of the chapters presented here emphasise assumptions that medicine, in the present, is influenced by the material histories of those tools and technologies used in its reproduction. Drawing on ideas borrowed from film theory – the related concepts of framing and gaze – Bonah and Danet (this volume) explore early autopsy films as a forerunner to the dematerialized teaching tools which have since become prominent in the material culture of medical education. Jessica M. Dandona (this volume) situates her chapter in a similar tradition, following scrap-book photographs and the gaze of some of the first women to receive medical training in the USA. The curious case of Phineas Gage's skull likewise allows for Elliott with Hall (this volume) to trace the history of Gage's improbable 1848 survival of a devastating brain injury, through to his skull's use in contemporary neuroscience and medical education. As with this chapter, Rachel Prentice (this volume), Kumoji and Nott (this volume) all also interrogate the enduring agency of the human body after death, contributing to a rich vein of research which considers human remains as a uniquely affecting epistemic tool (Alberti 2011; Hallam 2008; Wils et al. 2017). The enduring affect of historical materials is also especially apparent in the several chapters which consider medical museums (Elliott with Hall; Kumoji and Nott, both this volume) and libraries (Whiteley; Saward, both this volume). Once considered central to the material reproduction of knowledge, these spaces have become tangential to contemporary educative practice. As is especially apparent in the case of museum artefacts, material culture offers an insightful bridge between temporalities in medicine; the preservation, reappearance and reproduction of objects disrupts any linear, teleological narrative of biomedical progress.

Thematic essays

Beyond the alphabetical, temporal and geographical orderings of individual objects, five thematic essays are interspersed through the collection, also in alphabetical order. These help to collate the rest of the collection by theme and offer further introduction both to the individual chapters and to the ideas which bind them together. Organised by colour, many of the chapters in this collection speak to more than one of these themes. Sally Wyatt explores art and artistry in the reproduction of medical knowledge and, in particular, how material reproductions of the body make claims to scientific objectivity. Harro van Lente considers how the circulation of concepts, images and objects helps to standardise and legitimise practice, but also has the potential to constrain medical innovation. In a separate essay, Wyatt explores the various, often gendered forms of 'invisible' labour which are suggested by or have gone into the production of the various materials considered throughout the collection. Andrea Wojcik introduces the affordances provided by material simulations of the body. As a reflective attempt to recreate bodily function and reproduce embodied knowledge through practice, simulation has an important role in the reproduction of medical knowledge but also facilitates the uncritical transfer of potentially problematic concepts and practices. Attention to sensorality taps into tacit dimensions of learning and also helps evoke the atmospheres and affective dimensions of medicine. This is what Rachel Vaden Allison and John Nott also consider in their essay on the role of space, place and affect in the learning of medicine. Candida Sánchez Burmester's essay considers those materials which exist at the margins of or beyond the bounds of traditional biomedical frameworks. In doing so, she engages with postcolonial and decolonial critiques of medical epistemology and suggests that there may be some therapeutic value in embracing materials that buck epistemic convention.

Collaborations and conclusions

This collection traces an inherently collaborative and interdisciplinary endeavour, one which also helps to address the concerns of the editors' own project, Making Clinical Sense (MCS), a historically informed group ethnography based at Maastricht University in the Netherlands. The MCS team includes the editors and all of the authors of the thematic essays in this collection. Together, we focus on the materiality of medical education in three medical schools – Maastricht University in the Netherlands, Semmelweis University in Budapest, Hungary, and the University for Development Studies in Tamale, Ghana. Making Clinical Sense has been generously funded by the European Research Council and spans research conducted between 2016 and 2021. This collection includes contributions from the researchers directly engaged in the MCS project (see chapters by Craddock; den Harder and Harris; Kumoji and Nott; Wojcik et al.; and Allison for research drawn from this project); from colleagues and collaborators at Maastricht and further afield; and from many scholars whose work inspires these ideas, irrespective of discipline. This collaborative intent is apparent throughout the collection; authors have read each other's work, offered comments, suggested readings and made connections. In these various constellations of collaboration, we find new ways to focus on the materiality of medical knowledge and new forms through which we might express these ideas. While we cannot predict the afterlife of what is presented in this book, we hope that, by delving into the vibrancy and liveliness of these materials, these chapters might offer emotional, practical, moral, ethical, political, aesthetic and affective lessons for the future of medicine. Taken as a whole, we hope that this collection will reflect the work of an interdisciplinary array of scholars and practitioners considerate of the material conditions of biomedical understanding. By opening up conversations about materials and practices in medical education – previously the domain of a small group of practitioners, designers and educationists – each chapter makes an 'ethico-political commitment to neglected things, and the affective remaking of relationships with our objects' (Puig de la Bellacasa 2011: 100; also in in Belsky, this volume). Materials help make sense of medicine and their making bears relevance for medical practice, both now and in the future.

Acknowlegements

The production of this book was supported by the European Research Council under the European Union's Horizon 2020 research and innovation programme (Grant Agreement No. 678390). This grant also supported the editorial work; the research conducted in chapters authored by Allison, Craddock, Harris, Nott and Wojcik; and the writing of the introductory and thematic essays by Allison, Harris, van Lente, Nott, Sánchez Burmester, Wojcik and Wyatt.

European Research Council
Established by the European Commission

References

Alberti, Samuel J. M. M. (2011), *Morbid Curiosities: Medical Museums in Nineteenth-Century Britain*, Oxford: Oxford University Press.

Barad, Karen (2003), 'Posthumanist performativity: Toward an understanding of how matter comes to matter', *Signs*, 28:3, pp. 801–31.

Bennett, Jane (2010), *Vibrant Matter: A Political Ecology of Things*, Durham, NC: Duke University Press.

Bowker, Geoffrey C. and Star, Susan Leigh (2000), *Sorting Things Out: Classification and Its Consequences*, Cambridge: MIT Press.

Classen, Constance (1993), *Worlds of Sense: Exploring the Senses in History and Across Cultures*, New York: Routledge.

Clever, Iris and Ruberg, Willemijn (2014), 'Beyond cultural history? The material turn, praxiography, and body history', *Humanities*, 3:4, pp. 546–66.

Daston, Lorraine (2004), *Things That Talk: Object Lessons from Art and Science*, New York: Zone Books.

Daston, Lorraine and Galison, Peter (2010), *Objectivity*, New York: Zone Books.

Dumit, Joseph (2014), 'Writing the implosion: Teaching the world one thing at a time', *Cultural Anthropology*, 29:2, pp. 344–62.

Dupré, Sven and Lüthy, Christoph Herbert (eds) (2011), *Silent Messengers: The Circulation of Material Objects of Knowledge in the Early Modern Low Countries*, Berlin: Lit.

Fenwick, Tara (2013), 'Sociomateriality in medical practice and learning: Attuning to what matters', *Medical Education*, 48:1, pp. 44–52.

Fickers, Andreas and van den Oever, Annie (2011), 'Experimental medial archaeology: A plea for new directions', in A. van den Oever (ed.), *Techne/Technology: Researching Cinema and Media Technologies*, Amsterdam: Amsterdam University Press, pp. 272–78.

Gabrys, Jennifer (2019), 'Sensors and sensing practices: Reworking experience across entities, environments, and technologies', *Science, Technology, & Human Values*, 44:5, pp. 723–36.

Geissler, Paul Wenzel, Lachenal, Guillaume, Manton, John and Tousignant, Noémi (eds) (2017), *Traces of the Future: An Archaeology of Medical Science in Africa*, Bristol: Intellect.

Goodwin, Charles (1994), 'Professional vision', *American Anthropologist*, 96:3, pp. 606–33.

Guerrini, Anita (2016), 'The material turn in the history of life science', *Literature Compass*, 13:7, pp. 469–80.

Hallam, Elizabeth (2008), *The Anatomy Museum: Death and the Body Displayed*, London: Reaktion Books.

Hammer, Gili (2018), '"You can learn merely by listening to the way a patient walks through the door": The transmission of sensory medical knowledge', *Medical Anthropology Quarterly*, 32:1, pp. 138–54.

Haraway, Donna (1997), *Modest_Witness@Second_Millennium.FemaleMan_Meets_OncoMouse: Feminism and Technoscience*, New York: Routledge.

Harris, Anna (2016), 'Listening-touch, affect and the crafting of medical bodies through percussion', *Body & Society*, 22:1, pp. 31–61.

Heering, Peter (2008), 'The enlightened microscope: Re-enactment and analysis of projections with eighteenth-century solar microscopes', *British Journal for the History of Science*, 41:3, pp. 345–67.

Helmreich, Stefan (2019), 'Reading a wave buoy', *Science, Technology, & Human Values*, 44:5, pp. 737–76.

Hendriksen, Marieke M. A. (2014), *Elegant Anatomy: The Eighteenth-Century Leiden Anatomical Collections*, Leiden: Brill.

Hodder, Ian (2012), *Entangled: An Archaeology of the Relationships between Humans and Things*, Malden: Wiley-Blackwell.

Howes, David and Classen, Constance (2014), *Ways of Sensing: Understanding the Senses in Society*, New York: Routledge.

Ingold, Tim (2002), *The Perception of the Environment: Essays on Livelihood, Dwelling and Skill*, London: Routledge.

Ingold, Tim (2007), 'Materials against materiality', *Archaeological Dialogues*, 14:1, pp. 1–16.

Kemp, Martin and Wallace, Marina (2000), *Spectacular Bodies: The Art and Science of the Human Body from Leonardo to Now*, Los Angeles: University of California Press.

Kneebone, Roger (2020), *Expert: Understanding the Path to Mastery*, London: Penguin and Viking.

Krebs, Stefan (2017), 'Memories of a dying industry: Sense and identity in a British paper mill', *The Senses and Society*, 12:1, pp. 35–52.

Latour, Bruno (2000), 'On the partial existence of existing and nonexisting objects', in L. Daston (ed.), *Biographies of Scientific Objects*, Chicago: University of Chicago Press, pp. 247–69.

Latour, Bruno (2007), *Reassembling the Social: An Introduction to Actor-Network-Theory*, Oxford: Oxford University Press.

Latour, Bruno and Woolgar, Steve (1979), *Laboratory Life: The Construction of Scientific Facts*, London: Sage Publications.

Law, John and Lynch, Michael (1988), 'Lists, field guides, and the descriptive organization of seeing: Birdwatching as an exemplary observational activity', *Human Studies*, 11:2&3, pp. 271–303.

Lock, Margaret M. and Nguyen, Vinh-Kim (2010), *An Anthropology of Biomedicine*, Oxford: Wiley-Blackwell.

MacGregor, Arthur (2007), *Curiosity and Enlightenment: Collectors and Collections from the Sixteenth to the Nineteenth Century*, New Haven: Yale University Press.

Malafouris, Lambros (2013), *How Things Shape the Mind*, Cambridge: MIT Press.

Margócsy, Dániel, Somos, Mark and Joffe, Stephen N. (2018), *The Fabrica of Andreas Vesalius: A Worldwide Descriptive Census, Ownership, and Annotations of the 1543 and 1555 Editions*, Leiden: Brill.

Maslen, Sarah (2015), 'Researching the senses as knowledge', *The Senses and Society*, 10:1, pp. 52–70.

Miller, Daniel (2008), *The Comfort of Things*, Cambridge: Polity Press.

Miller, Daniel (2010), *Stuff*, Cambridge: Polity Press.

Miller, Daniel (2013), *Consumption and Its Consequences*, London: Polity Press.

Mol, Annemarie (2002), *The Body Multiple: Ontology in Medical Practice*, Durham: Duke University Press.

Nott, John and Harris, Anna (2020), 'Sticky models: History as friction in obstetric education', *Medicine Anthropology Theory*, 7:1, pp. 44–65.

Pasveer, Bernike (2006), 'Representing or mediating: A history and philosophy of x-ray images in medicine', in L. Pauwels (ed.), *Visual Cultures of Science: Rethinking Representational Practices in Knowledge Building and Science Communication*, New England: University Press of New England, pp. 41–62.

Prentice, Rachel (2013), *Bodies in Formation: An Ethnography of Anatomy and Surgery Education*, Durham: Duke University Press.

Puig de la Bellacasa, Maria (2011), 'Matters of care in technoscience: Assembling neglected things', *Social Studies of Science*, 41:1, pp. 85–106.

Rice, Tom (2013), *Hearing and the Hospital: Sound, Listening, Knowledge and Experience*, Canon Pyon: Sean Kingston Publishing.

Sappol, Michael (2017), *Body Modern: Fritz Kahn, Scientific Illustration, and the Homuncular Subject*, Minneapolis: University of Minnesota Press.

Saunders, Berry F. (2008), *CT Suite: The Work of Diagnosis in the Age of Noninvasive Cutting*, Durham and London: Duke University Press.

Schouwenburg, Hans (2015), 'Back to the future? History, material culture and new materialism', *International Journal for History, Culture and Modernity*, 3:2, pp. 59–72.

Sibum, H. Otto (1995), 'Working experiments: A history of gestural knowledge', *The Cambridge Review*, 116:2325, pp. 25–37.

Smith, Pamela H., Meyers, Amy R. W. and Cook, Harold J. (eds) (2014), *Ways of Making and Knowing: The Material Culture of Empirical Knowledge*, Ann Arbor: The University of Michigan Press.

Stoller, Paul (1997), *Sensuous Scholarship*, Philadelphia: University of Pennsylvania Press.

Taylor, Janelle S. (2011), 'The moral aesthetics of simulated suffering in standardized patient performances', *Culture, Medicine and Psychiatry*, 35:2, pp. 134–62.

Underman, Kelly (2020), *Feeling Medicine: How the Pelvic Exam shapes Medical Training*, New York: New York University Press.

Wils, Kaat, de Bont, Raf and Au, Sokhieng (eds) (2017), *Bodies Beyond Borders: Moving Anatomies, 1750–1950*, Leuven: Leuven University Press.

ARCHITECTURE

DESIGNING A DISCIPLINE: ARCHITECTURE FOR PATHOLOGY IN THE INTERWAR PERIOD

Annmarie Adams

'He is taken to the threshold of the subject and prepared to enter it himself', said pathologist Horst Oertel in describing his splendid new workplace in 1925 (Oertel 1925: 15). Oertel was referring to McGill University's Pathology Institute in Montreal, Canada, designed by Montreal architects Percy Erskine Nobbs and his partner George Taylor Hyde and opened the previous year on 6 October. For 30 years, pathology had been accommodated in the nearby Royal Victoria Hospital (RVH), first in ad hoc spaces and later in a purpose-built wing, but now it had its own entirely separate quarters. Dozens of dignitaries, including Quebec's 14th Lieutenant Governor Narcisse Pérodeau and the university principal Sir Arthur Currie, gathered to celebrate the momentous occasion. Funded in part by the prestigious Rockefeller Foundation, Currie expressed high expectations for the new facility's future: 'I am glad to witness the building of this Pathological Institute, of which so much good is anticipated' (Anon. 1924a: 16). Currie's expectations no doubt extended beyond the simple accommodation of pathologists and hospital casualties.

In this chapter, I show how the architecture did much more than simply accommodate. It bridged hospital and university; it linked the past and the future; it housed and enabled cutting-edge technologies; and according to Oertel, it even dissipated tensions within his growing medical field. In his exquisitely detailed description of the institute,

Oertel claimed that the building brought the two sides of his discipline together, 'the academic (university) and the practical (hospital) connections', which had previously 'retarded their development' (1925: 1). How does architecture define the reproduction of medical knowledge? In the case of pathology, how did architecture shape medical education? What and where is the threshold of a medical specialty, as Oertel describes? Does a separate building constitute a separate discipline? How does architectural evidence influence our understanding of pathology?

This contribution explores these themes of threshold, autonomy and disciplinary self-fashioning in the history of pathology and medical education. In particular, I probe the emergence of a separate, purpose-built architecture for pathology in the first half of the twentieth century as a measure of professional autonomy. My sources are mostly visual: architectural drawings, photographs and contemporary accounts. Although this material culture approach has been engaged to study other medical specialties – for example, we can read the history of paediatrics in the evolution of the children's hospital or responses to tuberculosis in the changing design of the sanatorium – the spatial history of pathology is unexplored.[1] Reading architecture as a primary source in the history of pathology allows us to see how a field established its self-identity, settled interdisciplinary tensions and drew disciplinary boundaries or thresholds. Focusing on a single, well-documented building for pathology – Oertel's Institute – permits us to assess architecture as an arena of decision-making that captures a particular time and place. Architecture registers historical nuances that are illegible in textual documents and destabilises the histories of medicine that rely so heavily on the work of individual physicians.

What is pathology? What was its particular historical situation in the early twentieth century? The history of pathology has been written by notable historians of medicine through the work of particular physicians, theories, procedures, and technologies.[2] A spate of recent books on pathology illuminate its cultural importance in the nineteenth- and the twentieth-century culture (Meli 2017; Sappol 2002). Although dissections were carried out as early as Greek antiquity, modern pathology as a discipline, not as a practice or theory, is often associated with the work of German physician Rudolf Virchow in the nineteenth century, particularly his cell theory and systematic method for autopsies. Many historians of medicine refer to Virchow as 'the father of modern pathology' (Eisenberg 1986: 243). Another crucial factor in the rise of the specialty of modern pathology was the development of the microscope, allowing scientists to see the growth and development of tissues and cells. 'Without the microscope, the cell could be considered in merely impressionistic terms. By emphasizing the role of the instrument, cellular pathology provided the focus for the development of pathology as a separate specialty', explains historian of medicine Russell Charles Maulitz (1993: 182).[3] James R. Wright, in probing the relationship of surgery and pathology, sees the proliferation of laboratory testing and community hospitals as key to the emergence of the clinical pathologist (Wright 1985: 319).

Connection

McGill University's Pathology Institute (sometimes called Pathological Institute) is an ideal case study for two reasons: it was a significant, even transformative building, and it is extraordinarily well documented. Oertel implied Montreal's Pathology Institute was among the earliest in North America to bring together the academic and practical sides of the specialty (1925: 1). Through its location and orientation, it united the concerns of the university and the hospital. Figure 1.1 illustrates how the Pathology Institute was strategically located close to both the Royal Victoria Hospital and McGill University, in between them in fact, almost like a hyphen connecting two words. An underground tunnel linked it to the hospital so that bodies could be moved to the new morgue easily and discreetly. A busy intersection linked it to the campus.

The form of the Pathology Institute also linked it to the university, through its architect, Percy Nobbs, who was responsible for many of the campus buildings and served as Director of the School of Architecture from 1903 to 1913. It is considered to be among Nobbs' finest projects. Architectural historian Susan Wagg, in her biography of the Scottish-born architect, points to its function as a connector as evidence of its success: 'When completed, the Pathological Institute served as the keystone in a gracefully descending architectural sequence that repeated the natural contours of the hill. Not only was the clash of scales beautifully resolved, but the whole area was visually enhanced' (1982: 42).

The design of the Pathology Institute also cued images of the lower campus by association. In particular, it closely resembled Figure 1.2, the Macdonald Engineering Building, also designed by Nobbs, a building

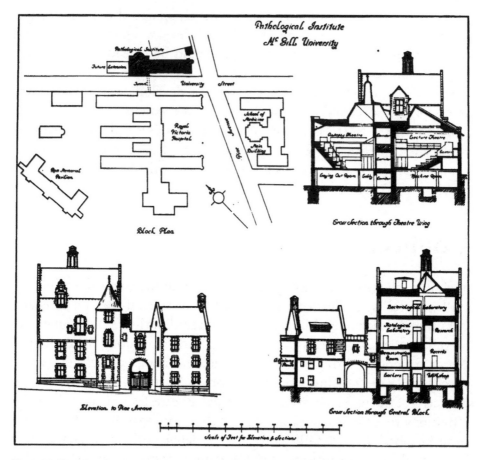

Figure 1.1: Site plan showing location, sections and elevation of Pathology Institute, published in 'Pathological Institute of McGill University' (Oertel 1925: 2).

with a particularly heroic past. An original Macdonald Engineering Building (designed by Andrew Taylor 1893) and the university's first, purpose-built building for medical education, known as Old Medical (designed by John William Hopkins and Daniel Berkley Wily 1872; subsequent additions by Andrew Taylor), were both lost in fires in April 1907, a mere eleven days apart (Adams 2016: 171–85). Nobbs built the new Macdonald Engineering Building in 1908 to replace the one lost in the fire. Because of its extraordinary genesis, the building has a rather heroic image, an aspect showcased by a stunning sculpture on the building's south side, showing a phoenix rising from the ashes. It follows, then, that subsequent buildings which echo its forms might share in this legacy. Wagg describes the Pathology Institute as a 'reduced version of

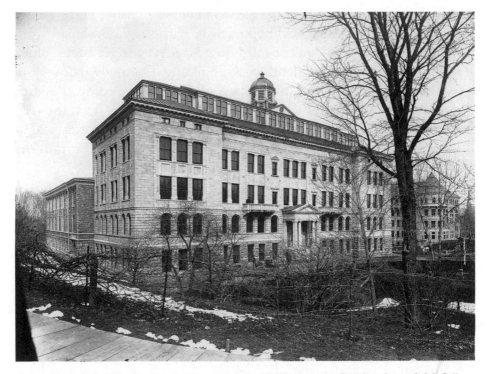

Figure 1.2: William Notman & Son, photo of Macdonald Engineering Building (*c.*1895). McGill University, Montreal, McCord Museum, VIEW–2538, http://collections.musee-mccord.qc.ca/en/collection/artifacts/VIEW-2538. Accessed 13 June 2022.

the Engineering Building without the central doorway', explicitly connecting the two buildings through their formal resemblances (1980: 90). By making the Pathology Institute look like Engineering, then, Nobbs linked the medical building to the heroic history of McGill University by association.

Three parts

Although the Pathology Institute is a relatively small building, its strong architectural statement counterbalances the effects of its massive neighbours, particularly the expansive, pavilion-plan Royal Victoria Hospital across the street. Figure 1.3 shows Nobbs' approach to the institute's scale was to divide it into three distinct parts. The main section of the limestone building, along University Street, is a three-storey, narrow, rectangular wing, with intersecting, steeply pitched roofs. This middle section includes the entrance; on the second floor is a massive, north-facing histology lab (the histological approach in pathology developed from microscopical anatomy); on the third floor is an even larger bacteriological lab, occupying the full depth of the building. Dormer windows and a pair of chimneys give this middle part of the institute complex something of a residential air. Figure 1.4's view of this section from the rear, however, was much more industrial than residential. Two-storey glazing distinguished the elevations of two major, stacked laboratories from the exterior.

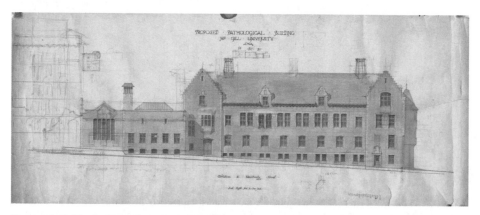

Figure 1.3: Nobbs & Hyde, Pathological Building, front elevation. John Bland Canadian Architecture Collection, McGill University.

To the north of this main section is a squarish block, that protrudes in back and front. This northernmost section included the building's three large gathering spaces: the medical museum, the lecture room and the autopsy theatre. In the basement were the morgue, preparation and delivery rooms. In the rear, the semi-circular seating of the autopsy theatre protruded from the square block. The bulbous, apse-like shape of this section – almost ecclesiastical in its form – clearly demarcated the location of the all-important autopsy theatre. Like the operating theatre is to surgery, the autopsy theatre is the centrepiece of the discipline.

Figure 1.5, showing the third and smallest section of the Pathology Institute, sited along Pine Avenue, is its most domestic. Oertel describes it as an 'attached cottage'. Linked to the main building only by an arched, overhead bridge on the second floor, the animal house of the Pathology Institute is sited at an acute angle to the rest of the building, following the orientation of Pine Avenue rather than University Street. Here two caretakers lived on the first two floors, with animals above. The gate of

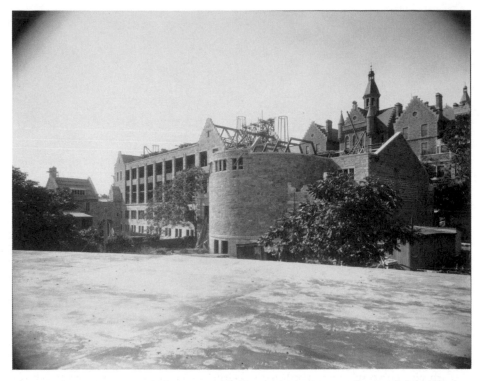

Figure 1.4: Exterior photograph, Pathological Building under construction (1922–24). John Bland Canadian Architecture Collection, McGill University.

the overhead bridge to the animal house leads to a generous courtyard, facing the university sports stadium and nearby park. Since this block of Pine Avenue, just east of University Street, were mostly picturesque Victorian houses, Nobbs' decision to locate the animal quarters there and to essentially camouflage the building as a regular family (i.e. human) home, was inspired. A baronial turret just to the east of the overhead bridge, containing a stair, is an overt nod to the turrets on the south end of the patient wards of the Royal Victoria Hospital, which contained toilets rather than stairs.

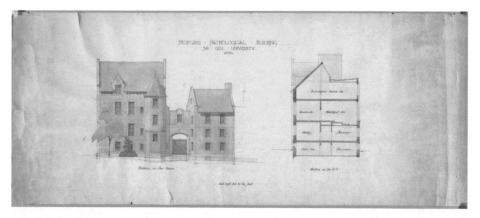

Figure 1.5: Nobbs & Hyde, animal house, Pathological Building. John Bland Canadian Architecture Collection, McGill University.

Separate architecture as disciplinary autonomy

Before the time when pathology merited separate quarters, what Maulitz calls the 'pre-professional' era, pathology was accommodated in general urban hospitals. It is difficult to pinpoint the exact date of this separation in different national contexts – in Germany it occurred during Virchow's time – but Oertel wrote in 1925 that 'the creation of pathological institutes [...] is, on the North American Continent, of very recent date' (Maulitz 1993: 169; Oertel 1925: 1). Some hospitals had a dedicated section or wing; sometimes pathology was in the basement. A good example of pathology integrated in the hospital, for Stevens, was Grace Hospital in Detroit, where pathology was located above the floor dedicated to surgery (Stevens 1928).

Some pavilion-plan hospitals that opened in the final years of the nineteenth century added a dedicated pathology wing. The Royal Victoria Hospital, Figure 1.6, which had been designed by British hospital specialist Henry Saxon Snell, for example, saw as its first addition a multi-storey Pathology Wing added to the north of its easternmost pavilion only five years after its opening. Designed by Andrew Taylor, the new wing was located just north of the surgical theatre, along University, and brought the lineup of hospital buildings to an elegant close, with its apsidal form. It even had a separate entrance on University Street,

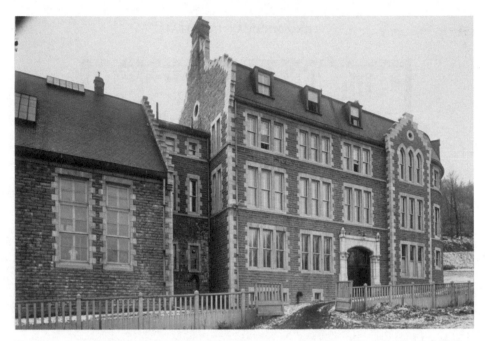

Figure 1.6: Andrew Taylor, photograph of old pathology wing of the Royal Victoria Hospital. Collection Royal Victoria Hospital, now McGill University Health Centre.

expressing its semi-separate status. The RVH example is an excellent illustration of the close spatial relationship of pathology and surgery, as it was located adjacent to and connected on three levels to Snell's surgical theatre. The addition of purpose-built architecture for pathology so soon after the opening of the hospital is evidence that the field was extremely important, and changing, perhaps even becoming a symbol of the up-to-date urban hospital and university. The important message is that it was stepping away from the hospital, and becoming visible as a distinct unit in the university. As guest-of-honour British pathologist Arthur Boycott said at the opening, 'pathology is a science which, by its achievement, has amply deserved the right to stand on its own feet' (Anon. 1924a: 16).

It thus follows that a significant moment in the history of pathology is when completely separate, purpose-built buildings for pathology appear, about 1906. In 1918, American architect Edward Stevens saw it as an issue of both location and scale, and said that a separate pathology department was commonplace in Europe by this time. 'In the larger hospitals in Europe', he says in the second edition of his classic text *The American Hospital of the Twentieth Century*, 'the pathological department is under separate management' (Stevens 1918: 142). Stevens illustrated

140   THE AMERICAN HOSPITAL

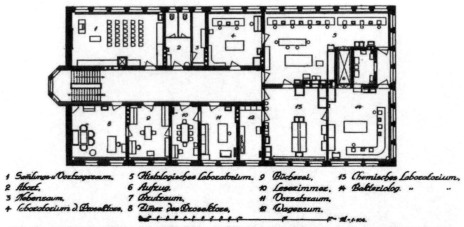

1 *Sämlings-Vorbereogszraum.*   5 *Histologisches Laboratorium.* 9 *Bücherei.*   13 *Chemisches Laboratorium.*
2 *Abort.*   6 *Aufzug.*   10 *Lesezimmer.*   14 *Bakteriolog.* ..
3 *Nebenraum.*   7 *Brutraum.*   11 *Vorratsraum.*   ..
4 *Laboratorium d Prosektors.*   8 *Zimer des Prosektors.*   12 *Wagraum.*

FIG. 211. MUNICH-SCHWABING HOSPITAL. PATHOLOGICAL BUILDING. SECOND FLOOR PLAN

Figure 1.7: Plan of Munich-Schwabing Hospital, Pathological Building (Stevens 1918: 140).

this concept of separation, which he said was 'self-explanatory', with plans of the Pathological Institute of the Munich-Schwabing Hospital in Germany (Stevens 1918: 139–40, 142). Stevens' plan, Figure 1.7, shows a modest rectangular building with rooms aligned along a double-loaded corridor. These room types represent the basic programme for a pathology institute after about 1906: museum, lecture room, laboratories, library and autopsy or dissection room or theatre. A photograph under the plan showed the all-important dissection room in Munich, with large, generous windows and two autopsy tables, suggesting simultaneous operations. The design of such buildings facilitated the movement of a pathological/morbid body from reception to dissection to preparation and segmentation and eventually to display in the museum (Alberti 2011; Adams 2016: 171–85).

Historians of medicine point to the Pathology Institute at Charité Hospital in Berlin, Figure 1.8, as the first separate institute in Europe, which appeared 50 years before the widespread trend of separating pathology from general hospitals. Virchow himself demanded the physical separation, seeing it as a mark of autonomy. Maulitz explains:

Ackerknecht noted a quarter century ago, Virchow demanded the establishment of a physically separate Pathological Institute: this was

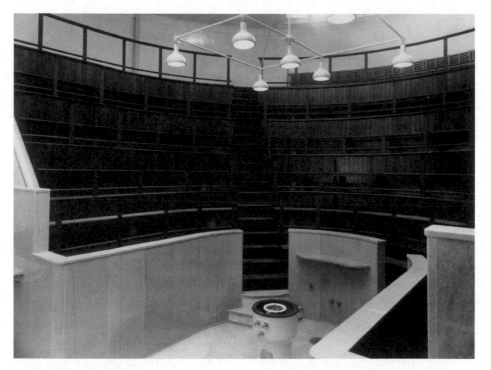

Figure 1.8: Interior photograph of the autopsy theatre. John Bland Canadian Architecture Collection, McGill University.

but one precondition he set before he would return to the scene of his colleagues' and his own political discomfiture of the troubled 1848–50 period. (1978: 167–68)

Given this politicised context, the location of the Pathology Institute across the street from the hospital was an expression of disciplinary autonomy. Boycott articulated as much in his speech on opening day, as noted by a newspaper journalist: 'if medicine and surgery were abolished, pathology would go on itself. "It no longer rests on these other studies", he said. "It has grown up and now demands an independent kind of existence"' (Anon. 1924b: 8).

What the plans tell us: Autopsy and labs

The correspondence between the architects reveals much about the design process for a medical building in the 1920s, particularly a building that needed to be 'one of the finest Pathological Departments in existence', as mentioned in the letter commissioning Stevens as consultant from the hospital superintendent H. E. Webster, 10 April 1922 (n.pag.). After an in-person meeting of the local and the consulting architects, Stevens wrote to Nobbs outlining what he and his partner Frederick Lee believed to be the important points for the Montreal-based architects to consider, based on their review of an initial plan (Stevens 1922). The Toronto office affiliated with the Boston-based firm also supposedly sent plans (these do not seem to have survived). Note that nearly all the consultants' comments focused on the plan, especially on adjacencies and circulation issues.[4]

The correspondence focuses on two key interiors, the autopsy theatre and the laboratories, which also nicely illustrate distinct traditions within the field. The architects' resolution of the two parts shows how the building served to unite these tensions. Historian of medicine Rue Bucher explains: 'If they saw pathology as a science, then its mission was investigation and communication of knowledge' (Bucher 1962: 42).

Those who saw pathology as a medical specialty might consider the autopsy theatre as the signature space of a pathology institute. Nobbs' design, which we know only from Oertel's description and one photograph in Figure 1.9 – it was demolished in 1971[5] – privileged light and view. Oertel's description in a piece for the Rockefeller Foundation third series on medical education is so sharp, it almost stimulating a tour:

> The main entrance hall opens to the left directly into the large lecture room and museum, and into the autopsy suite consisting of a large theater and two smaller private stops rooms. The lecture room is in the form of an amphitheater provided with a top gallery and from 130 to 150 seats, concentrated as much as possible around the lecture platform. [...] Daylight is furnished by skylight principally, and artificial light by twelve high-power incandescent lamps. (1925: 8)

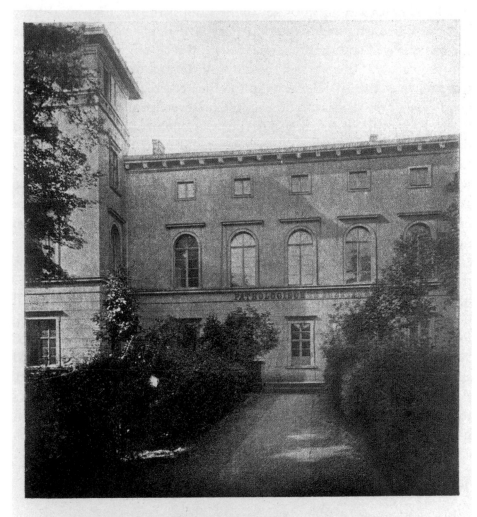

THE OLD PATHOLOGICAL INSTITUTE IN THE CHARITÉ

Courtesy of Prof. Otto Lubarsch

Figure 1.9: Photograph of old pathological institution in the Charité, Berlin. Credit: Wellcome Collection. Attribution 4.0 International (CC BY 4.0), https://wellcomecollection.org/works/yq37u3as?wellcomeImagesUrl=/indexplus/image/M0017266.html. Accessed 18 May 2022.

As Oertel notes, visibility was key in the autopsy theatre, Figure 1.10, for both the demonstrator and the students. The demonstrator needed to see the cadaver well and the students needed to see both the demonstrator and the cadaver. This area of the autopsy theatre, ostensibly the stage, was known as the pit. 'The seats in the theater rise abruptly, affording a good view of the demonstrations in the pit, even from the back benches' (Oertel 1925: 8–9). Artificial lighting was sophisticated: 'Attached to the ceiling is a special fixture, with seven 150-watt blue bulb lamps in focusing artificial daylight on the operating tables' (Oertel 1925: 9). 'The whole fixture is hung high enough not to interfere with the vision of the students and also to prevent the heat of the lamps from bothering the operator', reported Oertel (1925: 15). Students were expected to take notes while viewing an autopsy.

The second key space for early twentieth-century pathologists was the laboratory. Nobbs' Pathology Institute had two large labs, both facing the rear of the building, like the autopsy theatre, to receive optimal north light. The most significant of the labs was on the second floor, for pathological histology. We know from a letter written by Stevens to Nobbs that this long and narrow lab, 112 × 26 feet, was designed for 120 students to look through microscopes simultaneously (Oertel 1925: 9). As in the autopsy theatre, vision shaped the design. Figure 1.11 shows that floor-to-ceiling windows allowed a large amount of natural light into the spaces plus the architects specified twenty-three 300-watt lights.

Homage to Virchow

In case the physical separation of the department from the hospital and the deep investments in both spaces for autopsy and for laboratories were not blatant enough, Nobbs included two to three sculptural decorations in the design of the Pathology Institute that articulate the Institute's legacy. In addition, there are four Latin quotes.

'Sedibus et causis moriborum per anatomen et experimenta indagandis' (Seat and causes of diseases to be studied through anatomy and experiments); 'Hic est locus ubi mors resurgens rediviva est' (Here is the place where death arises to new life); 'Hic est locus ubi mors gaudet succerrere vitae' (Here is the place where death rejoices to be of service to life); 'Nihil sic revocat a pecato quam frequens mortis med-

itatio' (Nothing prevents error or sin so much as frequent contempla-
tion of death). (John Bland CAC Website 2002: n.pag., translation
on website)

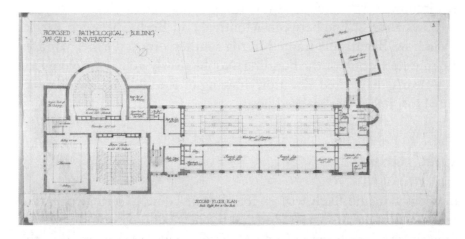

Figure 1.10: Nobbs & Hyde, plan of second floor, Pathological Building. John Bland Canadian
Architecture Collection, McGill University.

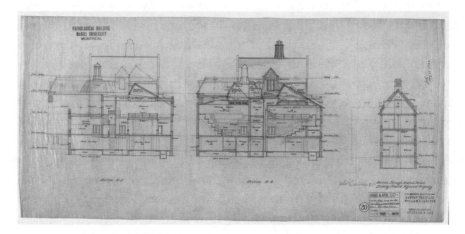

Figure 1.11: Nobbs & Hyde, section through Pathological Building. John Bland Canadian
Architecture Collection, McGill University.

Wagg links the inclusion of these Latin sayings to an explicitly Scottish architectural tradition. She says 'the old tower houses and castles
of Scotland had been embellished with pious mottos and with carved
crests and monograms, and Nobbs revived these traditional decorations
to convey a contemporary message of comfort' (Wagg 1982: 43–44).

Reading Nobbs' building as a politicised source in the history of pathology, however, compels us to a different sculptural moment in the building. Nobbs includes an emblem, Figure 1.12, that pays tribute to both Virchow and the architectural setting of his work in Berlin. Its presence draws a direct line between Montreal and Berlin, between Oertel and Virchow. Beautifully framed in the southern-most dormer window of the middle section of the building, Nobbs' nearly-round emblem features a clearly delineated elevation drawing of Rudolf-Virchow-Krankenhaus Hospital in Berlin-Wedding.

Conclusion

In an undated memo, likely written for a hospital donor, Oertel writes that there was a 'gentleman's agreement' that the new building would serve the 'routine work' of the hospital (n.d.: 4). Visual evidence suggests that the design of the building functioned as a powerful form of agreement, beyond the local issues discussed by Oertel. The building's location and form linked hospital and university. Communication between and among architects connected the building to others in Europe and the United States; Stevens' advice also ensured the Pathology Institute was up-to-date and of its time, while at the same time Nobbs' sensitive massing paid homage to the Scottish and medical traditions across the street. Remarkably, the front and the rear of the Pathology Institute expressed different but complementary architectural messages. While the 'front' was conservative and contextual, then, the rear exploded in functionalism, with the autopsy theatre and two cutting-edge laboratories calling for attention. Finally, sculptural detailing articulated a legacy that linked Montreal-based pathologists back to Rudolf Virchow, shrinking time and space.

The Pathology Institute thus shows how architecture contributes to a medical discipline. In pathology in the 1920s in Montreal, a separate building constituted a separate discipline. Architectural drawings, photographs and contemporary accounts allow us to begin a spatial history of pathology. Architectural history shows how a medical field established its self-identity, settled interdisciplinary tensions and drew disciplinary boundaries and thresholds.

Figure 1.12: Nobbs & Hyde, sculptural detail on Pathological Building. John Bland Canadian Architecture Collection, McGill University.

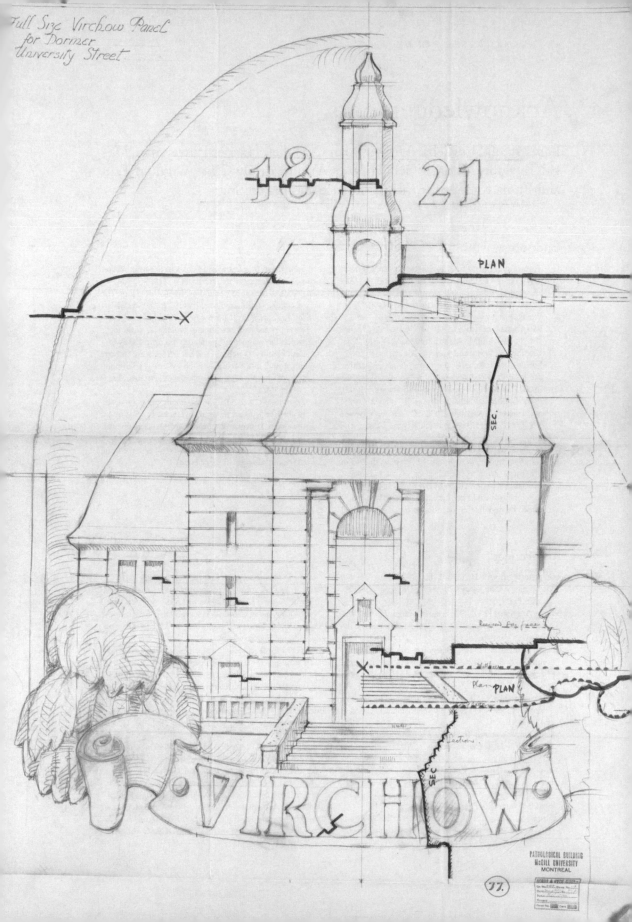

Full Size Virchow Panel
for Dormer
University Street.

18 21

PLAN

PLAN

·VIRCHOW·

PATHOLOGICAL BUILDING
McGILL UNIVERSITY
MONTREAL

77.

Acknowledgements

I am grateful to Richard Fraser, Joan O'Malley, Harriet Palfreyman, David Theodore, Thomas Schlich, Jim Wright, Emily Cline, Cigdem Talu and Fiona Kenney for their assistance and inspiration.

Endnotes

1. To me 'material culture' privileges the engagement of visual and spatial sources. As examples, see Adams and Theodore (2002), Adams and Schwartzman (2005), Adams (2007) and Adams et al. (2008).
2. For contributions of individual physicians, see Erwin Heinz Ackerknecht (1953), Russel C. Maulitz (1978), Harold M. Malkin (1993: 143–58), Paul Klemperer (1958) and George Androutsos (2005). For histories focused on theory and procedure, see Prüll Cay-Rüdiger and John Woodward (1998), Prüll Cay-Rüdiger and John Woodward (2003), Piers D. Mitchell (2012), James R. Wright (1975) and Hector O. Ventura (2000). On technology, see Maulitz (1993: 160–69), particularly the section 'The mid-nineteenth century: The microscope as authority'; and Malkin (1998).
3. See Maulitz, *Morbid Appearances*: 'Then, on the eve of the introduction of the microscope into pathology, the creation of new chairs began slowly to transmute this inchoate tradition into something like a discipline'; he says in the footnote to this, 'The implied contention should be made explicit: the microscope was instrumental in this process' (1987: 136n14). See also, for more general outline of development of cellular pathology, Maulitz (1978: 162–82). Also see Ackerknecht: '[Microscopy] proved to be the avenue toward this new system of cellular pathology, which has dominated pathology far into the twentieth century. [Virchow] and his school were to turn more and more from physiology and experiment toward morphology and microscopical pathology' (1953: 55).
4. See Adams (2007: 34): 'The argument, taken up again in chapter 4, is that planning overtook ventilation as the major concern of hospital architects about the time of World War I.'
5. A precious student paper indicates the arrangement of the building in 1977; see Soucy 1977.

References

Ackerknecht, Erwin H. (1953), *Rudolf Virchow, Doctor, Statesman, Anthropologist*, Madison: University of Wisconsin Press.

Adams, Annmarie (2007), *Medicine by Design: The Architect and the Modern Hospital, 1893–1943*, Minneapolis: University of Minnesota Press.

Adams, Annmarie (2016), 'Designing the medical museum', in S. Schrank and D. Ekici (eds), *Healing Spaces, Modern Architecture, and the Body*, UK: Ashgate, pp. 171–85.

Adams, Annmarie and Schwartzman Kevin (2005), 'Pneumothorax then and now', *Space and Culture*, 8:4, pp. 435–48.

Adams, Annmarie and Theodore, David (2002), 'Designing for "The Little Convalescents": Children's hospitals in Toronto and Montreal, 1875–2006', *Canadian Bulletin of Medical History*, 19:1, pp. 201–43.

Alberti, Samuel J. M. M. (2011), *Morbid Curiosities: Medical Museums in Nineteenth-Century Britain*, Oxford: Oxford University Press.

Androutsos, George (2005), 'Giovanni-Battista Morgani (1682–1773): Creator of pathological anatomy', *Journal of the Balkan Union of Oncology*, 11:1, pp. 95–1010.

Anon. (1895), 'Pathological department opened at the Royal Victoria Hospital', *Montreal Daily Star*, 26 January / June, n.pag. [from RVH scrapbook].

Anon. (1924a), 'Open pathology bldg. at McGill', *Montreal Daily Star*, 7 October, pp. 16.

Anon. (1924b), 'Pathology's scope needs broadening says Dr Boycott', *The Gazette*, 7 October, p. 8.

Adams, Annmarie, Schwartzman, Kevin and Theodore, David (2008), 'Collapse and expand: Designing for tuberculosis', *Technology and Culture*, 49:4, pp. 908–42.

Bucher, Rue (1962), 'Pathology: A study of social movements within a profession', *Social Problems*, 10:40, pp. 40–51.

Eisenberg, Leon (1986), 'Rudolf Virchow: The physician as politician', *Medicine and War*, 2:4, pp. 243–50.

John Bland Canadian Architecture Collection, McGill University (2002), 'History writ large: the architecture of Percy Erskine Nobbs', John Bland Canadian Architecture Collection, http://cac.mcgill.ca/nobbs/search/detail.php?projectid=244&mj=All&pn=All&mn=All&ct=Montreal&pro=QC&sta=All&cn=

Canada&key=&records=235&page=11. Accessed 1 June 2020.

Klemperer, Paul (1958), '"The Feilding H. Garrison Lecture": The pathology of Morgagni and Virchow', *Bulletin of the History of Medicine*, 32, pp. 24–38.

Malkin, Harold M. (1993), *Out of the Mist: The Foundation of Modern Pathology and Medicine During the Nineteenth Century*, Berkeley: Vesalius.

Malkin, Harold M. (1998), 'History of pathology: Comparison of the use of the microscope in pathology in Germany and the United States during the nineteenth century', *Annals of Diagnostic Pathology*, 2:1, pp. 79–91.

Maulitz, Russell C. (1978), 'Rudolf Virchow, Julius Cohnheim, and the program of pathology', *Bulletin of the History of Medicine*, 52:2, pp. 162–82.

Maulitz, Russell C. (1987), *Morbid Appearances: The Anatomy of Pathology in the Early Nineteenth Century*, Cambridge: Cambridge University Press.

Maulitz, Russell C. (1993), 'The pathological tradition', in W. F. Bynum and R. Porter (eds), *Companion Encyclopedia of the History of Medicine*, London: Routledge, pp. 169–91.

Meli, Domenico Bertoli (2017), *Visualizing Disease: The Art and History of Pathological Illustrations*, Chicago: University of Chicago Press.

Mitchell, Piers D. (2012), *Anatomical Dissection in Enlightenment England and Beyond: Autopsy, Pathology, and Display: The History of Medicine in Context*, Farnham, UK: Ashgate

Oertel, Horst (1925), 'Pathological Institute of McGill University', in *Methods and Problems of Medical Education*, 3rd series, New York: Rockefeller, offprint pp. 1–20.

Oertel, Horst (n.d.), Memorandum on the steps which led to the construction of the pathological institute and the relations of the Royal Victoria Hospital and University to it.

Prüll, Cay-Rüdiger and John Woodward (eds) (1998), *Pathology in the 19th and 20th Centuries: The Relationship between Theory and Practice*, Sheffield: European Association for the History of Medicine and Health Publications.

Prüll, Cay-Rüdiger and John Woodward (eds) (2003), *Traditions of Pathology in Western Europe: Theories, Institutions, and Their Cultural Setting*, Pfaffenweiler: Centaurus.

Sappol, Michael (2002), *A Traffic of Dead Bodies: Anatomy and Embodied Social Identity in Nineteenth-century America*, Princeton: Princeton University Press.

Soucy, Richard (1977), 'The Pathology Institute', student paper, Montreal: McGill University, Blackader-Lauterman storage, AS42M38 1977 S68.

Stevens, Edward Fletcher (1922), File of letters to Percy Nobbs and others, found at the Royal Victoria Hospital in the early 1990s (hospital closed 2015), Key letter is Stevens to Nobbs, 1 May 1922.

Stevens, Edward Fletcher ([1918] 1928), 'The Department of Research', in *The American Hospital of the Twentieth Century*, [2nd ed.] 3rd ed., New York: Architectural Record Publishing Co.

Ventura, Hector O. (2000), 'Rudolph Virchow and cellular pathology', *Clinical Cardiology*, 23, pp. 550–52.

Wagg, Susan (1980), 'Percy Nobbs at McGill', *Canadian Heritage*, August, pp. 14–5.

Wagg, Susan (1982), *Percy Erskine Nobbs: Architect, Artist, Craftsman*, Montreal: MQUP.

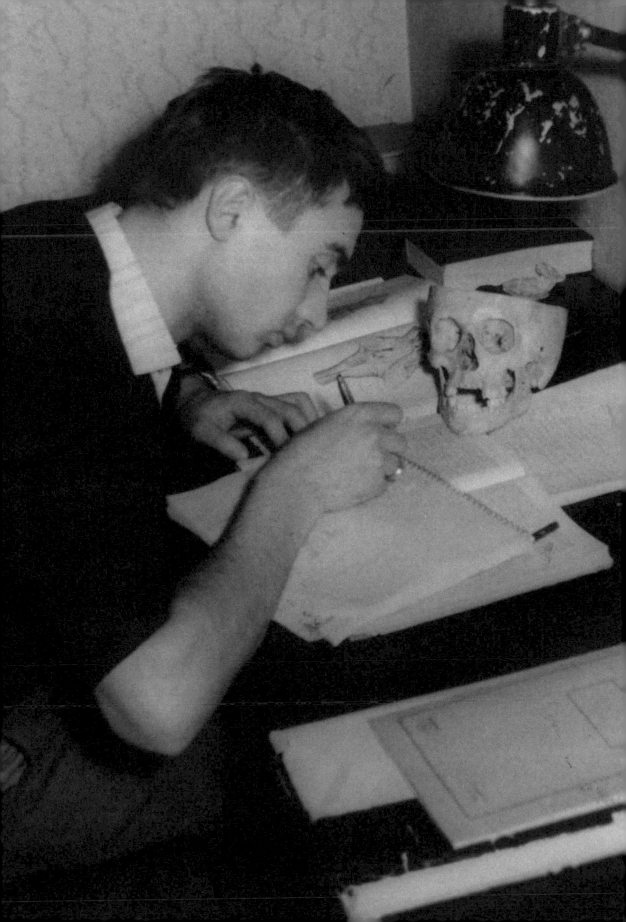

ART

OBJECTIVITY, ART AND MEDICAL IMAGES

Sally Wyatt

Objectivity is the cornerstone of modern science. It refers to the ideal and attempts to observe reality, free from emotion and bias. To achieve objectivity, scientists' observations should be conducted following the scientific method so that they can be communicated and shared with others in order to advance collective knowledge about the world. Objectivity is usually contrasted with personal subjectivity, in which people rely on their own experiences and feelings to make judgments.

The objective–subjective dualism is also present in medicine, with doctors and other medical professionals having access to objective knowledge which they apply to make sense of the subjective experience of patients. The experiences, feelings and symptoms of patients need to be linked to the shared, cumulative, objective knowledge of medicine so that doctors can make diagnoses and offer treatment.

Whether objectivity can ever be realised is much debated in the philosophy of science (Kuhn 1962), feminist science studies (Haraway 1988) and postcolonial histories of medicine (Vaughan 1991), though it remains an important regulatory ideal. Measurement and numbers are a particularly important source of claims to objectivity, in medical and other domains (Porter 1995). In historical, sociological and anthropological studies of health and medicine, the role of images in the production of knowledge and the disciplining of bodies has long been a topic of attention (Lynch and

Figure TE1: Student sketching while preparing for an exam at the Medical University of Budapest. Image courtesy of Semmelweis University Archives (HU-SEKL 49/a, Image gallery/ photos, I/2).

Woolgar 1990; Burri and Dumit 2008). For example, Stefan Hirschauer (1991) argues that much effort has gone into making images look like the body and the body like the image and that these mutually produce ways of seeing for both doctors and artists.

The tension between subjectivity and objectivity in medicine and in medical training and education is apparent in the images and illustrations that can be found in textbooks and in classrooms. Paintings, drawings, prints, etchings, photographs and other forms of illustration are central to medical education, as aspiring doctors learn about ideal, normal and pathological bodies and body parts.

Medical students are often expected to draw what they see as a way of developing their powers of observation, while the images in their textbooks and adorning the walls of classrooms are produced by professional artists and illustrators (with more or less formal acknowledgement – see also section on 'Invisible Work', this volume). Medical topics have long been the object of art, such as Rembrandt's *Anatomy Lesson of Dr Nicolaes Tulp*. In the European tradition, by the Renaissance and even more so during the Enlightenment, doctors and artists often worked together to produce stable and objective representations of the body that could travel between places and over time as part of the shared, collective knowledge that constitutes medicine. Lorraine Daston and Peter Galison (2007) explore in great detail how objectivity came to dominate ways of knowing and of seeing in medicine and other fields, especially with the introduction of technologies and techniques facilitating mechanical objectivity.

Jessica M. Dandona (this volume) examines the role of personal scrapbooks of photographs, produced in the United States in the second half of the nineteenth century by some of the earliest women medical students. She describes how the acquisition of anatomical knowledge involved at least three practices: the visual and haptic explorations of dead bodies, the study of anatomical illustrations in textbooks and elsewhere, and the women's creation of their own illustrations of what they observed. The goal was, through a recursive process of observing, cutting and drawing, to bring bodily structures and the illustrations into alignment.

Staying in the classroom, Rachel Vaden Allison (this volume) describes how chalkboards remain an essential pedagogical tool. Examining a book published early in the twentieth century about the technique of blackboard sketching, she explains how the ability to make anatomical drawings in real time in front of a class of medical students can be challenging for both teachers and students. Medical educators are trained in many things, but rarely in the effective use of a chalkboard. Even though there are many alternatives (including textbooks and photographs in both paper and digital form) that could provide immediate and accurate images, real-time drawing is still part of the repertoire of medical education, often dominating the space of the classroom. Students copy these drawings into their own notebooks, learning how to see and how to record.

A single drawing is the focus of Harriet Palfreyman's chapter (this volume), a drawing created by Dorothy Davison, an artist who worked closely with a surgeon, Geoffrey Jefferson, in mid-twentieth century England. They consulted each other extensively, negotiating their different ways of seeing, or 'four-eyed sight'. This is the term coined by Daston and Galison to capture how naturalists in the eighteenth century

> tried to guide the pencils, brushes, and burins [sharp tools used in engraving] of their artists [...] [T]hese collaborations aimed at a fusion of the head of the naturalist with the hand of the artist, in which the artist surrendered himself (or, often, herself) entirely to the will and judgment of the naturalist. (2007: 88)

There are many possible sources of tension that can occur when artists and scientists collaborate. Daston and Galison (2007) describe conflicts arising because of the usually higher social status enjoyed by scientists. Sometimes this involved the imposition of the scientist's will and way of seeing, and sometimes had more mundane manifestations, such as deferring payment or not acknowledging the work of the artists (again, see section on 'Invisible Work', this volume). Even though that social difference largely remains in the twenty-first century, the relationship between surgeon and artist or craftsperson does not have to be one of subordination. Roger Kneebone and Fleur Oakes (this volume) reflect on their own collaboration as, respectively, surgeon and embroiderer. Both are working with the grain of their own materials and not against it. Oakes, as an artist, remains committed to her aesthetic ideals, but in the process might see what surgeons are trained to overlook. Furthermore, by seeing through the eyes of the artist, and not aiming for 'four-eyed sight', the work of the artist can re-acquaint them with the wonders of the body.

Medical photography is the topic of Anne Katrine Kleberg Hansen's chapter (this volume). She is concerned with how medical photographs (of fatness in the early twentieth century) are simultaneously displays of data, diagnostic tools and instruments for knowledge creation. Photography is a particularly interesting technique, as it has always had a double identity. It is simultaneously seen as a tool to capture reality, and thus an aid to objectivity, but it is also an addition to the media and repertoires available to artists. In Jakob Lehne's chapter (this volume), he traces the early development of another related technology of medical imaging, the medical ultrasound. His careful historical analysis shows how a small group of researchers worked tirelessly on the ideas and materials involved in developing this tool, highlighting the importance of informal connections in the lead up to the more formalised teaching with this instrument. Facilitated by these educational practices, the ultrasound has now become one of the primary tools for creating 'objective' images in medicine today, from a baby's first photo to the portable version threatening to supersede the stethoscope at the bedside.

Drew Danielle Belsky (this volume) draws attention to the construction of 'accuracy' in biomedical images. She argues that this is not simply a matter of objectively depicting bodily structures, but is also the result of the possibilities offered by the tools and skills of people. These can include implements for drawing and painting, but increasingly also digital tools and medical imaging. Thus, accuracy for the medical illustrator is not only about precise measurement. It also involves aesthetic, moral and practical considerations, all of which change over time and across place.

These contributions remind the reader that images of many different sorts have long played a role in the practice of medicine and the training of doctors. But they also remind the reader that a picture is not always worth a thousand words and that sometimes more than a thousand words are needed to explain how pictures come into being and how they should be interpreted. The chapters mentioned above highlight the constructed nature of medical images, whatever the technique used to produce them. This directly challenges the notion that such images can ever be objective. But we also need to remember that notions of objectivity are themselves always in flux, as new techniques for producing knowledge and images emerge.

References

Burri, Regula Valérie and Dumit, Joseph (2008), 'Social studies of scientific imaging and visualization', in E. Hackett, O. Amsterdamska, M. Lynch and J. Wajcman (eds), *The Handbook of Science and Technology Studies*, 3rd ed., Cambridge: The MIT Press, pp. 297–317.

Daston, Lorraine and Galison, Peter (2007), *Objectivity*, Brooklyn: Zone Books.

Haraway, Donna (1988), 'Situated knowledges: The science question in feminism and the privilege of partial perspective', *Feminist Studies*, 14:3, pp. 575–99.

Hirschauer, Stefan (1991), 'The manufacture of bodies in surgery', *Social Studies of Science*, 21:2, pp. 279–319.

Kuhn, Thomas (1962), *The Structure of Scientific Revolutions*, Chicago: University of Chicago Press.

Lynch, Michael and Woolgar, Steve (eds) (1990), *Representation in Scientific Practice*, Cambridge: The MIT Press.

Porter, Theodore (1995), *Trust in Numbers: The Pursuit of Objectivity in Science and Public Life*, Princeton: Princeton University Press.

Vaughan, Megan (1991), *Curing Their Ills: Colonial Power and African Illness*, Cambridge: Polity Press.

BALLOONS

LESSONS FROM A BALLOON

Christine den Harder and Anna Harris

A balloon filled with water rests precariously on an office filing cabinet (Figure 2.1). The permanent marker features drawn on its green bulbous skin smile up to the fluorescent lights on the ceiling. The next day it has burst, seeping water over the edge of the metal drawers and onto a few papers lying on a desk. It has done its job anyway. It shared an important lesson with medical students about a symptom of many diseases, something they are likely to see in their future clinical practice. Our chapter focuses on this balloon and how it is used in medical teaching, drawing examples from the Skillslab, an institution within the medical faculty at Maastricht University where medical students are taught hands-on practical skills of clinical examination. This is where Christine works and Anna has conducted ethnographic fieldwork. During their fieldwork, Anna and Christine shared an office, their desks side by side and separated by the filing cabinet upon which the balloon burst. At the Skillslab, depending on the type of skill that is being taught, students either practice these skills by examining each other or by using mannequins and other tools. The balloon lesson features in a teaching session for the second-year medical students. After learning about the basic abdominal examination in their first year, they come to the Skillslab to learn about signs of underlying pathology. One of these is ascites.

Ascites means that there is fluid where it should not be in the abdominal cavity, and assessing its presence was part of the student's lesson on the abdominal examination. One of the ways to assess whether ascitic fluid could be present is to check for the so-called shifting dullness. The student (performing being doctor) percusses (taps) the abdomen and listens to the sound: dull sounds signify an underlying solid structure or fluid, whereas the gas-filled bowels produce hollow, drum-like tympanic

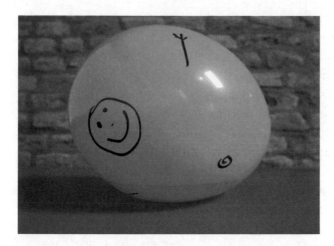

Figure 2.1: Replication of the green balloon. Image courtesy of author.

sounds. Ascitic fluid sinks with gravity, while the gas-filled loops of the bowel rise. Changing the patient's position will therefore cause free-flowing fluid to reposition as well, causing dullness to be heard where it previously was not: shifting dullness. Ascitis, however, is only present when there is an underlying medical condition. The causes are many, ranging from heart disease to malignancy. Shifting dullness will not be found by examining a healthy fellow student, making the concept rather illusive. That is why the balloon offers students something more tangible: it allows the teacher to show students what actually happens with ascitic fluid inside of a patient's abdominal cavity, in various positions.

How might this simple balloon, now shrivelled into sticky scraps, have taught so much? How does it open up doctors in training to a world of gastrointestinal diseases? In this chapter, we focus on three lessons that the balloon offers in regards to medical education as well as studies of simulation. In line with the anthropologist Elizabeth Hallam's (2013) call to pay more attention to locally made teaching materials in medical education, we suggest that the balloon not only provides an excellent pedagogical tool but also expands thinking about simulation. It does so, we suggest, by highlighting the power of sensory analogies that attend closely to the material properties of objects in simulation.

Lesson 1: Sensory (material) analogy

The balloon was a simulation. Many fields of practice have long used simulations, from the Ancients to contemporary times. Simulations are models based on what is known, projecting into situations where the conditions are not known. Simulations have long been used to teach doctors medicine, and nowadays the academic field of medical education even has a whole sub-field that specialises in the topic called 'simulation-based health professions education', with its own conferences and journals. Simulation in medical education may refer to things, people or events, depending on the learning purpose. In this chapter, we are interested in material simulation technologies, which mostly conjure images of plastic models and mannequins. We broadly define material simulation technologies as material objects which simulate a clinical situation.

Since the development of the first medical simulators which had moving parts and dynamic effects (Owen 2016), simulation-based health professions education has focused on issues of 'fidelity', that is, the extent to which the simulator 'looks, feels and acts like a human patient' (Hamstra et al. 2014: 387), often with the aim of trying to achieve 'high fidelity'. Rather than using the dichotomy between 'high' and 'low' fidelity (Tun et al. 2015: 168), Hamstra et al. prefer to differentiate between 'structural fidelity (how the simulator appears) and functional fidelity (what the simulator does)' as their starting points for distinguishing and evaluating teaching tools (2014: 388). They propose to shift the focus more to functional fidelity in regards to clinical task demands, rather than physical resemblance (structural fidelity), which they refer to as the 'tactile, visual, auditory, and olfactory features of the simulator' (Hamstra et al. 2004: 389). That is, they reject the growing importance placed on expensive and 'realistic' simulators and prefer those which focus on functionality, thus being potentially inexpensive, and, they argue, simple to make.

Rather than distinguishing between the functional and sensory properties of a simulation, we propose that the balloon is an example of how a combination of both can work very effectively. Put another way, we believe that a good teaching tool can attend to function through close attention to its sensory properties; how it feels, looks, sounds and smells. To think through these possibilities further, we introduce the term *sensory analogy*. Analogy, like simulation, is a term with a long theoretical and philosophical tradition. It is a way of comparing relations (Durrenberger and Morrison 1977), where the relation is between things which are comparable in significant ways. The challenge is in working out what counts as a significant feature that is comparable in making an analogy. What makes a good comparative feature seems hard to elucidate. In his article on using analogies in surgical education, Pamidi writes vaguely that a good analogy is 'similar in significant respects' (2020: 1). He mostly refers to visual similarities, using a halved cauliflower for example as a vegetable visually similar to brain anatomy. We find Mary Hesse's (1966) work in the philosophy of science more useful in developing an understanding of analogy here, for she uniquely focuses on *material analogy*. Material analogy refers to comparative features that are shared, and observable, features that often draw from personal and cultural experience.

We agree with others that finding such sensory analogies in simple objects takes a certain skill (Pamidi 2020), yet disagree with medical educators who suggest that simple simulations are easy to make (Hamstra et al. 2014). The teacher must know about the patient's clinical features they are trying to find a comparison to, to simulate and to be creative enough to explore the possibilities of alternatives that offer a connection and, at the same time, further the lesson's learning goals. The balloon lesson was developed by one teacher in the Skillslab and was shared in lesson preparation sessions and, less formally, in coffee break discussions. The lesson was not obvious, it needed to be learned, and the teachers learned something in the making of it too (Hallam 2013). It worked because it focused on what the materials could teach, how they highlighted and amplified and simplified, all at once, an aspect of something much more complex. We explore this in more detail in the next lesson, in regards to how the balloon offers spatial possibilities that other teaching objects do not.

Lesson 2: Attending to the body as a three-dimensional space

One of the great challenges of many traditional teaching technologies, such as textbooks or lecture slides, is trying to orientate medical students to the body as a three-dimensional space. Newer industries, such as haptics and virtual reality, are treating this challenge as a driving factor in their development of technology. Older techniques, such as blackboard drawing, also offer a three-dimensional rendering of the body (Harris 2015; Allison forthcoming) through layers of coloured chalk so medical students can draw and imagine the bodies being crafted in front of them.

In this same vein, we find that the simple balloon can help craft a sensory and spatial imaginary.

Because the balloon, when filled with air, is slightly transparent, the fluid inside is visible, and not only that, but dynamic as well (unlike e.g. chalk drawings). The transparency allows for a three-dimensionality that is not the same as in textbook diagrams. It thus attends to the spaces of the body in a different way, emphasising those spaces which often aren't recreated in plastic models – the absent spaces and voids – which is where ascites (fluid) collects (see also Dumit and O'Connor's 2016 work on fascia). These might be considered the in-between spaces of the body. As with other simple technologies – such as, a knitted uterus in the Skillslab, which offers a dynamic lesson for childbirth (Nott and Harris 2020) – the teacher can move the balloon around and show how ascites fluid shifts in the body. This helps simulate the classic but hard to conceptualise sign of shifting dullness. The actual contents of a fellow students' abdomen are not visible and looking at a static textbook picture doesn't visualise the positional changes of ascitic fluid. This is where the balloon proves helpful: it's partially filled with water to show an air–fluid level and can be moved around to simulate various patient positions.

In her work with surgeons, the anthropologist Rachel Prentice (2013) shows the importance of developing a three-dimensional spatial and sensory imagination when surgeons learn to use laparoscopic equipment. They have to imagine, she writes, that they are 'swimming in the joint', that is, that they are one with and inside the body (such as inside a joint during arthroscopy). The balloon invites such an imaginary, whether in an abdominal examination or in other lessons, such as the lesson crafted by teachers in a workshop, where they created a thoracic cavity with a balloon to practice percussion. The balloon, in all its simplicity, requires a certain 'leap' of the imagination, and it is precisely this work that is so crucial to developing a close understanding of, from inside, future bodies and future patients.

Lesson 3: Simple materials

Bought in a large packet, a balloon is, in most parts of the world, an inexpensive item, and, in many countries, is easy to source. We suggest that it is the availability as well as the simplicity of this object that contributes to making it such a successful teaching object. As our colleague and collaborator Marijke Kruithof has shown, over and over again in her workshops making and repairing Skillslab materials around the world, by using simple, locally sourced objects in simulation sessions, teachers and students alike can not only improvise but can also learn a lot from the work that goes into making these objects.

Hallam (2013) writes about the improvised use of simple materials in medical education as a form of improvised creativity. During her fieldwork in the University of Aberdeen Medical School, she became interested in the more eclectic use of ready-to-hand materials to make 'one-offs for local on-site consumption, rather than in high numbers for international distribution' (Hallam 2013: 103). She suggests that these purpose-made models have been largely under-researched, yet are 'crucial in facilitating and deepening anatomical understandings of the body' (Hallam 2013: 103), particularly because they are so integrated into local instruction and teaching practices.

We see local improvisation with materials over and over again in the Skillslab – a teacher pulls a curtain taught to make a heart sound, uses parts of their bodies to simulate others (one of our favourites being how teachers put their arms out as ovaries, see also Natasha Myers 2015 for bodily configurations in teaching, or squeeze a juice packet to simulate a jugular venous pressure examination). Teachers do not always stick to lesson plans, but rather they are constantly improvising with their own bodies and the materials that come to hand (Harris and Rethans 2018).

Our collaboration at the Skillslab developed these ideas concretely in a making workshop where we merely facilitated space, time and some simple craft materials and the teachers in the laboratory made their own teaching technologies. We offered balloons and teachers came up with wonderful ways in which they could be used. For example, they filled them with plasticine and different lumpy materials, to make a scrotum examination comparison chart. They critically engaged with their models, considering other materials they could use, and how they did or did not complement models already in use, wondering what they added to the lesson, if anything. Because the materials were simple and easy to source, prototypes could be made and destroyed without worry. It also worked outside the vast industry in commercially produced and ready-made materials that are so often used in medical education, which do not always fit easily into local teaching sites, whether due to the ways in which disease is materialised or the techniques and resources required for use. Yet, while the materials in the workshop were simple, as we suggested above, making these objects required experience and skill.

Conclusion

As the surgical education Roger Kneebone has discussed in his work on clinical simulation, too often in medical education emphasis is placed on technological sophistication 'at the expense of theory-based design' (Kneebone 2005: 549). While medical educators want to do away with distinctions between high and low fidelity, and lose terms like fidelity altogether, they still cling to the idea that expensive simulations are more 'sophisticated', as even Kneebone describes (2005: 549). We argue that cost does not equate to sophistication, and in fact the simplest, least expensive materials can be part of elegant clinical examination lessons. We suggest that the sophistication involved in making models is in considering their sensory analogical properties. We highlighted the importance of attending to the material possibilities of teaching objects, particularly their spatial dimensions, and suggested that simple and inexpensive forms of simulations can be easily used and adapted.

We do not believe that the learning possibilities for such simple models require, as Hamstra et al. write, the 'suspension of disbelief' (2014: 387), but rather that sensory analogies require a lot of work on behalf of the learner, in a way that exercises the imagination. Just as Hallam found in her fieldwork – that it was the movement between different models that drew students into 'a more concentrated visual exploration of both renderings' (Hallam 2013: 110) – so too do we believe that this comparative work, the movement between models and the imagination that is layered and built through engagement with them, is a crucial aspect of learning in medicine. In fact, these models come into their own for concepts that are particularly hard to grasp, concepts such as shifting dullness which relates to invisible spaces in the body. The simplicity of the models offers, as Hallam also found in Aberdeen, an on-the-spot solution for dealing with the conceptual puzzles which arise in local teaching situations at the Skillslab in Maastricht.

The medical educationalist and humanities scholar Alan Bleakley writes that 'analogies serve anticipatory functions in learning, preparing students for situations that are not readily experienced but may be simulated' (2017: 87). Working with analogies in medicine, in material forms, requires significant cognitive leaps (Bleakley 2017). As science educators Alan Harrison and David Treagust point out in their work on the use of analogies in science education, teachers must keep in mind that 'an analogy does not provide learners with all facets of the target concept' (2006: 22). It is precisely this extra work required that we suggest makes sensory material analogies such as the balloon, objects seemingly so far from resembling future patient bodies, so rich in terms of the lessons that they can offer.

Acknowledgements

The research conducted for this article was supported by the European Research Council under the European Union's Horizon 2020 research and innovation programme (Grant agreement no. 678390; awarded to Anna Harris).

References

Allison, Rachel Vaden (forthcoming), 'Crafting bodies: An anthropological exploration of the entanglement of technology and the senses in 21st century medical education', Ph.D. thesis, Maastricht: Maastricht University Faculty of Arts and Social Sciences.

Bleakley, Alan (2017), *Thinking with Metaphors in Medicine: The State of the Art*, Abingdon, Oxon: Routledge.

Dumit, Joseph and O'Connor, Kevin (2016), 'The senses and sciences of fascia: A practice as research', in H. Lynette, E. Krimmer and P. Lichtenfels (eds), *Performativity of Embodiment: Thinking Alongside the Human*, London: Lexington Books, pp. 35–54.

Durrenberger, Paul and Morrison, John W. (1977), 'A theory of analogy', *Journal of Anthropological Research*, 33:4, pp. 372–87.

Hallam, Elizabeth (2013), 'Anatomical design: Making and using three-dimensional models of the human body', in W. Gunn, T. Otto and R. C. Smith (eds), *Design Anthropology: Theory and Practice*, Oxford: Berg, pp. 100–16.

Hamstra, Stanley, Brydges, Ryan, Hatala, Rose, Zendejas, Benjamin and Cook, David (2014), 'Reconsidering fidelity in simulation-based training', *Academic Medicine*, 89:3, pp. 387–92.

Harris, Anna (2015), 'The blackboard anatomist', *British Medical Journal*, 350:h345, https://doi.org/10.1136/bmj.h345. Accessed 24 November 2021.

Harris, Anna and Rethans, Jan-Joost (2018), 'Expressive instructions: Ethnographic insights into the creativity and improvisation entailed in teaching physical skills to medical students', *Perspectives on Medical Education*, 7:4, pp. 226–27.

Harrison, Allan G. and Treagust, David F. (2006), 'Teaching and learning with analogies: Friend or foe?', in P. J. Aubusson, A. G. Harrison and S. M. Ritchie (eds), *Metaphor and Analogy in Science Education*, Dordrecht: Springer Netherlands, pp. 11–24.

Hesse, Mary B. (1966), *Models and Analogies in Science*, Indiana: University of Notre Dame Press.

Kneebone, Roger (2005), 'Evaluating clinical simulations for learning procedural skills: A theory-based approach', *Academic Medicine: Journal of the Association of American Medical Colleges*, 80:6, pp. 549–53.

Myers, Natasha (2015), *Rendering Life Molecular: Models, Modelers, and Excitable Matter*, Durham: Duke University Press.

Nott, John and Harris, Anna (2020), 'Sticky models: History as friction in obstetric education', *Medicine Anthropology Theory*, 7:1, pp. 44–65.

Owen, Harry (2016), *Simulation in Healthcare Education: An Extensive History*, Cham: Springer.

Pamidi, Narendra (2020), 'Use of essential analogies in clinical anatomy active learning curriculum: A personal reflection', *Translational Research in Anatomy*, 18, pp. 1–3.

Prentice, Rachel (2013), *Bodies in Formation: An Ethnography of Anatomy and Surgery Education*, Durham: Duke University Press.

Tun, Jimmy Kyaw, Alinier, Guillaume and Kneebone, Roger (2015), 'Redefining simulation fidelity for healthcare education', *Simulation & Gaming*, 46:2, pp. 159–74.

CADAVERS

THE GEOGRAPHY OF THE DEAD AND THE MOVEMENT OF THE LIVING: KINETIC CONSCIOUSNESS AND THE LIMITS OF THE CADAVER

Rachel Prentice

Two works of art, with not quite a century separating their creation, frame the contrast I explore in this paper. First, the man from Vesalius' 1543 *De Humani Corporis Fabrica* takes a step forward, his left arm raised and pointing toward the sky and the right pointing downward, see Figure 3.1. His eyes rise skyward, as if asking God in which direction he is headed. He has no skin. The Vesalian man's muscles are delineated and labelled. Yet there is something odd in that upraised left arm. A bent arm should have a flexed biceps brachii muscle (as any bodybuilder or Popeye watcher can attest). This one is slack. Similarly, the quadriceps and the gastrocnemius muscles of the left leg, the one rooted to the ground, should bulge more than the right as the leg takes all the man's weight, leaving the right leg unweighted and poised to leave the ground. As these slight inaccuracies reveal, Vesalius created history's most famous anatomical atlas by dissecting bodies of the dead, whose muscles no longer flex.

Figure 3.1: Andreas Vesalius, *De Humani Corporis Fabrica Libri Septem.* Courtesy of the Wellcome Collection, London, UK.

SECVNDA
MVSCVLO.
RVMTA
BVLA.

The second work is Rembrandt Van Rijn's painting, *The Anatomy Lesson of Dr. Nicholaes Tulp* from 1632, see Figure 3.2. In this painting, Tulp demonstrates the anatomy of a man's arm to a gathered group of observers. In his right hand, he holds what is likely to be a pair of forceps with which he grasps a tendon of the cadaver's arm. He holds his left hand up making a gesture that echoes the Vesalian man's hands. The gathered men look at Tulp or off into the distance. Only one observer looks at the tendon that Tulp holds up to view. In a living body, a tendon stretched like this would flex the fingers, not leave them extended as depicted. But the fingers' stiffness may indicate a body in a state of rigor mortis. Tulp's left hand and red-cheeked face jump out of the painting. His liveliness and mobility present a marked contrast to the cadaver, whose face and feet recede into shadow and whose skin is the chalk-pale colour of the dead. Whereas Vesalius posed his skinless man like a man in motion, Rembrandt took pains to emphasise the corpse's deathly pallor. The body stretches out before the gathered audience, his abdomen available for and vulnerable to dissection.

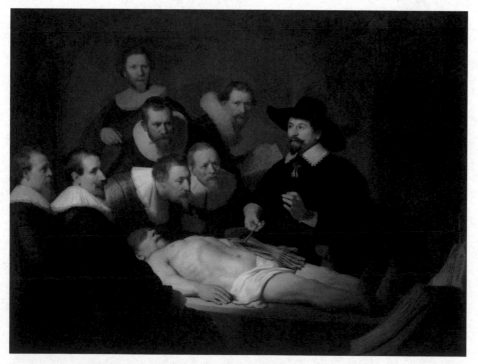

Figure 3.2: Rembrandt van Rijn, The Anatomy Lesson of Dr Nicolaes Tulp, 1632. Courtesy of the Mauritshuis, The Hague, The Netherlands.

These two depictions of bodies reveal the difficulties of using the dead to model the living. Vesalius tried to portray the moving body's dynamism and complex interplay of muscles, but the Vesalian man's flaccid muscles reveal the limitations of his source material. Rembrandt painted the inanimate cadaver, which has been the standard reference for biomedicine's *lingua franca* and its most formative teaching object for two centuries. But the fingers on the cadaver's hands do not move as living flesh would move. This is a difference between the person who is, from before birth until death, a body in motion and the body as a scientific object that is fixed and immobilised, akin to a dead insect pinned to a mat. I contend that biomedical practitioners have built their epistemology on examining and teaching the immobile body of the dead at the expense of the lessons that moving bodies could provide. Kinetic consciousness, the ability to analyse motion and link pathological effects to distant causes, allows practitioners to address the causes of maladaptive movement and can have profound consequences for rehabilitation. Yet, as I show, kinetic consciousness remains at biomedicine's margins.

Anatomists select each teaching cadaver from elderly bodies (far in age from most medical students). Technicians shave, embalm, and place the body, naked, on a dissection table in a body bag. The dissection table typically sits in an inner room within a larger laboratory space that contains other dissection tables, sinks for handwashing, bright red bio-waste bags, the occasional wired-together skeleton, and other signs that mark the space as laboratory space and focus the eye and attention on the body bag and its contents. I did participant observation in two anatomy laboratories during eighteen months of ethnographic research into North American anatomy and surgery education. I observed that the laboratory setting and the cadaver's preparation help beginning or future medical students to relate to the cadaver as a medical object. But, as the body that once housed a living, agential person, the cadaver is never ontologically stable: it is always person and thing. Contemporary anatomists make use of this duality to teach lessons about medical care and respect for bodies (Prentice 2013). After orientation to the laboratory, students cut the bag open as a first intimate revelation that prepares them for more significant revelations to come. Over the course of weeks or months, students dissect the cadaver in layers, usually following the body's 'natural compartments' (Good 1994: 73), departing from those compartments towards the end, when the cadaver ceases to resemble anything human, but still holds significant lessons about the structures hidden inside.

The cadaver is the prime object of ritual initiation into the mysteries of biomedical practice and what a medical student might call a 'high-impact' learning tool. As a teaching tool and introduction to clinical practice, the cadaver offers emotional lessons about death and dying, moral lessons about respect for and handling of human bodies, practical lessons about opening the body in layers and dissecting some of the body's 50,000 named parts as they appear in embalmed human tissues, perceptual lessons in the art of visualising the body's structures in three dimensions, and clinical lessons about correlations and pathologies that might present in the clinic.

In contrast, kinetic consciousness typically develops among practitioners at biomedicine's outer edges where it is found in some engineers, coaches, physical therapists, martial artists and other movement experts. When I discussed knowledge of movement among medical practitioners with a physician–ethnographer who had given a talk at my home institution, he said physicians are 'very bad' at what he called 'functional anatomy'. I prefer to call this kind of knowing 'kinetic consciousness' to emphasise the acquired nature of this skill, which can range from understanding of the physics of bodies in motion to trained mastery of the interplay of body parts built from years of careful observation and manipulation. This is the ability to recognise the effects of maladaptive movement on the body, even or especially at sites distant from an injury. The idea is easy in principle. Any reader can experience this: sit straight, become aware of the two bony protrusions at the bottom of your pelvis as they make contact with the chair (it helps if the chair is not too soft) then drop your chin to your chest. Feel how that movement affects your head, neck and back. Then raise your chin toward the sky (gently) and feel how this movement travels down the front of your abdomen to your pelvis. An injury along one of these pathways could lead to compensations and eventual dysfunction anywhere along these expanses and beyond. Yet recognition of the interconnected nature of bodily movement often is missing at the heart of biomedicine. In this chapter, I look at how one object – the cadaver – supports an atomistic epistemology that seeks answers in ever-finer resolution of the nature of tissue damage, leading to increasingly powerful visualisation techniques and resolution of molecular mechanisms. This geographic approach, akin to repeatedly hitting the '+' button on a digital map, assumes that the answers to clinical problems will be found at specific sites of injury, rather than in the complex interplay of bodily structures in motion.

A closer look at the material affordances of the cadaver in its role as a teaching tool reveals an object that is uniquely and poorly suited to teaching the dynamics of movement, especially whole-body movement. At the most superficial level, this is crassly obvious: the cadaver is, quite simply, too stiff. It does not bend. Embalmed tissues do not stretch. It cannot be used to demonstrate more than the most minimal movements. Examining movement requires a practiced eye, which can be aided by video recordings, treadmills and other special equipment. Movement problems may involve multiple compensations that require interpretation. The study of movement is the product of experience and expert judgment and is, thus, not amenable to the 'fierce *yearning* for clarity' that Shigehisa Kuriyama marks as a founding concern of Euro-American medicine (2002: 64, original emphasis). In this chapter, I treat the dissection of cadavers as a formative experience for biomedical trainees (Good 1994) that privileges the search for and treatment of the site of disease and marginalises more dynamic rehabilitation approaches to disordered movement.

From muscles to tissues to cells

Although dissection has been widely practiced among peoples worldwide, only the Greeks and their European successors felt compelled to develop detailed knowledge of 'somatic structure' (Kuriyama 2002: 120). Despite this interest, the science of clinical correlation only began to develop in earnest in the late eighteenth century. Prior to the late eighteenth century, physicians saw no connection between the histories they took in the clinic and the bodily geography that others were mapping in the anatomy laboratory (Foucault 1973). In the late eighteenth century, pathological anatomists began to seek anatomical lesions inside the deceased that corresponded to symptoms seen in the living. Michel Foucault quotes physician René Laënnec's early nineteenth-century entry on pathological anatomy in his *Dictionary of Medical Sciences* (*Dictionnaire des sciences médicales*): 'pathological anatomy is a science whose aim is the knowledge of the visible alterations produced on the organs of the human body by the state of disease' (Laënnec cited in Foucault 1973: 135). Early pathological anatomists sought to understand how disease manifests at specific sites in specific types of tissue. Surgery at the time was relegated to butchers and barbers, so focus remained on elaborating disease mechanisms rather than on repair.

As John Nott and Anna Harris (2020) remind us, material histories can be sticky, keeping objects clinging to past practices. Clinical correlations remain an important part of anatomy education and clinicians in many fields told me that clinical discoveries made in the anatomy laboratory remain the most memorable moments of their anatomy education. But the primary focus of dissection for medical students is naming and identifying structures.

> The majority of the time is spent trying to separate natural surfaces, to distinguish the boundaries of gross forms and identify tiny nerves, veins, lymph glands, and to match these to the relation to each other but in finer and finer detail, revealing the natural body. (Good 1994: 73)

The students Good describes likely learned to see and to name even smaller structures in a histology class, where microscopes and stains would help them examine cells and cellular abnormalities. There is an assumption in this method that Good does not question, which is that the secrets of the body's functioning reside in understanding the body's workings at ever-smaller levels, leading ultimately to cellular-level visualisations and molecular-level analyses. I do not dispute the power of this method. Instead, I contend that this pushes young physicians to look for solutions by looking at bodies at increasingly high resolutions, often neglecting solutions that might ask them to seek answers in relations among structures in motion. Object and method work together to produce this atomistic approach: cadavers are vastly better for exploring structures than they are for modelling how structures work together to produce living movement.

Biomechanics researchers trace the origins of their field to Aristotle's *The Movement of Animals* (Martin 1999). *Mosby's Medical Dictionary* defines biomechanics as the study of mechanical laws and their application to living organisms, including the body and its locomotor system. Nineteenth-century biomechanics is typically equated with the work of E. J. Marey and Eadweard Muybridge. This work was obsessed with the gaits of horses. Yet the movement traces Marey developed were largely rejected by the medical establishment of his day as too abstracted from direct observation of the body (Mayer 2010). Today, biomechanics research encompasses a huge range of topics and disciplines, including anatomy, physiology, several areas of engineering, orthopaedics, rehabilitation science, sports science, ergonomics, kinesiology and others.

Biomechanics, especially understanding of the extended linkages of tissues across the whole body, often is absent in biomedical practice. Analysis of human movement is a 'subjugated knowledge' in the Foucauldian sense; that is, a knowledge that remained underdeveloped or was buried when a field coalesced, especially if it challenged institutional or formal knowledges (1997: 7). Movement analysis pushes away from anatomy, a science largely dedicated to discovery and description of body parts, toward physics, which few biomedical practitioners study in depth. But specific practices matter here. As Janelle Taylor writes, 'The interesting question [...] is exactly how, in any given instance, representational, social, material and other practices may work together to materialize bodies in very particular ways within specific kinds of relations' (2005: 746). In this case, anatomy's historical place at the beginnings of the explosion of medical and other sciences in the nineteenth century and the relative ease and precision of studying dead bodies and their parts, has locked biomedical scientists into an epistemology built on increasingly atomistic understandings of bodies rather than broad understanding of functional relations that might lead to rehabilitative solutions.

Veterinary medicine has largely followed the biomedical model, but limited treatment options for some common conditions have led some animal researchers to collaborate with trainers on movement rehabilitation. A pathologist and a comparative anatomist, who are working to bring stronger understandings of movement pathologies into veterinary medicine, wrote a study guide for veterinary students at the University of Georgia (Uhl and Osborn 2016) that follows principles intended to help students begin to develop kinetic consciousness. Packed biomedical and veterinary curricula likely cannot sustain extensive movement education, but these principles are intended to start the process:

1. *Pathomechanical forces can cause injury and pain in humans and animals. Correcting mechanics may lead to relief.* This statement seems obvious, but the authors are acknowledging that many practitioners have a weak understanding of pathomechanical forces, making this perhaps the most radical provocation to practitioners on this list.
2. *Biomechanical awareness takes time to develop and biomechanical issues take diligence to correct.* The authors note that kinetic consciousness requires 'trained judgment' (Daston and Galison 2007: 309),

the accumulation of years of practice at reading bodies, injuries and compensations. Fixes are not necessarily quick, which would make them unattractive to medical systems dedicated to cost containment. Further, this requires patience and compliance on the part of animal handlers and injured humans.

3. *Human patients and animal handlers can learn to evaluate their own or their animals' movement and suggest corrections.* The suggestion that lay experts can contribute to rehabilitation pushes against a biomedical epistemology built upon the patient's objectification and compliance (or, in the veterinary case, the compliance of human handlers).

4. *The idea that drugs and surgery are the only solutions is a common misunderstanding that needs correction.* This principle challenges two centres of biomedical money and power. As importantly, the authors advocate for solutions that seek an injury's cause in pathological movement mechanics, rather than surgical intervention or chemical palliation that treats lesions that result from that movement.

Efforts to bring kinetic approaches into biomedicine also are emerging from fields at biomedicine's margins. For example, several areas of recent work, such as Thomas W. Myers *Anatomy Trains: Myofascial Meridians for Manual and Movement Therapists* (2014), seek to demonstrate the significance of fascia and a whole-body understanding of movement. Approaches that adapt W. Buckminster Fuller's tension-and-compression models known as 'tensegrity' to body movement urge practitioners to take seriously the physics of all tissues, including connective tissues (Scarr 2018). 'Biotensegrity' treats bodily structures like the cables and struts of a suspension bridge, rather than the beams and cantilevers of a medieval cathedral. Traditional approaches to biomechanical movement often isolate body parts:

> Motion is then analyzed through a system of joints and levers that are frequently considered in isolation from one another and without the connective tissues that surround and link them together, but such analysis is a gross simplification, always incomplete and in some cases absurd. (Scarr 2018: 41)

Biotensegrity and fascial approaches to human motion ask practitioners to consider connective tissue as significant in functional analyses of human anatomy. But as the subtitle for Myers's book suggests, this knowledge exists primarily at the margins of biomedical practice. Biotensegrity experts utilise the physics of movement to examine how structures interact without assuming that movement is primarily a function of a structure's relation to gravity.

Stephen M. Levin is an orthopaedist who began exploring the structures of natural bodies – plants and animals – as tensegrity structures. Levin contends that clinical experience led him to look for the internal organising forces of a body that can 'function at sea, in air, on land or in space, right side up or upside down and not be dependent on outside forces to maintain its structural integrity' (Levin cited in Scarr 2018: xiii). The physics of biotensegrity are considerably more complicated than solid-body mechanics, which might be a hindrance to their adoption in biomedicine. And, as occurred with Marey's traces in the nineteenth century, I have seen contemporary practitioners reject models that look too abstracted from the body. Biotensegrity models look very abstract, indeed.

> The resolution of a 'local' condition can then require a whole-body approach to treating it, or vice versa, particularly if tissues some distance away have become chronically adapted to changes in the structural balance and an understanding of biotensegrity provides the rationale for this. (Scarr 2018: 130)

Scarr argues that practitioners can initiate changes in the body, but then must allow the body's systems to move toward a different state of 'health'. Intriguingly, in a footnote, he suggests that treatment could include drugs or surgery, but also could include 'yoga, tai chi, exercises, postural and movement advice, etc.' (Scarr 2018: 130). He advocates a range of therapeutic possibilities that extend well beyond biomedicine and advocates an approach that suggests that practitioners do not fix bodies, bodies fix themselves when pointed in a more functional direction.

Annemarie Mol (2002) demonstrates ethnographically how a disease (atherosclerosis) can be enacted in different ways through different practices. This important approach shows the heterogeneity of practices and the ways they mostly hold together in clinical settings, even when information given by the varying practices conflict. However, Mol's ontological approach flattens the institutional and educational structures that may give one practice hegemony over others or may make some practices difficult for practitioners to understand or accept. An approach that asks practitioners to move from identification and description to physics, from dissection of the dead to analysis of the living, and from practices like surgery, which renders the living closer to the dead, to practices that enrol the living in their own rehabilitation asks much of contemporary biomedical institutions and practitioners.

A journey into dynamic movement

The development of my own biomechanical consciousness is relevant because it took place outside the anatomy laboratory. While doing ethnographic research into anatomy and surgery education, I took an anatomy course at a Boston-area medical school in 2001 and then spent autumn 2001 and most of 2002 doing participant observation in a medical school that I call Coastal University and another round of fieldwork in 2006 at a Canadian University that I call Urban University. I observed anatomy classes (both lectures and dissections), observed surgeries, worked with a group building digital tools for medical education, spent an afternoon dissecting an elbow and had many formal and informal talks with anatomists. During this anatomy training, I developed structural knowledge and the ability to visualise structures in three-dimensional space. But my understanding of biomechanics did not begin until three things converged: my own long-term rehabilitation from a badly broken ankle, my attempts to understand my horse Shantih's problematic movement and the start of a research project that examines the scientific and aesthetic dimensions of horse and human movement. When I began this project, I met a trio of researchers that included a high-level dressage trainer and two scientists. The group had worked on rehabilitation of horses deemed crippled by traditional veterinarians. The dressage trainer used careful training to make these horses sound again, not by resolving lesions, but by retraining the horses' movement to reduce maladaptive mechanical stresses.

Their work got me thinking about problems I had with my own horse, who tended to dive onto her left front leg when doing left turns. When I began thinking about her movement issues holistically, I realised that she was diving onto that leg to avoid putting weight on her right hind leg, which was weak and possibly damaged. Left uncorrected, the excessive forces on her left front leg could lead to damage in that leg. As I developed whole-body awareness, I realised that the three-dimensional understanding of structures I had developed in anatomy classes made the structural and three-dimensional aspects of kinetic consciousness easier to develop. But none of my anatomy classes focused on movement. One digital application under development analysed the movement of the finger joints. I also witnessed only one demonstration of human movement in the anatomy laboratory, as I recount in the next section. But neither the application nor the demonstration examined distant effects of maladaptive movement.

As I became attuned to mechanics in humans and horses, I learned about many failures to consider movement. For example, the orthopaedist who put my shattered ankle together conducted follow-up exams by looking at an X-ray and, occasionally, manipulating my foot. He remained wholly focused on the site of injury and never once asked me to walk, an act that would have revealed a significant limp and compensations in my hip and back that persisted until I found two holistic bodyworkers, a Rolfer and an Alexander Technique teacher, who addressed the movement of my entire body. A different orthopaedist told a friend's husband he wanted to operate on his back for back pain. My friend said the back problem was caused by two failed knee surgeries he had in his twenties. She remained unconvinced that surgically altering his back would fix the problem or whether it would provide short-term palliation and long-term problems. I convinced her to find a different orthopaedist. In a third case, a chiropractor told me about a woman who had a hip replaced at a relatively young age. She knew the damage to her hip originated with an imbalance in her knee. She asked the surgeon how to prevent degradation of the artificial hip (one does not get infinite replacements). The surgeon said he didn't know: She would have to consult a knee specialist. These cases may be specific to biomedicine in the United States, where physical therapy is atrophied in relation to other countries and hyperspecialisation among physicians prevails. But in each case, the surgeons involved remained overly focused on the site of injury and failed to consider the bodies involved as complex kinetic systems whose problems might originate far from the local site of injury or pain or might originate at a local site and migrate elsewhere.

Damaged structures versus dynamic movement

Two ethnographic examples from the anatomy laboratory at Coastal University illustrate the different ways bodies are learned and known in universities. On a late winter day, a group of six undergraduate students taking an anatomy course had a problem. Charged with opening up the chest cavity and finding the heart, this particular group followed their instructor's guidelines to the letter, but found only a chest cavity filled with clotted blood. They spent much of the hour removing the blood then got frustrated and asked their instructor for help. After removing more blood, the instructor asked the entire class to gather around. He showed everyone what he could find of the heart and aorta. He explained that the patient, an elderly man, had a dissecting aneurysm in his aorta: the tissues of the largest blood vessel in his body had split, allowing blood to fill his chest cavity, killing him. The moment contained an unstated lesson: disease occurs at specific sites in the biological body and evidence of that disease can be found after death. When one finds the lesion, one finds the problem. The students, most of whom planned to go to medical school, learned that the lesion – the site of injury – and the pathology are co-located.

Later that spring, I watched a hand surgeon demonstrate the mechanics of the human hand and forearm to a group of medical engineering students. She used a fresh-frozen (not embalmed) cadaver arm, which looks and behaves more like a living body part than an embalmed arm would. The arm, severed at the humerus, rested on a stainless-steel tray and initially was delicately swathed in a white cloth. After some nervous jostling and nudging, the students settled in to watch the demonstration. The surgeon dissected the forearm, revealing the long thin tendons that link the finger joints to the strong muscles of the forearm. Much like Dr. Tulp in Rembrandt's painting, the surgeon grabbed a tendon near the elbow and pulled, flexing the corresponding finger. She grabbed another tendon and pulled, flexing a different finger. When she released the tendons, the corresponding fingers relaxed into their normal, not-quite-extended state. During the demonstration, the surgeon talked about how robotics engineers need knowledge of anatomy to reproduce human-like movement. This was the only demonstration of human movement that I

witnessed in the anatomy laboratory during eighteen months of participant observation. And it was for engineers, not medical students. Further, it explored only the movement of the fingers and the forearm, not
how, for example, movement in the shoulder might affect the wrist or,
with an unsevered arm, how movement of the elbow could affect the
low back. The engineering students were learning to think of the body
as muscular and tendinous pulleys that flex the hand. This lesson would
help them, eventually, to design assistive technologies, prosthetics or robots. The unstated message was that the causes of bodily action may be
several joints away from physical effects.

From objects of inquiry to subjects in rehabilitation

Biomechanical and biotensegrity approaches to understanding and re-
habilitating bodies have remained at biomedicine's margins, hampering
approaches that work more from the movement of the living than from
the dissection of the dead. I have argued that the atomistic approach to
the body begins with the cadaver, inert bodily matter that can be dissected into its tiniest parts. The cadaver acts as a kind of gravity well, drawing practitioners into its secrets, but is much less amenable to studies of
movement and movement pathologies. The cadaver's immobility lends
itself to treatment of bodies as objects to be scrutinised at high levels of
resolution, perhaps contributing to the biomedical objectification of patients (Thompson 2005; Prentice 2013). Seen in this light, Scarr's comments about initiating changes that let the body heal itself and Uhl and
Osborn's four principles of rehabilitation look more radical, particularly
the statement that patients and animal handlers can learn to evaluate
movement and help with corrections.

At the beginning of this chapter, I called out some ways that Vesalius' and Rembrandt's images reveal differences between dead and
living bodies. These differences do not detract from the scientific and
artistic achievements of the two works. But they do reflect the problem
with studying the dead to understand the living: the dead are no longer
self-organising systems able to respond and adapt to external forces. Altered by gravity and chemistry, cadavers lend themselves to exploration
of immobilised structures but not to discovery of how bodily structures

respond to inputs at a distance. The biomedical epistemology that seeks knowledge in ever-greater fragmentation of parts down to cellular and molecular components has produced many of biomedicine's most significant treatments. But it is possible that future discoveries in rehabilitation sciences will come from those who leave the anatomy laboratory for the physics department, the martial artist's dojo, or the trainer's gym. Put differently, it may be time to study moving bodies to understand and correct pathomechanical abnormalities in living beings.

Acknowledgements

I'd like to thank María Fernández, who read an early version of this chapter.

References

Daston, Lorraine and Galison, Peter (2007), *Objectivity*, New York: Zone Books.

Foucault, Michel (1973), *The Birth of the Clinic: An Archaeology of Medical Perception* (trans. A. M. Sheridan), New York: Vintage.

Good, Byron J. (1994), *Medicine, Rationality, and Experience*, Cambridge: Cambridge University Press.

Kuriyama, Shigehisa (2002), *The Expressiveness of the Body and the Divergence of Greek and Chinese Medicine*, New York: Zone Books.

Martin, R. Bruce (1999), 'A genealogy of biomechanics', *Lecture Presented at the 23rd Annual Conference of the American Society of Biomechanics*, University of Pittsburgh, Pittsburgh PA, 23 October, http://courses.washington.edu/bioen520/notes/History_of_Biomechanics_%28Martin_1999%29.pdf. Accessed 17 May 2017.

Mayer, Andreas (2010), 'The physiological circus: Knowing, representing, and training horses in motion in nineteenth-century France', *Representations*, 111, pp. 88–120.

Mol, Annemarie (2002), *The Body Multiple: Ontology in Medical Practice*, Durham: Duke University Press.

Myers, Thomas (2014), *Anatomy Trains: Myofascial Meridians for Manual and Movement Therapists*, London: Churchill Livingstone.

Nott, John and Harris, Anna (2020), 'Sticky models: History as friction in obstetric education', *Medicine, Anthropology, Theory*, 7:1, pp. 44–65.

Prentice, Rachel (2013), *Bodies in Formation: An Ethnography of Anatomy and Surgery Education*, Durham: Duke University Press.

Scarr, Graham (2018), *Biotensegrity: The Structural Basis of Life*, Edinburgh: Handspring Press.

Thompson, Charis (2005), *Making Parents: The Ontological Choreography of Reproductive Technologies*, Cambridge: MIT Press.

Uhl, Betsy W. and Osborn, Michelle L. (n.d.), 'The pathomechanics of degenerative joint disease: A one-health comparative case study approach', *Student's Guide*, http://www.aavmc.org/data/files/case-study/uhl%20-%20djd%20-%20student%20materials.pdf. Accessed 14 May 2017.

CHALKBOARDS

ANATOMY OF
THE CHALKBOARD

Rachel Vaden Allison

Part I: Chalkboard sketching

Frederick Whitney's *Blackboard Sketching*, an early twenty-first century guide to the charm and effective use of chalk and chalkboards, begins with the following reflection:

> [The] ability to draw easily and well on the blackboard is a power which every teacher [...] covets. Such drawing is a language which never fails to hold attention and to awaken delighted interest. (1909: n.pag.)

Written for educators and novice chalkboard illustrators, Whitney's compendium provides explicit direction as to the selection of chalk colour, length and width; the manner in which to handle a piece of chalk and the angle at which it should meet with the board; the speed and direction of both wrist and hand movement; and the pressure and accents one should apply to generate different strokes throughout the illustration. Imparted throughout the course of 29 illustrated and annotated plates (see Figures 4.1 and 4.2), these lessons are built around step-by-step instruction and describe the ever-many 'possibilities of chalk' for educational illustration – the intention here being that the educator, once versed in the basic strokes, should not merely copy the drawings provided, but might instead develop the skills to appropriate these techniques in a diverse array of pedagogic pursuits.

Whitney's compendium highlights two interwoven puzzles at the heart of chalkboard praxis: *how does one use a chalkboard effectively as an educational tool* and *how (and by whom) are these skills taught and learnt?*

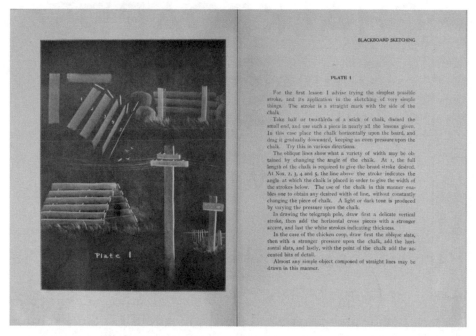

Figure 4.1: Plate 1 from Whitney's *Blackboard Sketching* (1909), demonstrating the general layout, approach, and relationship between all 29 plates.

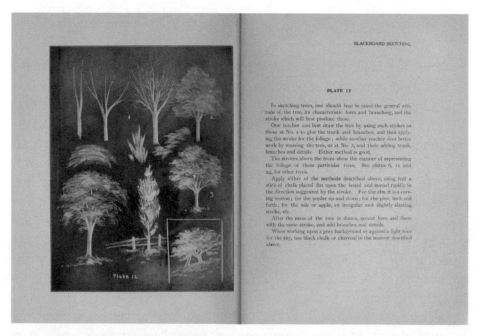

Figure 4.2: Plate 12 from *Whitney's Blackboard Sketching* (1909).

This is to say that, the chalkboard, a globally ubiquitous technology syn-onymous with classrooms, teaching and learning, is itself a relatively under-theorised pedagogical tool whose self-effacing materiality often goes unnoticed (Barany and MacKenzie 2014: 107) and whose practical use in illustration (as opposed to script or numerals) is seldom explicitly taught or examined. As the introduction to *Blackboard Sketching* laments, '[chalkboard illustration] has been considered impossible for most of us, because we have never done it. It has been strongly recommended, but no one has really shown us how' (Whitney 1909: n.pag).

Inspired by Whitney's compendium, in this chapter I explore the use of chalk and chalkboards for illustrative purposes within anatomy edu-cation, further asking: *what does the chalkboard provide its users (both edu-cators and students)?* And, *why does the chalkboard persist as an educational tool in the twenty-first century?* I consider these questions in relation to my ethnographic fieldwork in a medical school in Budapest, Hungary, alongside James Gibson's ([1979] 2015) theory of affordances. I do so first in conventional academic prose and then more speculatively in the second half of the chapter, using instructional, illustrated and annotated, plates, inspired by ethnographic excerpts, which enact the affordances with which I am concerned. Here, I am specifically interested in the par-ticular and unique *materio-pedagogic* qualities of chalk and chalkboards and the way in which these affordances contribute to anatomical illus-tration and the translation of anatomical knowledge between educator and student.

In keeping with the theme of this collection, I work from the un-derstanding that pedagogical tools and the practices they afford matter when it comes to students' learning behaviours and attitudes (Clinton and Wilson 2019: 326). The materiality of classroom technologies there-fore serves as a significant and inextricable factor within education – one that is thoroughly implicated in both the creation and translation of knowledge. In focusing on the use of chalk and board within anato-my training, I contend that it is not students' 'behaviours' and 'attitudes' alone, which are entangled with the materio-pedagogic qualities of the chosen teaching tool, but also the nature of the knowledge that is trans-lated. My work suggests that the use of chalkboard illustration with-in anatomy education aids in the translation of embodied and sensory knowledge, which, in turn, encourages in students a bodily orientation within the human anatomy. My hope is that these insights might also push back against the 'supremacy of the digital' (see, e.g. Baumgartner

2009; Al-jibury et al. 2015) within much contemporary medical education discourse and resource allocation.

The use of chalk and chalkboards in (anatomy) education

This chapter draws on ethnographic fieldwork conducted at Semmelweis University's Department of Anatomy, Histology, and Embryology, during the 2017–18 academic year. Throughout this time, I attended lectures, laboratory dissection classes, and histology lessons, along with observing practical and written examinations in both histology and gross anatomy. In all areas of Semmelweis' anatomy programme, I was struck by the consistent use of, and reliance on, chalk and chalkboards in the translation of anatomical knowledge. At Semmelweis' anatomy department, chalkboards maintain a prominent position in all places of learning. They appear in every dissection laboratory (both old and those recently built), sharing quarters with skeletons, cadavers, plastic models and other anatomical specimens; they hang alongside whiteboards and interactive whiteboards (or 'smartboards'), in front of rows of computers in digital histology classrooms; and they take centre stage in the two grand lecture theatres of the department (see Figures 4.3 and 4.4). This is not to say, however, that educators at Semmelweis' anatomy department did not have access to, or failed to incorporate newer (often digital) technologies within their teaching, but rather that, in many instances, the chalkboard was selected as the most appropriate and useful teaching tool – most often incorporated alongside, and in relation to, the use of cadavers and other anatomical specimens.

Though chalkboard use at Semmelweis was considered essential to learning (and employed in almost every lecture and lesson that I attended), I had difficulty throughout my fieldwork generating explicit discussion regarding the use of chalkboards within anatomy training. While the anatomy educators whom I researched alongside were all highly skilled practitioners of pedagogic chalkboard illustration, there was little obvious reflection concerning the medium itself and the practices related therein. This lack of instruction and reflexivity related to the materiality of chalk and chalkboards is made all the more intriguing given the revolutionary nature, proliferation and subsequent long-lasting supremacy of these objects within educational settings. Today, though the chalkboard endures as an iconic educational tool (albeit, with substantially less of a global classroom monopoly), it is doubtful that many chalkboard users continue to conceive of the technology as the 'cutting

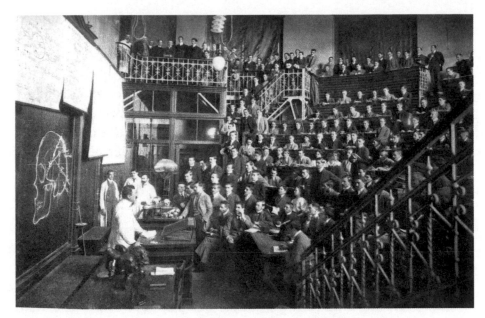

Figure 4.3: Chalkboard use in the main lecture theatre of Semmelweis' anatomy department in the early twentieth century (International Medical Congress, 1909).

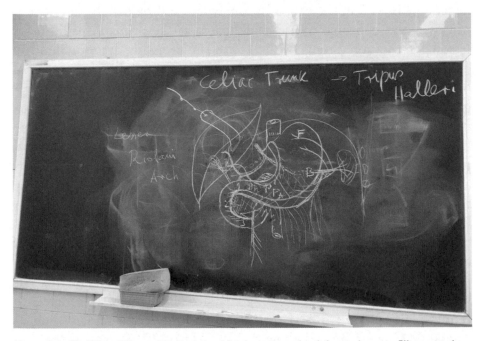

Figure 4.4: Chalkboard illustration depicting blood supply to the abdominal organs. Illustration by a Semmelweis tutor; photo by author, 2018.

edge' innovation it once was and, consequently, many fail to reflect on its use and unique materiality.

Introduced by school teacher James Pillans in a Scottish classroom at the turn of the nineteeth century, chalkboards (then made of slate and called 'blackboards') quickly made their way to, and first flourished in, places of elite military education (Barany and MacKenzie 2016) before becoming commonplace in classrooms throughout the world by the mid 1800s (Bumstead 1841). Praised for their ability to facilitate larger class sizes and collective learning (Krause 2000: 9), chalkboards reconfigured both the space of the classroom and the attitudes of and relationships between, teachers and students (Barany and MacKenzie 2016: 2–3). These technologies remained the dominant tools of teaching throughout most of the twentieth century, their monopoly only diminishing with the introduction of the whiteboard in the 1980s and the interactive whiteboard in the early 1990s.

However, the continued prevalence of chalk and board in certain educational spheres suggests that there is more than nostalgia or (an assumed) lack of resources at play when it comes to the contemporary use of these tools. One example of the chalkboard's enduring scholastic hegemony is seen in the case of Japan, where approximately 75 per cent of classrooms continue to use chalkboards as the primary medium for lesson presentation (report by the Tokyo Broadcasting System; Sankyuu cited in Emerling 2015); a position which reflects both a rejection of haphazard technology adoption and thoughtful decision making regarding which pedagogical tools might best support particular learning opportunities within classrooms (Emerling 2015). Another prominent sphere in which chalk and chalkboards have maintained a central presence is the world of mathematics. According to Michael J. Barany and Donald MacKenzie (2014: 112), though there is nothing about the chalkboard which is strictly essential to a mathematician, they nevertheless dominate in classrooms and seminars – the materials and methods of chalk and chalkboards serving a crucial role in the materialisation of abstract mathematical concepts (Barany and MacKenzie 2014: 123).

Within anatomy education, the use of chalk and chalkboards has been an important global teaching practice since the early nineteenth century, led by the work of distinguished artistic anatomists such as England's Charles Bell (Berkowitz 2011; Harris 2015). As was the case at Semmelweis, in French medical schools introduction to anatomy is taught by 'building' the body (or parts thereof) on the chalkboard, and is regarded as an 'excellent means of non-verbal expression' (Clavert et al. 2012: 787). In one 2013 study conducted in India, in which researchers analysed 200 anatomy students' perspectives in relation to the use of 'chalk and board' or 'PowerPoint', it was found that, in all parameters – including conceptual understanding, reproducibility and memorisation – the chalkboard was preferred by two-thirds of respondents. In their reasoning, researchers cited the superior teacher–student interaction and 'collective think' fostered by the chalkboard, which the authors contend allows for increased classroom 'spontaneity, flexibility and nonlinearity' (Rokade and Bahetee 2013: 839).

As is common, with the advancement of technology (and particularly digital technologies), the suitability of chalkboard use in the twenty-first century has been called into question – many institutions of higher education replacing these tools with, what Tim Ingold (2013: 124) has critically branded, 'sleek white screens'. I, like Ingold and others, see this as a rather short-sighted move which fails to consider what is lost when chalk and chalkboards are removed from places of learning. While the aforementioned qualities have been demonstrated as pedagogically significant, they can, in theory, be achieved with other 'visual aid' technologies and deal more with the interactive or relational potential of the medium, as opposed to the material specifics of chalk and board. For this reason, Part II of this chapter turns to a closer consideration of the precise illustrational opportunities that the chalkboard provides anatomy educators and students; qualities that I contend are unique to chalk and chalkboards, and that cannot be replicated using other tools, no matter how sleek. Before continuing to the second section of this chapter, however, I first draw on the work of Gibson ([1979] 2015) to help better theorise, and make sense of, the way in which the chalkboard remains an irreplaceable technology, as a result of its specific materio-peadogogic *affordances*.

The affordances of chalk and chalkboards for anatomy training

Working from the existing verb 'to afford', Gibson introduces the noun 'affordance' to refer to the relationship between the environment and the animal in a way, which he contends, no existing term had previously. Here, his intention was to describe what the environment – its medium, substances, surfaces and objects – affords human and non-human animals. For Gibson, the affordances of the environment are 'what it offers the animal, what it provides or furnishes' ([1979] 2015: 119). For instance, in speaking about the affordances of 'objects' Gibson provides the example of 'trace making' tools, which, when applied to surfaces leave traces and thus afford 'trace-making'. These marks on a surface may be used to 'depict and to write, to represent scenes and to specify words' (Gibson [1979] 2015: 125).

This is true of chalk and chalkboards. Used in combination, chalk and chalkboards afford the representation of numbers, scripts and illustrations, and, with the addition of the substance water and/or a soft, absorbent object (like a cloth), they allow for the erasure of depictions and for the surface to again be used in countless more representations. Furthermore, the surface of a chalkboard may vary greatly in size and may afford viewing in both the front row of a small dissection laboratory, or when sitting at the back of a grand lecture theatre, for instance. Chalkboards are durable and, with a little care, may remain in good working condition for decades. Chalk is a relatively cheap substance and both tools may be employed (in combination with natural light) without electricity, both in and out of doors, in the middle of a city or in rural areas, during blackouts, and so on. Chalkboards may be hung on a wall, or, in addition to a stand, may be positioned in the centre of a room, moved and angled at will. What's more, chalkboards require no internet connection, thus evading the various struggles that this utility too-frequently entails. These are some of the, more obvious, material affordances of chalk and chalkboards.

These affordances are not those unique to the chalkboard (all but the relative cheapness of chalk compared to non-permanent markers may also be said of the whiteboard), though they undoubtedly contribute to its historical innovativeness and contemporary usefulness. However, there are more precise and unique affordances of the chalkboard for education, which result from its specific materiality – what I am here calling its *materio-pedagogic affordances*. As Barany and MacKenzie (2014: 118) have noted in their consideration of chalkboard use in mathematics, chalk and board evoke a valuable sense of ephemerality that is unlike their twenty-first century counterpart, the interactive whiteboard, whose traces may be saved, shared and uploaded, as digital files; '[chalk] board writing does not move well from one place to another', the authors highlight. This is one example of the unique material affordances of chalk and board. I contend, however, that, when considering the specifics of sensory and embodied knowledge translation within anatomy education, the chalkboard offers its users much more. For example, chalk and chalkboards allow for a layering of traces, not possible with markers on a whiteboard; the friction of their meeting produces a rough sound and chalk dust, which may contribute to the multisensory translation of knowledge; and, chalk furnishes its user with the ability to produce both line and shade, a quality not provided by whiteboard markers and only clumsily and cumbersomely replicated by the interactive whiteboard.

Part II of this chapter is then devoted to a consideration of the unique affordances of the chalkboard for illustration in anatomy training. The format applied is inspired by Whitney's (1909) compendium and the anthropologist Kathleen Stewart's approach to, and writing on, affect. In particular, I draw on Stewart's monograph *Ordinary Affects* (2007), which argues for greater explicit attention to be paid to the affective, sensory and material dimensions of ethnographic research. Through a series of 'affective excerpts' and theoretically informed 'instructional plates', I tease out some of the possible materio-pedagogic affordances of chalk and chalkboards. The excerpts presented are taken from my fieldnotes and I have drawn the complementary illustrations using photographs I took during my fieldwork. I follow Whitney's plate-annotation format, in an attempt to think and draw about how the specifics of chalkboard illustration might be communicated to anatomy educators, with the explicit intent to highlight the affordances inherent within particular practices. The affordances I present are: *multisensoriality and traces of engagement*; *line and shade*; and *colour and layering*. My hope is that in following Whitney and Gibson's lead, and in taking Stewart's experiment in ordinary affects seriously, I too might 'provoke attention' (Stewart 2007: 1) in relation to the commonplace pedagogical practices of anatomy training, and might, more effectively, translate the affective, sensory, and material dimensions of chalkboard praxis.

Part II: Lessons in chalkboard sketching

What follows is an exploration of practices related to the use of chalk and chalkboards within anatomy training. Three 'lessons' are presented. Included in each is an 'affective excerpt', a snapshot of an anatomy class which I attended whilst at Semmelweis, and an instructional 'plate', in the manner of Whitney (Figures 4.1 and 4.2). The plates, made up of a chalkboard illustration, reproduced from photographs taken during my fieldwork, and an instructional text, explain the practices inherent in the illustration and work as a speculative teaching tool for anatomy educators. The lessons have each been crafted with the intent to highlight the unique materio-pedagogic affordances of chalk and board, with consideration to the translation of sensory and embodied anatomical knowledge between educator and student. The bracketed numbers found in both the ethnographic excerpts and instructional text, correspond with those found in the lessons' illustration.

Anatomy of the Eye: Multisensoriality & traces of engagement

Standing at the chalkboard, our teacher begins speaking about the sclera. As she talks, she reaches for a piece of yellow chalk and, pressing it firmly against the board, starts her illustration with a smooth, curved and continuous, yellow line [1] [2]. Turning to look at the class – the students and I, huddled on stools and wearing white lab coats – she makes a point of telling us that 'the outline should be white', but that she's drawing it in yellow, as 'it's the best piece [of chalk]' she can find.

Continuing the drawing – now swapping her yellow chalk for blue – she makes a small, rushed and jagged detail, and labels it 'CB' (or, 'ciliary body') [5] [6]. Then, head tilted and eyes squinting, she rubs at the lines with her finger, telling us, 'I didn't mean to draw it there, it's here instead'. She points a few centimetres to the left, leaving a number of chalky fingerprints on the board's surface [12], before delicately redrawing the small, mountain-peak-like zigzags of the ciliary body [6] – her chalk softly tapping as she creates each line. *Tap-tap, tap-tap, tap-tap.*

On the chalkboard, the original location of the ciliary body remains partially visible [10], as ad hoc finger-chalk-erasure usually is.

She returns to the thin, yellow outline of the sclera, telling us that she needs to 'fill it in a little'. Yellow chalk, again in hand, she says, 'it's just so fatty, that's why I'm drawing it so thick'. Here, she makes sure that the students note the purposeful and corresponding use of chalk and anatomy; that they can decipher the lines which detail 'characteristic' anatomy, from those which are unique to the specific chalkboard illustration. To make the 'fatty' sclera she turns the chalk on a slight angle and scrapes it horizontally across the board's surface, scratching it back and forth. *Scratch–scratch, scratch–scratch.* The sound is loud as she pulls and pushes the chalk, filling in the now thick layer of sclera with both colour and noise. As she does so, chalk particles fall from the chalkboard and settle in a thin, dusty yellow layer beneath – a third, material marker of the 'fatty', 'thick' sclera.

Our teacher takes a step back and pauses to allow the students to finish their own, copied, drawings.

Coming back to the chalkboard, she picks up a small piece of orange chalk. Gauging the size of her illustration, she makes a dashed, yet steady line, one-third of the way into the drawn eye – her chalk tapping down the chalkboard with metronomic regularity [7]. *Tap, silence, tap, silence, tap, silence.* Once more, she turns to the class and says, 'I do this [dashing] on purpose [...] so that you can see that this junction [the ora serrata between the ciliary body and retina] is serrated, it's not the same [type of structure] as this [pointing once more to the sclera]'.

She takes a few steps back from the chalkboard to give the students better vantage and reiterates, 'I make the thick layers of chalk on purpose, and this line [gesturing to the ora serrata], I made that serrated [dashed] on purpose too. Make sure you know that'.

The students nod and continue to copy her illustration into their notebooks.

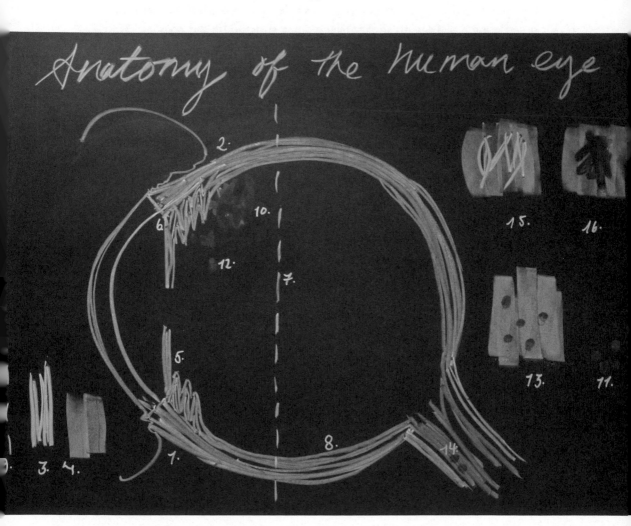

PLATE 1

The first lesson I advise for the use of chalkboards in anatomical illustration is to work with the tools' specific material qualities in mind. The advice given in this lesson pertains to any and all chalkboard illustrations, though is easily identifiable when considering the illustration of the human eye depicted in this plate.

Most contemporary chalkboards are made from a porcelain-enamel paint applied to a steel base, making the chalkboard's surface uniform in colour and texture and far smoother than its slate predecessor. Even so, there remains a reasonable degree of friction between the board's surface and a user's piece of chalk, which, in combination with an understanding of the textural consistency of chalk, may be deployed to the anatomy educator's advantage.

At nos. [1] and [2], the build-up of the yellow sclera may be observed, produced by the repeated pull and push movement of a single piece of chalk, applied at a slight angle and using a mid-length stroke. Filling out a structure in this manner [3] (as opposed to shading [4], introduced in Plate 4.2) helps to facilitate the translation of the 'thick' and 'fatty' nature of the structure (in this instance, the sclera), as students receive both visual and auditory input from the chalkboard.

In the same manner, the light tapping of chalk applied to create the blue ciliary body at nos. [5] and [6], and the ora serrata at no. [7], indicate the different physical nature of the anatomical structures – the ora serrata, for instance, being a serrated junction between the retina [8] and ciliary body [5] [6].

At nos. [5] and [6], a series of simple strokes were made by placing a piece of chalk in a vertical position and drawing it down and up in a zig-zag pattern, a number of times. At no. [7], the chalk was held in the same vertical position, then drawn down the board, top to bottom, breaking at regular intervals by lifting the chalk from the board's surface. Here, dashing [9] has been used to indicate structural serration.

Note that with these examples, one's approach should be informed by an understanding of the practical functioning of the human sensorium, specifically as pertains to the integration of perceptual information taken from different and multiple sensory modalities – here demonstrated in the entanglement of visual and auditory sensory stimuli, both of which (or, more accurately, the combination thereof) contribute to the anatomical knowledge translated between educator and student. *[For scholarship that deals with the 'multisensory' nature of the human sensorium see, among many wonderful examples, Marks 2002 and Pink 2011].*

When considering the nature of chalk (both pigment and tool), one must keep in mind the difficulty of total chalk erasure, when working within an existing illustration (as opposed to cleaning the entire board with a wet cloth). This material quality may also be used to the educator's advantage, as it creates a record of working and, importantly, mistakes, which enables students to better understand and record the build-up of the anatomical illustration. This affordance also helps students discern which structures must be drawn with accuracy, seen at nos. [6] and [10], where the position of the ciliary body was amended, mid-illustration.

In the same manner, the material nature of chalk allows for a record of 'traces of engagement'. By this I mean, for example, that the educator's chalky fingerprint [11] may become part of the illustration, revealing where she has pointed, or lingered, creating a parallel representation of the conversation which occurred during the production of the illustration, partially visible at no. [12]. The converse is also true, as fingertip traces may appear as small cleared spaces within a shaded area [13] or a single stroke of chalk [14].

Here, we see that while the majority of chalkboard traces made with chalk (or chalky fingers) are *additive* [15], in that they form an extra layer, which is superimposed upon the board's surface, the chalkboard also allows for the inscription of a type of *reductive* [16] trace (be it purposeful or accidental), a unique quality that anatomy educators should consider in their practice. [*Regarding the concepts of 'additive-' and 'reductive trace', see* Ingold 2007.]

Anatomy of the pelvis: Line and shade

For today's revision of the female pelvic region, our teacher first asks the students to make a drawing of the pelvic inlet. The students work together in small groups, discussing and sharing their illustrations.

Several minutes later, two students move to the chalkboard to replicate their joint illustration for the rest of the class. The students working at the board have a different approach than their teachers'. Educators press firmly and have a steady, confident stroke – one stroke of chalk per line or shaded area, is all that is usually needed. The students, however, hold the chalk tentatively and pull it lightly across the board, making multiple joining and overlapping strokes per structural line – they appear cautious, unsure of grasp or necessary pressure.

The students finish and our teacher moves to the chalkboard to correct a few minor structural lines. Her strokes are firm and easily distinguished from the students'.

We move to a second drawing, a lateral view of the pelvic bone.

Our teacher begins by making a firm, white outline, which generally indicates bone [7]. She continues to work on the chalkboard, as the rest of the class watches on.

As she moves to the pelvic muscles, she tilts the chalk on its side and scrapes it down the board making a thick, shaded pink area, indicative of muscle [14]. When shading, she applies a smaller amount of pressure, leaving the firmly pressed bone outline beneath still visible [10] [11] [12] [15] [16].

She carries on, now with a small piece of green chalk, which she uses to fill in the connective tissue [8]. These strokes have a lighter touch and are not shaded; instead, the area is furnished with a number of finely drawn lines [9].

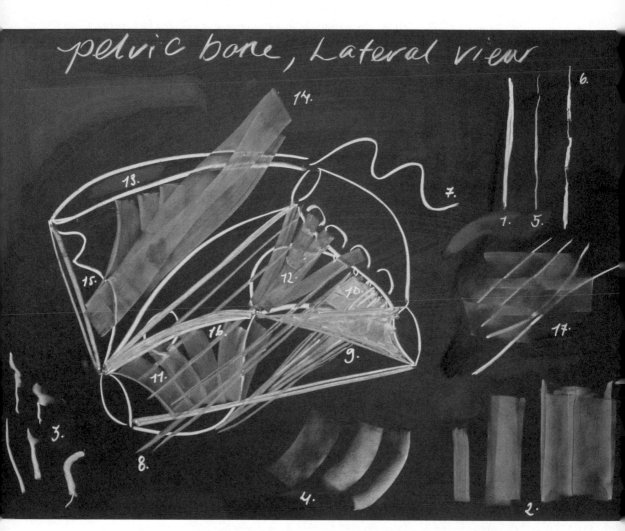

PLATE 2

With this plate, a lateral illustration of the pelvic bone is used to show the practical application of line [1] and shade [2] for anatomical chalkboard illustration. The strokes depicted in this plate are considered the basic building blocks of any chalkboard illustration. It is wise to practice these strokes in many directions and with different amounts of pressure [3] [4], before applying them in the service of one's own anatomical structures.

One piece of common advice relates to the particular handling of chalk, which, for the best illustrative results, ought to be firmly held in one's dominant hand and should be applied to the board's surface with enough pressure as to transfer a solid layer of chalk pigment, seen at nos. [1] vis-à-vis [5]. In general, one should use a small piece of chalk (⅓ – ½ a single piece) and hold it between the tips of the thumb, and pointer and middle fingers. The pressure applied should be greater than that given to a pen or pencil. Chalk grip and pressure should, as a rule, be applied uniformly, unless in the service of a particular and uneven detail. For some illustrations, a darker or lighter tone may be necessary, and this is produced by varying one's pressure on the chalk [6].

The anatomical structure to be drawn will dictate the kind of strokes one should employ, along with the manner of chalk handling. Here, it is important to understand that the choice of line [1] versus shade [2] can serve to indicate to students the material nature of the structure and, more fundamentally, allow for differentiation in the illustration. Note that consistency in these decisions, and across lessons, is important for inspiring in students an intuitive and bodily sense-memory of structural natures. [On 'body memory' see, as one example, Casey 1987.]

Line [1] should be engaged for the outlines [7] of illustrations and the (potential) structures within – for example, connective tissue, shown at nos. [8] and [9]. To produce a uniform line, one should hold the chalk piece vertically at one end, pulling it across the board in the desired direction, with an even pressure. The pressure given to an outline is generally greater than that given to internal structural lines, distinguished at nos. [7] vis-à-vis [8] and [9]. [For a comprehensive consideration of the 'history and life of lines', see Ingold 2007 and 2015.]

Shade [2] [4] is best employed in the service of more encompassing structures like muscle or fascia, as shown at nos. [10] and [11]. Here, the shaded stroke is produced with the side of a piece of chalk. In the case of no. [11], for instance, place the chalk horizontally upon the board and drag it gradually downward, keeping an even pressure on the chalk. The width of a shaded area is dictated by the size of chalk, so breaking a piece of chalk into two or three parts may be necessary, as seen at nos. [12] and [13]. The thickly shaded muscle at no. [14] has been made by using a full (long) piece of chalk and keeping a smooth, even pressure throughout.

Lastly, observe that the combined use of line and shade aids in the pursuit of layering. Here the pressure used when shading should be gentle enough so as to not completely obscure the line(s) beneath, seen at nos. [15], [16] and [17].

Anatomy of the abdomen: Colour and layering

Class begins with everyone gathered around an empty gurney in the middle of the laboratory. Our teacher arrives and asks us to move towards the front wall for today's 'mostly theoretical' lesson; 'we'll be working on the blackboard for now', she says. Our metal stools screech as we drag them across the tiled flooring, eventually settling in a semicircle, notebooks on laps and pencil cases in hand.

Our teacher starts with a brief 'rundown' of the layers of the abdominal wall to 'jog the memory'; 'skin, subcutaneous tissue, superficial fascia, external oblique muscle, internal oblique muscle [...], and peritoneum'.

As she speaks, she occasionally touches her own abdomen.

She picks up a yellow piece of chalk and, before beginning the illustration, says, 'I'm going to do a series of drawings on top of one another'. She explains that her illustration is a combination of three drawings, which she has merged to give the students a more complete and clear sense of the layers of the abdomen before we 'take a look at them on the cadaver'. She also tells us that she is going to keep the same colour system throughout today's series of drawings so that we can follow along without the need for continual labelling.

She moves to the chalkboard and begins to draw. Pulling the chalk down the board, she makes an initial, thick vertical line. As she fills in the layers of muscle, she works from deep to superficial and swaps between differently coloured pieces of chalk, telling the students, '*yellow* shows the transversus abdominis muscles [11]; *orange* is the internal oblique [12]; *green* is for the external oblique' [13]; and, lastly, 'I'll use *pink* for the rectus abdominis muscles' [14].

I hear the students heeding our teacher's instructions as they rustle around in their pencil cases for the requisite coloured pens.

The different colours of chalk crisscross over one another; each remaining visible, distinguished by both colour and direction.

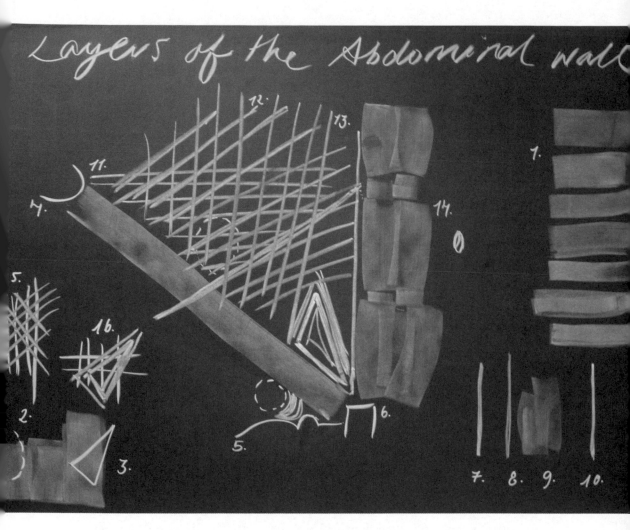

PLATE 3

Today the majority of contemporary chalkboards are no longer made of slate, but painted steel. This materiality (while also reducing glare) allows for a wider range of chalk colours to remain distinguishable on the board's surface.

The ventral illustration of the abdomen depicted in this plate provides a clear example of the effective use of chalk colour and layering in the service of an intricate depiction of complex anatomical structures, and builds on knowledge of line and shade presented in the previous plate. By employing multiple-coloured chalks [1], anatomy educators maintain the ability to depict, and differentiate within, complicated three-dimensional structures on the low-tech, two-dimensional chalkboard.

Note that, alongside the varied use of line and shade, the application of colour and layering helps facilitate clearer and more sophisticated student understanding, even as an illustration accumulates detail, as demonstrated in the basic examples at nos. [2] and [3].

In making this sketch, one should note that chalkboards offer users a degree of flexibility and control over their illustrations, which is not always available when using other visual aids (or, at least, this may be a more cumbersome process that requires access to, and a good grasp of, computer programs). This is demonstrated with this illustration, which was crafted from three separate abdominal representations, layered on the chalkboard in real-time and with a specific pedagogic outcome in mind. This practice of layering may be pre-planned by the anatomy educator or performed in a spontaneous manner, usually in response to student questions or difficulties.

When selecting the appropriate chalk colour, educators should consider the general attitude and characteristics of the anatomical structure they wish to depict, selecting a colour that might best, and most intuitively, represent this. In general, bones, seen at nos. [4], [5], and [6], should be drawn in white, veins in blue [7], arteries [8] and muscles [9] in red or pink, and nerves [10] in yellow.

In this illustration (which does not include veins, arteries, or nerves), yellow has been used for the transversus abdominis muscles [11], orange for the internal oblique [12], green for the external oblique [13], and pink for the rectus abdominis muscles [14]. Here, differentiation of the abdominal layers is further supported by varying the directionality of one's chalk strokes, as demonstrated in the examples at nos. [15] and [16]. This practice is not always suitable (either anatomically correct and/or intuitive, for instance), but should be employed where possible.

Lastly, educators should observe that the use of colour is most effective when each piece of coloured chalk has been selected for a precise purpose, and where this selection remains consistent throughout, and even across, lessons. This practice, along with adding layered elements in a strategic and *logical* sequence (here seen in the drawing of the abdominal muscles from deep to superficial) helps to bring coherence to the lesson, and to the students' bodily understanding of the anatomical structure depicted. In this way, the chalkboard allows an educator to build-up an illustration in a fashion consistent with the physical and layered nature of the human body. *[For a short discussion on the logic and discovery of the human body's 'natural compartments', 'boundaries', 'layers', and 'three-dimensional organisation', from the perspective of anatomy training and medical education, see Good 1994: 72-73].*

Conclusion

There is a tradition in medical anthropology which emphasises the role of dissection in anatomy education, that 'medical education begins by entry into the human body' (Good 1994: 74). This chapter, however, considers the materials which illustrate and guide students' entry into the anatomical bodies of their patients. Student's entry into the body is mediated by all of the materials that complement introductions to anatomy. The longstanding use of chalk and chalkboards is one example which shows how medical knowledge is tangled up in the material specificities of the technologies used in its teaching. These tools afford – alongside, and in relation to, the use of cadavers and other anatomical specimens – a sensory and embodied entry into the human body through its anatomical structures and their connections.

The few studies of chalkboards as a teaching technology have emphasised that, as with other visual aids in education, chalkboards contribute to increased student engagement, to collective think, spontaneity and flexibility, and ephemerality. Chalkboards are clearly far more than mere writing or notetaking tools, however. They focus student attention on the task at hand; they display history and sequence, affording the making of connections; and they strike a balance between commitment and experimentation (Barany and MacKenzie 2014; O'Hare 1993: 246).

However, as our anatomy lessons have shown, chalk and chalkboards do more still. These tools offer particular and unique *materio-pedagogic affordances* which contribute similarly unique understandings of anatomical knowledge. It is only through ethnographic reflection, and the exploratory practice encouraged by the above lessons, that the slippery material, sensory, affective affordances of chalk and chalkboards begin to emerge. These include the multisensory manner in which chalkboards communicate ideas, and the curious role of chalky traces in detailing the precision of anatomical structures; the various affective compositions of line and shade; or the role of colour and its layering in the representation of complex, three-dimensional structures. Although not all of these affordances are necessarily unique to chalk and chalkboards, when considered in combination, this incomplete taxonomy of chalkboard affordances highlights the distinctive and invaluable materio-pedagogic nature of this obdurate feature of medical education. While dissection may offer students entry to the anatomical body, chalkboards can help supplement its colours, textures and complexities.

Acknowledgements

All insights developed in this chapter are thanks to the expert pedagogical practices and skilled illustrations of the anatomy educators at Semmelweis University, to whom this research material, thinking, and illustrating is indebted. Specifically, I would like to thank Dr. Andrea Székely (MD/Ph.D.), associate professor at Semmelweis' Department of Anatomy, Histology, and Embryology, who facilitated my fieldwork, and whose teaching on the anatomy of the eye (Lesson 1), first ignited by interest in the unique materio-pedagogic affordances of the chalkboard in relation to the translation of sensory and embodied knowledge within anatomy training. Many thanks to Dr. Bianca Fiorentino Slotfeldt (MD), Dr. Dushyant Mukkamala (MD/Ph.D.), Dr. Danial Safavi (MD), and Dr. Arvin Shahbazi (DMD/Ph.D.), who spoke with me throughout my fieldwork and who kindly invited me into their lectures and laboratory lessons; and to the first- and second-year anatomy students at Semmelweis who welcomed me into their classrooms and shared their experience of learning anatomy with me. This work was supported by the European Research Council under the European Union's Horizon 2020 research and innovation programme (Grant agreement no. 678390; awarded to Anna Harris).

References

Al-jibury, Osama, Ahmed, Maroof, Najim, Muhammad, Rabee, Riham, Ashraf, Muhammad, Sherwani, Yusuf and Anjum, Osama (2015), 'The trend toward digital in medical education – playing devil's advocate', *Advances in Medical Education and Practice*, 6, pp. 581–82.

Barany, Michael J. and MacKenzie, Donald (2014), 'Chalk: Materials and concepts in mathematics research', in C. Coopmans, J. Vertesi, M. Lynch, and S. Woolgar (eds), *Representation in Scientific Practice Revisited*, Cambridge and London: The MIT Press, pp. 107–29.

Barany, Michael J. and MacKenzie, Donald (2016), 'A dusty discipline', in M. Pitici (ed.), *The Best Writing on Mathematics, 2015*, Princeton: Princeton University Press, pp. 1–6.

Baumgartner, Fritz (2009), 'Human medicine versus techno-medicine', *Texas Heart Institute Journal*, 36:3, pp. 268–69.

Berkowitz, Carin (2011), 'The beauty of anatomy: Visual displays and surgical education in early-nineteenth-century London', *Bulletin of the History of Medicine*, 85:2, pp. 248–78.

Bumstead, Josiah F. (1841), *The Blackboard in Primary School*, Boston: Perkins & Marvin.

Casey, Edward S. (1987), *Remembering: A Phenomenological Study*, Bloomington and Indianapolis: Indiana University Press.

Clavert, Philippe, Bouchaïb, J., Duparc, F. and Kahn, J. L. (2012), 'A plea for the use of drawing in human anatomy teaching', *Surgical and Radiologic Anatomy*, 34, pp. 787–89.

Clinton, Virginia and Wilson, Nicholas (2019), 'More than chalkboards: Classroom spaces and collaborative learning attitudes', *Learning Environments Research*, 22:3, pp. 325–44.

Emerling, Bradley (2015), 'Lessons learned from a chalkboard: Slow and steady technology integration', *Larry Cuban on School Reform and Classroom Practice*. https://larrycuban.wordpress.com/2015/04/26/lessons-learned-from-a-chalkboard-slow-and-steady-technology-integration-bradley-emerling/. Accessed 16 May 2022.

Gibson, James J. ([1979] 2015), 'The theory of affordances', in J. J. Gibson (ed.), *The Ecological Approach to Visual Perception, Psychology*, New York and East Sussex: Psychology Press, pp. 119–35.

Good, Byron (1994), 'How medicine constructs its objects', in B. Good (ed.), *Medicine, Rationality and Experience: An Anthropological Perspective*, Cambridge: Cambridge University Press, pp. 65–87.

Harris, Anna (2015), 'The blackboard anatomist', *British Medical Journal*, 350: 10 (February), p. 345.

Ingold, Tim (2007), *Lines: A Brief History*, London and New York: Routledge.

Ingold, Tim (2013), *Making: Anthropology, Archaeology, Art and Architecture*, London and New York: Routledge.

Ingold, Tim (2015), *The Life of Lines*, London and New York: Routledge.

International Medical Congress (1909), *Les Facultés de Médecine Des Universités Royales Hongroises de Budapest et de Kolozsvár*, Budapest: Imprimerie de la Société Anonyme Franklin.

Krause, Steven D. (2000), '"Among the greatest benefactors of mankind": What the success of chalkboards tells us about the future of computers in the classroom', *The Journal of the Midwest Modern Language Association*, 33:2, pp. 6–16.

Marks, Laura U. (2002), *Touch: Sensuous Theory and Multisensory Media*, Minneapolis and London: University of Minnesota Press.

O'Hare, Michael (1993), 'Talk and chalk: The blackboard as an intellectual tool', *Journal of Policy Analysis and Management*, 12:1, pp. 238–46.

Pink, Sarah (2011), 'Multimodality, multisensoriality and ethnographic knowing: Social semiotics and the phenomenology of perception', *Qualitative Research*, 11:3, pp. 261–76.

Rokade, S. A. and Bahetee, B. H. (2013), 'Shall we teach anatomy with chalk and board or power point presentations? – An analysis of Indian students' perspectives and performance', *Scholars Journal of Applied Medical Sciences*, 1:6, pp. 837–42.

Stewart, Kathleen (2007), *Ordinary Affects*, Durham and London: Duke University Press.

Whitney, Frederick (1909), *Blackboard Sketching*, Springfield: Milton Bradley Company.

CIGARETTE PAPERS

THE CIGARETTE PAPER, THE EMBROIDERER AND THE GENDERED CRAFT OF VASCULAR SURGERY

Paul Craddock

'The first row is the hardest', Fleur Oakes explained to me as she brought her needle through the corner of a cigarette paper. I had asked Oakes – one of the UK's most well-regarded embroiderers – to put 500 hundred stitches into a cigarette paper to recreate an exercise performed by Alexis Carrel, the so-called 'father' of vascular surgery. Carrel had been induced to improve his needle-and-thread skills after the fatal stabbing in 1894 of the French president, Sadi Carnot. Stab wounds were treated, at the time, by identifying and ligating severed blood vessels, tying a suture around them to stop the bleeding. The assassin had severed the president's portal vein, however, and his panicked surgeons were helpless. Though only a medical student at the time, Carrel presumed to criticise his superiors, insisting that Carnot might have been saved had they been able to *repair* the vessels. He practiced on cigarette paper – which, as Oakes pointed out to me, simulated the paperiness of an artery – aiming to cram in as many stitches as possible to develop the intricacy and delicacy required to work on tiny vessels (Anon. 1894; Tilney 2003: 36; Hamilton 2017: 12). Oakes was, I felt, best placed to help me re-enact this task. Not only was she a professional embroiderer, she had also accrued scores of hours in the

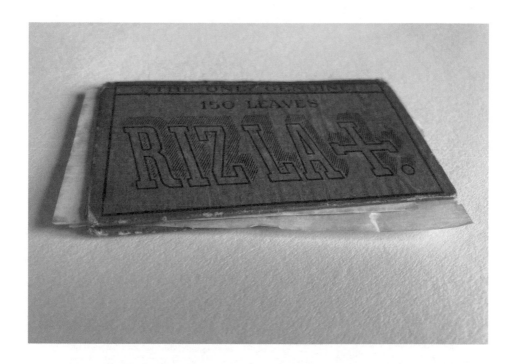

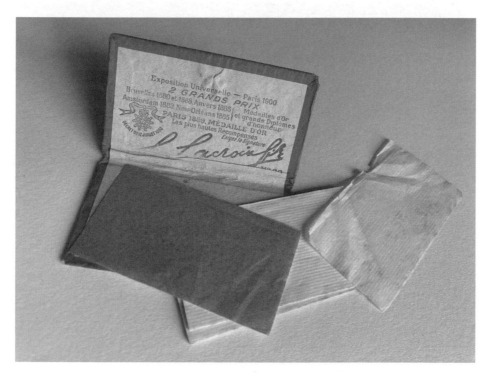

Figure 5.1 and 5.2: Turn of the century cigarette papers. Courtesy of author.

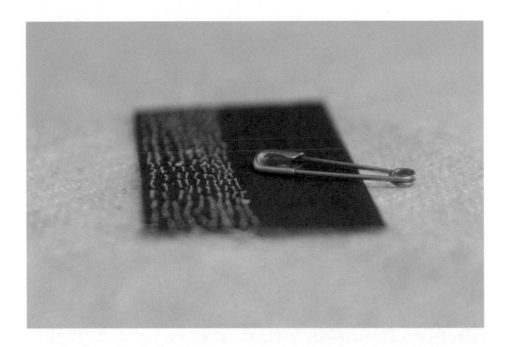

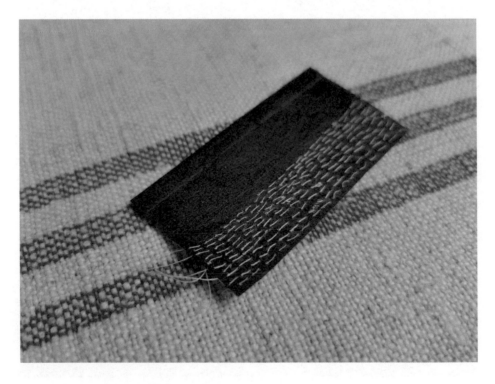

Figure 5.3 and 5.4: Oakes's half-finished, stitch-filled cigarette paper. Courtesy of Matt Redman.

operating theatre as the embroiderer in residence at Imperial College, London's vascular surgery department.

A cigarette paper is about the size of a small bar of hotel soap and it seemed unbelievable to me that anyone could fit *500* stitches into that tiny space. But, as Oakes pierced the paper for the first time, it emerged that the greater challenge was knowing how to manage the needle and thread. The exercise was not about filling space but placing tension in a material as thin and flimsy as tissue paper. Finishing her first row, Oakes counted fifteen stitches. Into the next row, she squeezed eighteen, which she offset to break up the pattern of perforation she had established. The cigarette paper had something to teach about the material integrity of the body: a cigarette paper, much like a blood vessel, is not a woven fabric; there is no warp and weft to keep her thread in place. In this way, the cigarette paper had lessons to impart.

I could hear the thinness of the material rasp as she pulled the thread through. 'It's very easy to tear', she explained – she actually did tear a tiny hole once or twice – 'and you have to bring the needle straight down, not at an angle or you'll create a bigger hole'. There was no going back once the paper had been punctured, however, so to minimise the damage her actions necessarily imparted, she had to commit to her mistakes. Whether a hole she made adhered to the patterns of tension she had established or not, she had to follow through every blunder, recalculating and recalibrating her approach after each puncture.

She had to, as she described it, 'take a reading' of the material and establish the most stable pattern for her stitches, staggering them to impart strength. Oakes described the entire exercise as a masterclass in managing tension; by puncturing the paper, she was 'setting up a pattern of weakness'. And with such lightweight thread and almost weightless paper, her usual relationship between body and materials was disrupted. She could not read the tension as she tightened the stitch, for example, and to compensate she had to use her fingers to feel for the needle's point in order to get some sense that the paper was piercing safely.

When Carrel performed the same exercise as a surgeon, he made two substantial imports from the professional world of textiles. First, he found his needle and thread at a haberdashery in Lyon. Surgeons' needles were far too thick and their sutures much too heavy to be effective on a material as thin as tissue paper. Regardless of the operator's skill, they would tear it as they would the vessels it represented. Second, he imported processes and techniques. Medical students at the turn of the twentieth century were expected to learn their needlecraft from wives, sisters or mothers. But unlike most mothers, Carrel's owned a lace factory (Levin 2015). No doubt using family connections, he supplemented this considerable head start with lessons with one of Lyon's most accomplished embroiderers: the world-renowned Marie Anne Leroudier.

Biographers tend to skim over Carrel's relationship with the female-dominated textile industry. And, despite being central to the surgical skills Carrel developed, Leroudier herself is often completely ignored or, worse, her employment leveraged as evidence of the man's genius. Taking three of Carrel's most recent profiles, for example, we learn that he had merely 'seen' needle and thread 'used in Lyon' (Ellis 2019: 256), that he 'was inspired' by 'watching' Leroudier (Kneebone et al. 2019: 23) and that he 'was taught' by her (Vernon 2019: 352). Only the last reference hints at an in-depth relationship, though as is invariably the case with references to Leroudier, it is a mere sentence long.

In a way, it is understandable that historians have overlooked Leroudier, though historical accounts unproblematically recognise earlier surgical (and male) innovators who worked on needlework techniques, such as Mathieu Jaboulay and his student Eugéne Briau (Cusimano et al. 1984). These men, like Carrel, expressed their contributions through the long-established means of academic papers and conferences. Such means of representing intellectual claims – deliberately recorded and citable – have made it easy for historians to account for them. And for Carrel, prizes and plaudits followed; he even won a Nobel Prize for work stemming from his manipulation of thin, papery materials. It has been comparatively far more difficult to work with, or even recognise, what Ursula Klein termed 'ineffable bodily skills' and 'connoisseurship of materials' (Klein 2008: 781), though several traditions have emphasised the role of the body in the creation of knowledge in the sixteenth, seventeenth and eighteenth centuries (see, e.g. Roberts 1995; Klein 2008).

The difficulty with writing about Leroudier is amplified because, aside from a collection of her work in Lyon's *Musée des Tissus* and a few scattered references, very little remains of Leroudier's legacy in any medium. Her influence in surgery is almost completely unacknowledged, veiled behind references to being Carrel's 'teacher' (Vernon 2019: 352), or to use Ellis's passive phrase, a woman he 'had seen' (Ellis 2019: 256). It is difficult, after all, to find the words to express that which cannot be put into words. But the tiny brown rectangle of paper that Oakes slipped into a stiff envelope at the end of our re-enactment suggested a more active engagement; it was no longer an everyday object, but an artefact marked by expert hands, the 'silent, brute remainder', to use Latour's term (1993: 82), of a practical investigation into hands, tools, and materials.

That paper stood witness to the knowledge Oakes produced and expressed through manipulating the thin, papery, non-woven material. When Oakes took the paper, needle and thread into her hands, she knew how to position her fingers, ascertained how much pressure to use to puncture the paper. When she'd been slightly too rough with her materials and ripped the paper a little, her experienced hands knew how to recover and to strengthen the ruptured area, or at least how not to weaken it further. The constellation of knowledge and competencies she drew on went beyond language – a capacity she has recognised and developed with Professor Roger Kneebone in their collaboration examining the material and performative dimension of surgery. Through developing a competence with similar tools and materials, Carrel would have evolved a comparable ability to manipulate non-woven fabrics in collaboration with Leroudier. He would have learned how to manage their delicacy and flimsiness, and he would have learned how far he could push his tools and materials.

By applying the lessons he learned with Leroudier to the human body, Carrel would go on to innovate the surgical technique of vascular anastomosis (the process of connecting two blood vessels using needle and thread). Without it, surgeons could not perform bypass operations, transplants or effectively treat stab wounds like the one that killed President Carnot. Undoubtedly, vascular anastomosis owes much to his drive and vision. When we account for the procedure, though, might we also emphasise the materials and processes it shares with embroidery: the singular challenge involved in manipulating non-woven materials, the intricacy required, the placement of tension and management of thread, working with one hand; the material and sensory engagement involved in the manipulation of arteries and veins (and cigarette papers). By engaging embroiderers like Oakes into conversations, drawing their insights into our historical accounts, we might better appreciate the material, performative dimension of surgical procedures like anastomosis. In the textual tradition of the history of medicine, I suggest, we have privileged Carrel's intellectual claim, neglecting to even mention how privileged he was to have learnt with Marie Anne Leroudier.

Acknowledgements

I would like to thank Fleur Oakes for her invaluable expertise in staging this re-enactment, and Professor Roger Kneebone for his years of unrelenting encouragement and support for my work in this area. Writing of this chapter was supported by the Making Clinical Sense project with funding from the ERC under the European Union's Horizon 2020 research and innovation programme (Grant agreement no. 678390).

References

Anon. (1894), 'Caserio struggled for life; the assassin's courage failed him in the end', *New York Times*, 16 August, p. 5.

Cusimano, Robert, Cusimano, Michael and Cusimano, Steven (1984), 'The genius of Alexis Carrel', *Canadian Medical Association Journal*, 131:9, pp. 1142–50.

Ellis, Harold (2019), 'The story of peripheral vascular surgery', *Journal of Perioperative Practice*, 29:8, pp. 245–56.

Hamilton, David (2017), *The First Transplant Surgeon: The Flawed Genius of Nobel Prize Winner Alexis Carrel*, New Jersey: World Scientific.

Klein, Ursula (2008), 'The laboratory challenge: Some revisions of the standard view of early modern experimentation', *Isis*, 99:4, pp. 769–82.

Kneebone, Roger, Oakes, Fleur and Bicknall, Colin (2019), 'Reframing surgical simulation: The textile body as metaphor', *The Lancet*, 393:10166, pp. 22–23.

Latour, Bruno (1993), *We Have Never Been Modern*, Cambridge: Harvard University Press.

Levin, Sheldon Marvin (2015), 'Alexis Carrel's historic leap of faith', *Journal of Vascular Surgery*, 61:3, pp. 832–33.

Roberts, Lissa (1995), 'The death of the sensuous chemist: The "new" chemistry and the transformation of sensuous technology', *Studies in History and Philosophy of Science*, 26:4, pp. 503–29.

Tilney, Nicholas (2003), *Transplant: From Myth to Reality*, New Haven: Yale University Press.

Vernon, Gervase (2019), 'Alexis Carrel: "Father of Transplant Surgery" and supporter of eugenics', *British Journal of General Practice*, 69:684, p. 352.

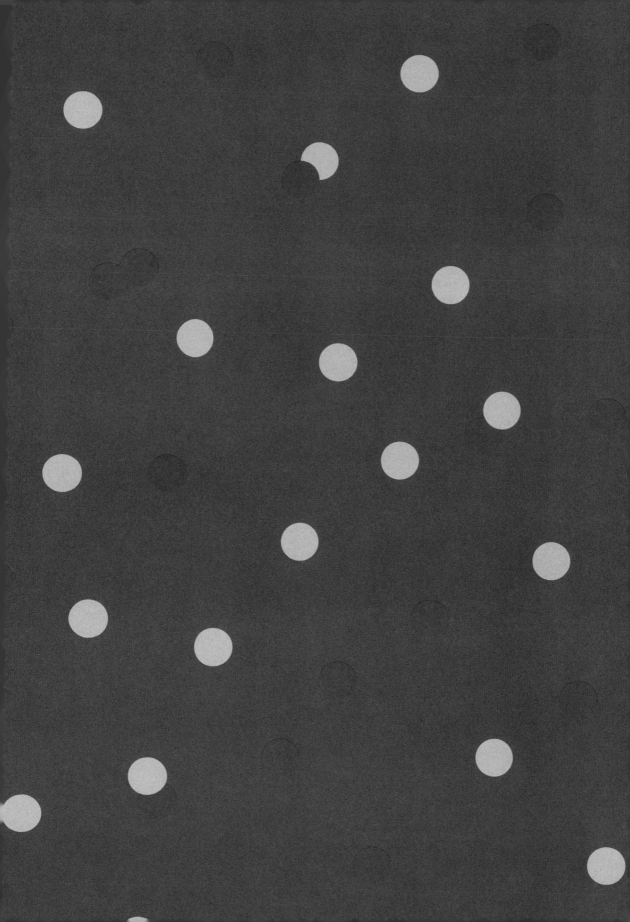

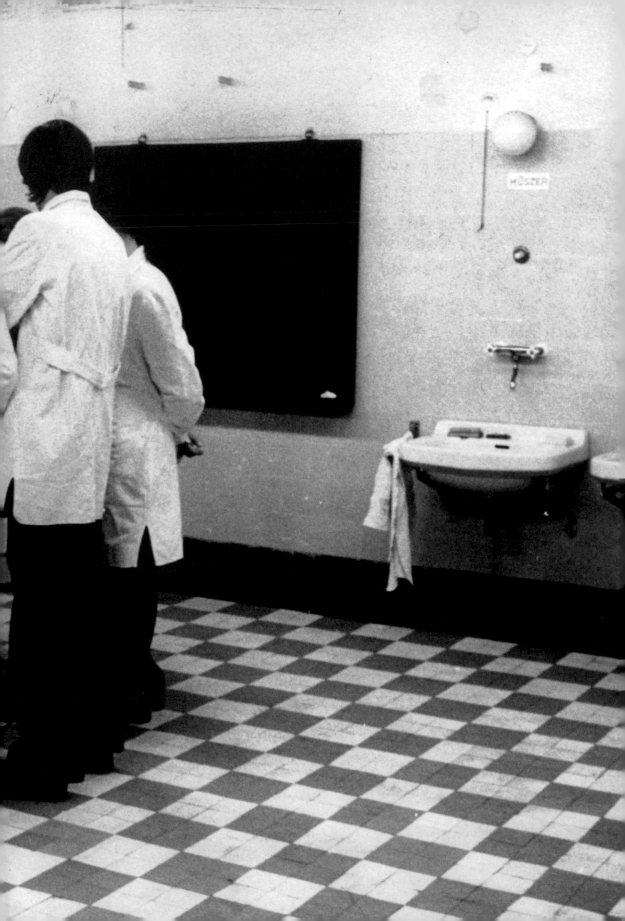

CIRCULATION

CIRCULATED CONCEPTS, IMAGES AND OBJECTS

Harro van Lente

C irculation is the secret of medical success. Medical professionals around the world are connected through the circulation of concepts, images and objects. While at different locations, different languages will be spoken and local practices will prevail, some words, some images, some instruments will be shared with professionals elsewhere – words defining a disease, films showing a diagnosis or objects affording an intervention (Pols 2012). Textbook images of ailments, treatments or medical approaches circulate and allow students to connect to the cosmopolitan world of medical expertise.

Mundane objects, like latex gloves, for instance, circulate around the globe to signify a truthful form of medicine. Kelly Underman (this volume) studies the fate of gloves in the pelvic exam. She shows how they facilitate and allow a professional form of touch, as they add legitimacy to the encounter and script the non-sexual touching of genitals. Likewise, Claire Wendland (this volume) shows how the stethoscope, as an iconic artifact, denotes and defines a medical professional. The object stands for biomedicine itself, she argues. Meanwhile, it also does things: it brings two people together, the listener and the person being listened to. And, she adds, when stethoscopes circulate they serve as unexpected homes for drug-resistant bacteria.

Those collectively shared images and objects signify medical expertise and summarise histories on their own. Medical students learn with them,

Figure TE2: Medical students gather in a dissection theatre at the Semmelweis University of Medicine, Budapest, Hungary, c.1970s. Image courtesy of Semmelweis University Archives.

they organise the profession and they convey specialism and trustworthiness to outsiders. Kaisu Koski and Kirsten Ostherr (this volume) analyse the props in the so-called 'breaking bad news' simulations. In the learning of a profession, the role of props like chairs, tissue boxes, a sheet with test results, but also the spatial qualities of the clinic door, have been overlooked, they argue. They help develop professional performance as they provide proximity and orientation. The circulation of such set-ups helps medical students in all corners of the world to practice problem solving skills. The circulation of concepts, images and objects thus expresses that local medical practices are part of a global constellation, even when they are, indeed, local.

Yet the phrase that concepts, images and objects 'circulate' is somewhat misleading, as it suggests that the circulating thing is the same everywhere. That is not the case: a concept, an image, an object will not be the same at different locations. Annemarie Mol and John Law (1994) detailed how the disease 'anaemia' is connected to technologies and skills and when these travel, for instance with western doctors working in tropical countries, is enacted with different skills, places, technologies, and that these do travel – the tropical medicine doctors from the Netherlands take the methods they learned abroad back to their clinics. Likewise, Marianne Boenink and colleagues (2016) showed how 'Alzheimer's Disease' has a different meaning in Northwestern Europe than in Canada, Mexico or South Africa. While in Western Europe it denotes a dreadful disease taking away autonomy and thus the core of one's identity, elsewhere a family member's loss of autonomy might also pose a significant financial threat to the family itself. Concepts mean and imply different things at different locations; the entity that travels changes its character.

The theoretical approach of Actor Network Theory (ANT) emphasises the importance of circulation. The approach follows the genesis of networks of humans, artefacts, rules and institutions – and how these networks build and change the world, that is, how they gain agency (Callon 1998). People and things are able to achieve something, according to ANT, through and in the networks that constitute them (Latour 2018). The necessity of networks in education can, for instance, be seen in Angela Saward's (this volume) history of educative film in medicine. Circulating physically through networks of learned institutions and libraries, but also reliant on related networks of technology which allowed for the production and projection of film, the emergence of medical film was wholly reliant on the networks which supported its development. ANT also stresses that when networks expand and when the concomitant concepts, images and objects travel, their character and meaning changes (Star and Griesemer 1989). This dual move – a spatial journey is accompanied by a change in meaning – is labelled as 'translation'. And, as the French know, *traduire c'est trahir* – translation also is betrayal.

Images, too, will change their message when circulated: graphs, figures, pictures, films and drawings will be interpreted differently. Claire Aland et al. (this volume), for example, show how digital images of human microstructures circulate. By using the concept of 'tracing', they analyse how medical students make a mental model of the bodily processes, based on those images. The so-called virtual microscope allows students to manipulate a digital file, as if it were an object. Aland and colleagues note how this also may confuse students.

When objects travel, they have to be made meaningful by a gradual uptake in daily routines and in professional practices – a phenomenon that has been described as domestication. And when they come to life in this way, their existence needs continuous maintenance and care (Pluig de la Bellacasa 2011). Concepts travel alongside these objects and also benefit from this care. In Lan Li's (this volume) chapter, for instance, the contentious circulation of social modernisation in communist China is traced through material changes in mid-century acupuncture manuals.

The circulation of concepts, of atherosclerosis for instance, brings together lessons and insights on how arteries may suffer from the deposition of fatty materials in the inner walls. It also points to networks of activities in clinical laboratories, in meeting rooms of committees, in board rooms of hospitals and in the consultation rooms of general practitioners (Mol 2003). When the concept of atherosclerosis travels around, the experiences, insights, approaches and preferences travel with it, but not in the same way and not leading to similar outcomes. Concepts circulate, between universities and hospitals, between patients and doctors, between the Global North and South. In this way, medical practices around the globe are connected, aligned and often largely standardised.

The circulation of concepts, images and objects also brings *standardisation*. When concepts, images and objects travel to a remote hospital, when they are taken up in local activities, when they become part of the routines of doctors and nurses, they change the activities and routines as well – in such a way that these are more or less aligned with practices elsewhere. That is, hospital routines, professional behaviour and local understanding are standardised. Anne Katrine Kleberg Hansen (this volume) looks, for instance, at the representations of fatness in photography. When such pictures become medical photographs they bring along a particular gaze and implicit instructions how to see and use them. The famous example of the distinction between endomorphy, mesomorphy and ectomorphy, described in the *Atlas of Men* by Herbert Sheldon at Columbia University, showed many young male students in the same postures. When circulated, the *Atlas of Men* defined and standardised the notion of fatness.

Not only has the language been adapted to the global, cosmopolitan reservoirs of knowledge and expertise but also the skills, the assessments, the approaches on how to manage patients and hospitals. In this way, circulating concepts, images and objects also introduce *norms*. Drew Danielle Belsky (this volume) focuses on how accuracy is performed in medical illustration. Accuracy, she shows, is less a measure of similitude, but rather a measure for how much it affords medical students to develop skills. In other words, illustrations do not just picture the worlds, but also introduce values and hierarchies. Circulated images and objects introduce a yardstick to measure how well the hospital is doing according to this global standard (Espeland and Sauder 2007). Such yardsticks help medical professions to organise themselves and, at the same time, measure the profession as well. They come with an invitation to reshape and do better. Christian Bonah and Joël Danet (this volume) for instance look at how autopsy films were used to transmit learning experiences in the mid-twentieth century; they show how the viewers' attention is guided and disciplined from afar. The circulation of these films also allowed for the circulation of autopsy as a highly regulated exercise, with autopsy rooms and dedicated theatres as performative settings. Bonah and Danet stress the role of 'framing', in this case, the framing of the corpse, and how it structures and evaluates the handling of professionals and students.

To conclude, when concepts, images and objects circulate a global network of thinking about and working on healthcare is mobilised and sustained. Circulation feeds and changes local practices and norms regarding good practice. This, of course, is a great good. The wonders of circulation also add a vulnerability to medical practices and learning. This circulation provides an infrastructure for expanding and feeding healthcare – it constitutes, as it were, the rails on which the trains of healthcare travel. This circulation also brings legitimation, standardisation and certain yardsticks. But, in the same way that trains do well on rails and poorly outside them, healthcare is also bounded by the circulation of concepts, images and objects. Circulation is not only the secret of medical success, but also its limitation.

References

Boenink, Marianna, van Lente, Harro and Moors, El-len (eds) (2016), *Emerging Technologies for Diagnosing Alzheimer's Disease: Innovating with Care*, London: Pal-grave Macmillan.

Callon, Michel (ed.) (1998), *The Laws of the Markets*, Ox-ford: Blackwell.

Espeland, Wendy Nelson and Sauder, Michael (2007), 'Rankings and reactivity: How public measures recre-ate social worlds', *American Journal of Sociology*, 113:1, pp. 1–40.

Latour, Bruno (2018), *Down to Earth: Politics in the New Climatic Regime*, Cambridge: Polity Press.

Mol, Annemarie (2003), *The Body Multiple: Ontology in Medical Practice*, Durham: Duke University Press.

Mol, Annemarie and Law, John (1994), 'Regions, net-works and fluids: Anaemia and social topology', *Social Studies of Science*, 24:4, pp. 641–71.

Pols Jeannette (2012), *Care at Distance: On the Closeness of Technology*, Amsterdam: Amsterdam University Press.

Puig de la Bellacasa, Maria (2011), 'Matters of care in technoscience: Assembling neglected things', *Social Studies of Science*, 41:1, pp. 85-106.

Star, Susan Leigh and Griesemer, James R. (1989), 'In-stitutional ecology, translation and boundary objects, amateurs and professionals in Berkeley's Museum of vertebrate zoology, 1907–39', *Social Studies of Science*, 19:3, pp. 387–420.

DISSECTING ROOMS

'THE LADY ANATOMIST': FRAGMENTED BODIES, PHOTOGRAPHIC ASSEMBLAGE AND THE 'ART' OF DISSECTION AT WOMAN'S MEDICAL COLLEGE OF PENNSYLVANIA, 1895–98

Jessica M. Dandona

In western medical practice, the study of human cadavers has long functioned as one of the primary means by which knowledge of the body is produced – and reproduced. Well before the nineteenth century, the practice of dissection had become coded as an implicitly gendered one – male 'science' uncovering the secrets of a female 'nature'. Yet as women entered medical schools in increasing numbers during this period, they engaged not only in anatomical study but also in the wide array of visual and material practices associated with this science, disrupting the longstanding association of the female form with mute matter.

This chapter examines two scrapbooks created by students at Woman's Medical College of Pennsylvania (WMC) in the late 1890s. In these albums, students' intimate relationship with the dead body is highlighted in ways both earnest and, at times, humorous. In his study of dissecting room photographs, John Harley Warner persuasively argues that such portraits commemorate a shared rite of passage, one that was integral to the professional self-fashioning of nineteenth-century medical students. 'As visual memoirs of a transformative experience', he writes, dissection room 'photographs are auto-biographical narrative devices by which the students placed themselves into a larger, shared story of becoming a doctor' (Warner 2009: 15). At the same time, however, by visually transforming living students into ghostly, inanimate images and cadavers into potentially animate subjects, the photographs restore a measure of agency to the nameless dead upon whose bodies the text of anatomy is written. These images thus trouble the conventional relationship between medicine's subjects and its objects, highlighting connections between the living and the dead, and blurring the lines between 'science' and 'nature'.

Life at Woman's Medical College

While numerous photographs survive in the archives of Woman's Medical College, these two scrapbooks compiled by students in the late 1890s stand out for their complexity and visually striking character. Created by Alice Evans (WMC 1898) and Laura Heath Hills (WMC 1896), the albums provide an intimate glimpse into daily life at a woman's medical college, as seen in Figures 6.1 and 6.2. Both Hills and Evans went on to have long and successful careers as physicians and later donated their albums to the WMC archives. They would have overlapped by at least two years in their studies, 1894–95, but as dissection was confined primarily to the first two years of study, 1894 is the most likely year in which their photographs were made. The precise author of the photographs is unknown – it may have been one or both students. At least eleven photographs, Figures 6.3 and 6.4 for instance, are common to both albums, suggesting that the process of constructing the books was founded on exchange, emulation and shared experience.

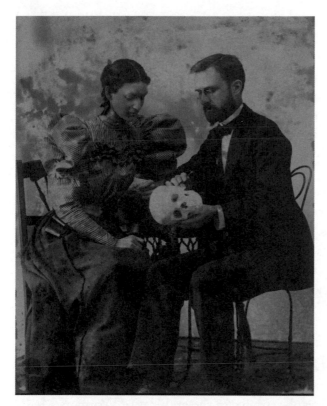

Figure 6.1: Scrapbook of Laura Heath Hills: Alice R. Evans and Dr. Hill, Eye, Ear, Throat Dr., *c.*1896, p. 7. Laura Heath Hills, M.D. Papers ACC-126. Woman's Medical College of Pennsylvania Photograph Collection, The Legacy Center, Drexel University College of Medicine.

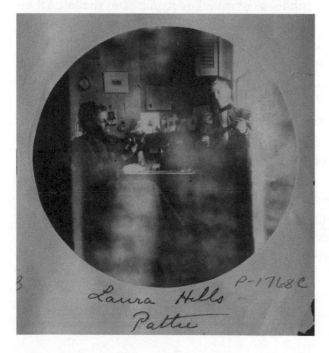

Figure 6.2: Alice Evans Scrapbook, *c.*1895–98, p. 13. Alice R. Evans-Miller, M.D. Papers ACC-221. Woman's Medical College of Pennsylvania Photograph Collection, The Legacy Center, Drexel University College of Medicine.

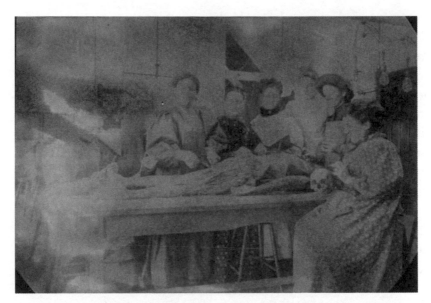

Figure 6.3: Scrapbook of Laura Heath Hills: Dissecting Room, c.1892–96, p. 15. Laura Heath Hills, M.D. Papers ACC-126. Woman's Medical College of Pennsylvania Photograph Collection, The Legacy Center, Drexel University College of Medicine.

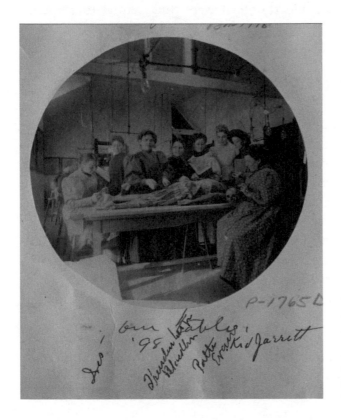

Figure 6.4: Alice Evans Scrapbook, c.1898, p. 10. Alice R. Evans-Miller, M.D. Papers ACC-221. Woman's Medical College of Pennsylvania Photograph Collection, The Legacy Center, Drexel University College of Medicine.

The majority of photographs in the Evans album are cyanotypes of a deep indigo hue. Their round format and lack of crisp detail suggest that they were made using one of the early portable cameras manufactured by Eastman Kodak in the 1890s. The Hills album likewise contains early snapshots but also includes personal correspondence, cards and other documents. The photographs document a pivotal moment for women in the history of medical education. Between 1850 and 1882, five medical schools devoted exclusively to educating women physicians opened in the United States. An increasing number of medical schools offered co-educational training beginning in the 1890s and, by 1900, women would make up 5 per cent of the American medical profession (Kaiser et al. 1984: 218). In the period when these photographs were made, WMC offered an unusually rigorous four-year curriculum, with opportunities for clinical work at nearby hospitals. Anatomical dissection was a central component of this curriculum and extended over a two-year period. Courses on 'Operative Obstetrics and Operative Gynaecology', offered in the third and fourth years, extended this experience through surgical practice on cadavers (Anon. 1894: 11). Encounters with the bodies of both the living and the dead were thus central to students' medical training.

In the dissecting room

Among the 74 photographs extent in the Alice Evans scrapbook, a surprisingly large number are devoted to images of the dissecting room – eleven in total. Six of these reappear in the much larger Hills scrapbook. These photographs, I would argue, do important work in normalising and documenting the students' access to human remains at a time when the study of medicine by women continued to be highly controversial (Wells 2001). Not surprisingly, given both its centrality to medical education at this time and the continuing controversy over anatomy's association with grave-robbing and desecration of the body, the act of dissection often formed the central focus of debate concerning medical education for women.

In an address delivered to the students of the Massachusetts Medical College in 1850, for example, Professor John Ware warned that undertaking dissection could lead male medical students to 'forget that the object before us is anything but a mere subject of our art' (Ware 1850: 24). Ware argued that the danger was even more pronounced, however, for *women* medical students, who risked not only losing their 'reverence for the inanimate body of a fellow being' but also 'tarnishing that delicate surface of the female mind', leading to its 'defilement' (Ware 1850: 24–25). In short, Ware made an argument that was echoed many times over the course of the century: women studying medicine and engaging in dissection, in particular, were in danger of *unsexing* themselves by destroying the very characteristics – delicacy, intuition and tenderness – that were understood to define their gender (Sappol 2002: 62, 90; Wells 2001).

This was an argument that the faculty of WMC soon grew used to refuting in their public defence of medical training for women. Thus, in 1858, Professor of Anatomy and Histology E. H. Cleveland addressed dissection directly in her introductory lecture to the incoming class. Drawing on many of the same arguments as male writers opposed to medical education for women, but turning them to a different purpose, Cleveland writes,

> We know it has been objected that familiarity with such subjects as belong properly to the science of medicine, with anatomy and kindred studies, cannot fail to injure or destroy those feelings of delicacy and refinement which add peculiar lustre to the character of woman. [...] We strenuously advocate the necessity of giving to all women a knowledge of the human body, 'with its marvelous beauty of structure and office,' and we do it remembering their high vocation as nature's appointed guardians of childhood and youth. (1858: 10–11)

By evoking contemporary concepts of women's role as deeply linked to care for others, Cleveland recasts the practice of medicine as the natural extension of labor in the home, extending the maternal metaphor to the protection of society itself. The reference to the beauty of the body, meanwhile, operates at the intersection of Christian belief, evolutionary theory and aesthetics, while also distancing the process of gaining 'knowledge' from the abject materiality of anatomical dissection.

The 'Lady Anatomist'

Anxiety over the participation of women students in the act of anatomical dissection extended beyond the medical profession. Appearing in a number of publications in the early 1880s, for example, the satirical poem 'The Lady Anatomist' parodies the misdirected passions of a student more interested in her beau's anatomy than his loving charms. The woman medical student in the poem, who remains 'cold' in the face of affection and whose lips utter not terms of endearment but rather 'scientific' words, abruptly comes to life when her suitor offers her his 'heart' (Anon. n.d.: n.pag.). 'Tis' just what I wanted – blood-vessels and nerves, / And muscles contracting in regular curves', she exclaims, before offering to examine his 'auricles [and] ventricles, too' (Anon. n.d.: n.pag.).

The woman medical student appears here as a *femme fatale* – the examination of her suitor's heart must, necessarily, be post-mortem – but, through its structure and sequential enumeration of body parts, the poem also enacts the disarticulation and segmentation of the corporeal form entailed in the act of dissection. Such popular sources demonstrate a pervasive anxiety regarding the ways in which women's intellectual curiosity – and pursuit of a medical education in particular – might displace or even pervert the 'natural' course of human affections, effecting a transformation of the female body from erotic object to investigating subject in search of a cadaver. The students of WMC would take on this theme quite directly in *Daughters of Aesculapius* (1897), a compilation of stories and photographs published to familiarise the public with daily life at Woman's Medical College. In the story 'A Maiden Effort', a student wryly recounts, 'One afternoon [Sidney Brooke] called for me at college, [and] as bad luck would have it […] I appeared with a handful of scalpels which belonged to different girls, and which I was taking to have sharpened. I shall never forget that man's face' (*Daughters of Aesculapius* 1897: 48–49). Any direct visual representation of students engaging in dissection, however, is carefully omitted from the book, in favour of Figure 6.5, a photograph depicting classmates gathered around the anatomy demonstrator, Elizabeth Bundy, as she dissects a brain. Taken together, text and image thus seek to capitalise upon the public's fascination with the taboo subject of dissection but also to contain the threat posed by the investigation of male bodies by female students. The dissection of a brain – the organ most associated with humankind's higher faculties, rather than its baser instincts – likewise helps to allay fears that women medical students might explore more controversial areas of human anatomy, such as the reproductive system.

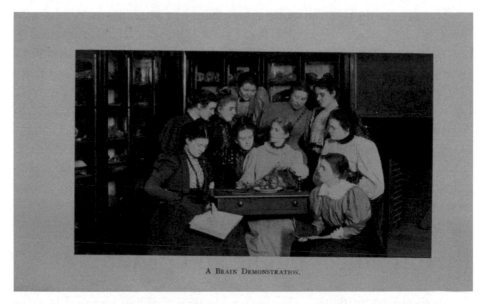

A Brain Demonstration.

Figure 6.5: A brain demonstration, frontispiece from *Daughters of Aesculapius: Stories Written by Alumnæ and Students of the Woman's Medical College of Pennsylvania* (Philadelphia: George W. Jacobs & Co., 1897). Woman's Medical College of Pennsylvania Photograph Collection, The Legacy Center, Drexel University College of Medicine.

Anatomy's subjects

The act of dissection performed by women medical students not only violated societal expectations of gender roles but also contravened centuries of tradition that linked anatomical investigation, metaphorically, with male penetration of the female body. As Katharine Park has documented in her history of the origins of dissection, beginning in the early modern period 'the female figure [came] to illustrate internal anatomy in general, apparently by association with the uterus: where the male bodies are mostly surfaces, the woman is identified with a visualizable inside' (Park 2010: 27). The era in which Hills and Evans created their scrapbooks saw a proliferation of heavily eroticised images of male anatomists preparing to dissect female cadavers. Scholars such as Ludmilla Jordanova have analysed in detail the ways in which such images cast dissection as a process of unveiling, one that associates the feminine with passivity and death, while linking masculinity with the active penetration of the female body (Jordanova 1989: 99, 104; Bronfen 1992: 3).

The dissecting room photographs created by students at WMC and the performance of dissection itself thus represent a transgression of both historical and contemporary boundaries that defined women (and symbolically feminised male bodies) as the *object* of the anatomist's exploration, but never the anatomist herself. The stakes of this debate were high: as Michael Sappol and others have noted, by the mid-nineteenth century, the practice of anatomical dissection and ready access to cadavers had become one of the primary means by which American medical schools distinguished themselves from their rivals, associated their programme with the authority of European tradition and sought to attract new students (Sappol 2002: 2, 55; Jordanova 1989: 100).

Performances public and private

By representing students at Woman's Medical College engaged in anatomical dissection, the photographs in the scrapbooks speak to the establishment of professional identity by commemorating a shared rite of passage. However, a comparison of the photographs from WMC with examples from other institutions, Figures 6.6 and 6.7, respectively, reveals significant differences between standard tropes found in images of the dissecting room and those produced by Evans and Hills.

In a photograph from the University of Maryland, for example, male medical students line up facing the camera, with the cadaver laid before them. Painted markings on their lab coats identify the students' home states, while the Socratic epigraph 'Know thy Self' lends an air of classical authority to the proceedings. A skull and bones arranged into an artful *memento mori* below the cadaver, meanwhile, evoke the precedent of countless oil portraits of anatomists and physicians, inserting the men into a long lineage of distinguished anatomical investigation. While the students pose with scalpels in hand, their attention is focused on the photographer, not the cadaver. It is not the *performance* of dissection, in other words, that is here commemorated but rather the students' shared identity as members of the medical confraternity. While the lifeless body of the cadaver is displayed for the viewer, little information can be gleaned from its contours. Rather, its presence serves to affirm male medical students' privileged access to the body, here presented as passive, inert flesh upon which the students' scalpels will record the twin passage of both time and discovery.

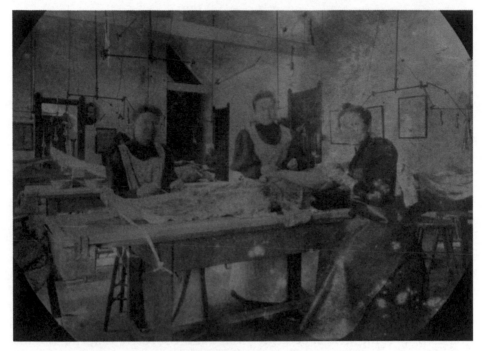

Figure 6.6: Scrapbook of Laura Heath Hills: Dissecting Room, *c.*1895, p. 15. Laura Heath Hills, M.D. Papers ACC-126. Woman's Medical College of Pennsylvania Photograph Collection, The Legacy Center, Drexel University College of Medicine.

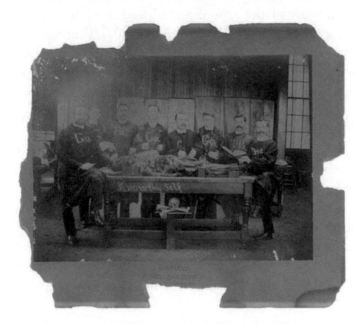

Figure 6.7: University of Maryland School of Medicine, Baltimore, *c.*1890. Photograph. Collection of John Harley Warner.

In contrast, in a photograph from the Hills scrapbook, students appear caught in mid-motion as they glance at the photographer. The presence of a student seated on the same side of the dissection table as the photographer establishes a sense of shared identity even as it invites the viewer to imagine that they, too, are engaged in dissection. The composition is crowded with additional tables and students in the background, framed anatomical prints and the tools of dissection: it is, above all, *a working space*. What is celebrated, in other words, is not students' privileged access to the body per se, but rather access to medical study itself.

As visual representations, the photographs created by Evans and Hills give form to the potentially transgressive and secretive ritual of dissection, what one contemporary called 'an abomination to the popular mind' (Dwight cited in Warner and Rizzolo 2006: 404; Dwight 1896: 75), but they do so in ways that normalise, contain and shelter it from prying eyes. The scrapbooks are intensely personal, by design made to close and hide their contents, and they record intimate details of the students' lives. By pairing images of the dissecting room with photographs of evening meals, bedtime rituals and collective toil, the albums fold both the space and the work of dissection into a form at once shared and private.

According to the WMC Faculty Minutes, the dissecting room was separate from the main part of the school and closed to male visitors with the exception of William Henry Parish (1845–1903), Professor of Anatomy from 1881 until his death (Wells 2001: 215). Even at co-educational schools of medicine, it was common practice for there to be separate dissecting rooms for male and female students. The hidden space of the dissecting room thus finds its echo in the closed pages of the album – like the room itself, available to only a limited circle of the 'initiated'.

In contrast, the photograph from Maryland and many others like it circulated in a more public context. Printed in a large format and mounted on cardboard, reproduced in college annuals or even mailed as postcards to friends and family, such dissecting room photographs served to enhance the prestige of the college and lend authority to those initiated into the rites of passage they commemorate. In such images, anatomical dissection functions as a kind of synecdoche for medical training itself, representing at once its philosophical basis and its most controversial act.

The anatomist as artist

If the construction of a scrapbook entails creating meaning through the making, collecting and assembling of photographs and other ephemera, the dissection and preservation of the human body likewise explore the relationship between part and whole through a process of making, unmaking and display. Students at WMC often discussed their work in terms that strongly evoke these aesthetic and material dimensions of anatomical study. Writing in 1893, for example, Mary McGavran (WMC 1895) confided to her diary, 'I have commenced my fourth part in dissecting. It is Dr. Parishes [*sic*] arsenic subject – the arteries are beautiful – we can trace them out to the finest hair-like branches – the anastomosing about the shoulder and elbow is *very* interesting' (McGavran cited in Kaiser: 230; McGavran n.d.: 31). McGavran here expresses a keen aesthetic appreciation of the body's structures and the unique variations found within individual cadavers, both brought to light by anatomical science.

Dissection consists of more than the visual and tactile exploration of the body: its end goal is the display of the muscles, arteries, veins, joints and tendons of the body. It thus constitutes a process of gradual and methodical *transformation*, one that is nearly sculptural in both its tools and its products, as students excise skin, fat and excess tissue to reveal the underlying structures of the body 'laid bare'. Scholars such as Mary Hunter have pointed to the ways in which the act of dissection also bears a strong resemblance to the process of drawing: in both, it is the skilled hand of the operator which delineates structure, echoing the lines of the body through his or her own movements (Hunter 2015). Drawing was also a common practice in the dissecting room. Although there is no evidence that this practice took place at WMC, at many schools, including the nearby University of Pennsylvania, prizes were awarded for the best notebook documenting anatomical anomalies uncovered in the dissecting room.

As students undertook dissections, then, they simultaneously engaged in an act of creation – the transformation of a body into an object of display – *and* in an act of destruction, for that transformation required the gradual fragmentation of the body until its form became nearly unreadable as human. As Helen MacDonald has argued, 'Learning anatomy was always as much about destroying as creating' (2006: 38). It was this labour that made the body 'speak': 'the work of seeing', Susan Wells writes, 'was supported by the work of arranging and constructing; the opening of the body revealed nature, but the labor of the student rendered it intelligible' (2001: 217).

The curriculum at WMC, like other institutions of its time, thus placed a premium on the skills involved in the preservation and display of the body. Students in the dissecting room were being trained to be anatomical makers even as they unmade the body. While they struggled against the inevitability of corporeal entropy, students sought ways to remake the body in an incorruptible form – much as the photograph seeks to preserve a singular moment in time. The process of transforming a cadaver into either an ephemeral or a more permanent spectacle involved making injections to 'color and harden veins, arteries, lymphatics' and other structures, with the goal of rendering bodily structures visually distinct and legible – making them match, in other words, the colourful anatomical illustrations in textbooks and prints (Ponce 2013: 351).

In preserving the body, students commemorated and safeguarded the results of their labours as a mark of their new professional identity. The college's annual announcement for 1894 draws attention to the importance of this process, stating, 'The College possesses an excellent museum of specimens. [...] Alumnae are specially invited to send to it any specimens which they may be able to procure. Each specimen will be suitably mounted and *labeled with the name of the donor*' (Anon. 1894: 20, emphasis added).

Like the photograph, the anatomical specimen functions to preserve the appearance of life – and, like the photograph, is subject to its own inevitable corruption. Both commemorate their maker as well as their subject, and both suggest that the dissecting room remained a space in which power relations were explored in ways both profound and disconcerting. The long and persistent association of anatomical dissection with the appropriation of the bodies of the poor, the destitute and the socially marginal casts a long shadow over these images, as specimens created from the unclaimed bodies of the dead were used to celebrate the legacy of women medical students (Richardson 1987; Hurren 2012). Moreover, at a time when physicians routinely created, collected, exhibited and even sold specimens, this practice – like that of dissection – likely served to strengthen women medical students' claim to professional standing in their field.

The book of the body

The practice of dissection was deeply informed by the abundance of images and objects that surrounded students in the dissecting room. Framed anatomical prints, teaching charts, specimens and texts provided both an overview of the *process* of dissection and, in many cases, a visual model for its finished product. Photographs of the dissecting room at Woman's Medical College offer glimpses of framed works similar to George Viner Ellis and George Henry Ford's enormously popular folio of large-format lithographic plates (Ellis and Ford 1882) as well as several hanging charts and an articulated skeleton. Their presence highlights the important role played by such images and objects in teaching students not only how to present, but also how to *read* the dead body.

This abundance of anatomical imagery led some authors, such as the Scottish anatomist John Cleland, to warn students of the dangers of over-reliance on the text: 'The student ought to study the "subject" in the dissecting-room, and his books at home', Cleland argues, 'and he ought never to be encouraged in the too common error of looking on his dissections as mere illustrations for the statements of the text-book' (Cleland 1888: v). The anatomist attempted to solve this problem by omitting illustrations from his manual and urging students to make notes and sketches based on their direct observation of the body. Cleland writes,

> It is expected of the student that before coming to the dissecting-room he should glance over, each evening, a portion of work in this book, and consult his descriptive manual sufficiently to have an intelligent idea of what he is to exhibit on the subject the next day. Taking with him this book to the dissecting-room, he will with its aid cultivate his manipulative powers and his observations; and on his return home he will recur to his text-book, and find how far his own observations agree with those of more experienced men. He will find it also an invaluable habit, of more than mere anatomical advantage in later life, to devote a short time each day before he quits his dissection to taking written notes and sketches of what he sees before him. (1888: vi)

The process of acquiring anatomical knowledge, then, involved a complex interweaving of sources both the first- and the second-hand. These include not only the visual observation and tactile exploration of the cadaver itself but also the work of memory, the study of anatomical illustrations and descriptions in dissection manuals and textbooks and the creation of images and objects made *by* students, including the photographs in these albums. Each in turn draws upon the other for its meaning. In each case, the body is presented piecemeal – as a composite of isolated parts, united only by the conceptual framework of dissection itself. Like a scrapbook, then, anatomy creates meaning through the logic of adjacency and analogy, and like the reading of an album, the book of the body unfurls its pages over time.

In creating their scrapbooks, Evans and Hills both emulate and transform the anatomical treatise. In effect, the students create a *new* book of the body, one based on their personal and shared experience of dissection and presented from the point of view of a student in their midst. In this process, they had many models to draw on: beginning with Vesalius, Figure 6.8, many anatomical atlases prominently featured an illustration of the anatomist engaged in the act of dissection. If anatomical prints, manuals and textbooks offered students a model for how to dissect the human body, these representations of respected anatomists served as a model for how to be a student of anatomy. Surrounded by iconic representations of and by male anatomists – not least of which was a reproduction of Rembrandt's famous painting, *The Anatomy Lesson of Dr. Nicolaes Tulp* (1632), which hung in the dissecting room at Woman's Medical College – Evans and Hills assert their own status as icons of a new age. In doing so, they mark the double trespass of their engagement in anatomical dissection – at once crossing the boundary between the living and the dead and entering spaces reserved for anatomy's time-honoured rituals of male homosocial bonding (Hunter 2015).

Death and the photograph

We have established, then, that the scrapbooks produced by students at Woman's Medical College in the 1890s constituted a form of professional self-fashioning, one defined through artistry as well as labor and study. In the process, the photographs made by women medical students challenged long-held beliefs regarding anatomy's ideal practitioners and their relationship to the objects of anatomical study. The rewriting of this narrative did not end there, however: in these works, photography's own

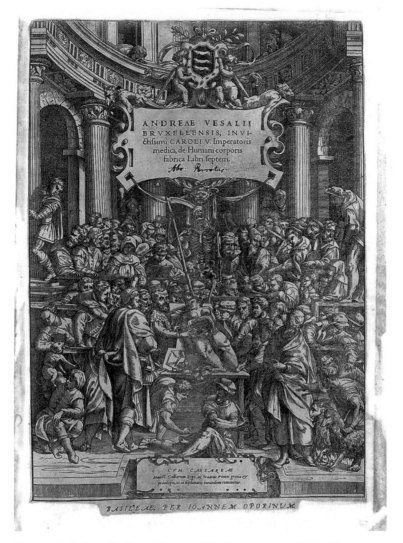

Figure 6.8: Andreas Vesalius, title page of *De Humani corporis fabrica libri septem*, 1543, engraving. Wellcome Collection, London. Attribution 4.0 International (CC BY 4.0).

'deathlike' nature lends complexity to the process of both studying the body *and* representing it.

In *Camera Lucida*, the French structuralist Roland Barthes argues, 'the photograph's immobility is the result of a perverse confusion between two concepts: the Real and the Live' (Barthes 1980: 79). 'By attesting that the object has been real', he contends, 'the photograph surreptitiously induces belief that it is alive' (Barthes 1980: 79). Throughout the scrapbooks, as in Figure 6.9, numerous details help to create this confusion, whether it is the white head-scarves worn by both a cadaver and the student dissecting her body; the rhyming of three hands – two belonging to a student and one to a corpse; or the way in which the patterned draperies covering a dead body begin to resemble a woman's fashionable gown. The medium of the photograph thus threatens to 'reanimate' the bodies of the dead, troubling the sense of mastery that helped secure a professional identity premised upon medical authority over both the living and the deceased.

The photograph's tendency to enact a kind of symbolic death creates another level of ambiguity in the relations between dissector and dissected. Captured and displayed in one frozen instant, the students in these photographs are rendered as deathlike as the objects of their scrutiny, the ghostly blur of their features evoking the same process of decay that will beset the bodies before them. Barthes again highlights the dual nature of the photographic portrait. 'There is always a defeat of Time [...] *that* is dead and *that* is going to die', he writes of the photographic subject, 'They have their whole lives before them; but also they are dead (today), they are then *already* dead (yesterday)' (Barthes 1980: 96). Through the play of time and the gaze, the photographs in these scrapbooks thus break down the boundaries between subject and object and between the seer and the seen.

In this sense, the works created by Evans and Hills offer an alternative understanding of the entangled histories of photography and medicine. For the late-nineteenth century physicians, photography appeared to offer an objectivity that was quickly becoming the defining goal of 'scientific medicine' (Daston and Galison 2007; Amirault 1993–94: 57). In the photographs discussed here, however, the works' indeterminacy, ambiguities and lack of clarity do not reaffirm the power relations established by the clinical gaze but instead reveal its instability. In these images, the students of Woman's Medical do not assume the identity of their male peers as much as unsettle that identity, opening up new spaces of possibility and meanings in the process.

In photographs of their fellow students, Alice Evans and Laura Heath Hills offer viewers a valuable record of the ways in which fin-de-siècle women medical students broke with historical precedent and transgressed cultural boundaries in their relationship to the human body and its remains. Through the creation of their scrapbooks, I have argued, these two students author a new book of anatomy: one that highlights the intimacy between the living and the dead in the study of medicine,

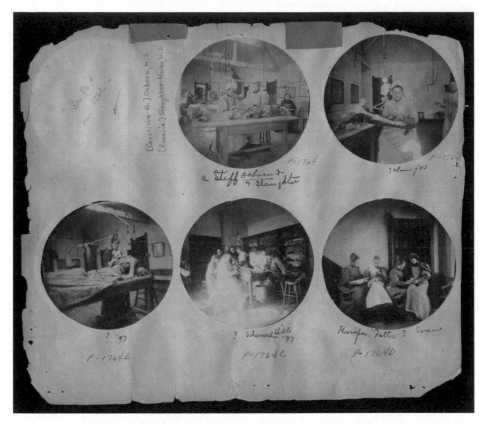

Figure 6.9: Alice Evans Scrapbook, *c.*1898, p. 9. Alice R. Evans-Miller, M.D. Papers ACC-221. Woman's Medical College of Pennsylvania Photograph Collection, The Legacy Center, Drexel University College of Medicine.

celebrates the artistry of anatomical dissection and explores the complexities of scientific investigation. In the process, they create a work that is both a monument to memory and a *memento mori*.

Acknowledgements

Research for this chapter was supported by a Fellowship in the History of Women and Medicine, funded by the Drexel University College of Medicine Legacy Center and the Library Company of Philadelphia (2018).

References

Alumnæ and Students of Woman's Medical College of Pennsylvania (1897), *Daughters of Aesculapius: Stories Written by Alumnæ and Students of the Woman's Medical College of Pennsylvania*, Philadelphia: George W. Jacobs & Co.

Amirault, Chris (1993–94), 'Posing the subject of early medical photography', *Discourse*, 16:2, pp. 51–76.

Anon. (1894), *Forty-Fifth Annual Announcement of the Woman's Medical College of Pennsylvania, North College Avenue and Twenty-First Street, Philadelphia: Session of 1894–95*, Philadelphia: The Jas. B. Rodgers Printing Co.

Anon. (n.d.), *The Lady Anatomist*, MS 135639, Pasadena: The Huntington Library, George Dock Papers.

Barthes, Roland (1980), *Camera Lucida* (trans. R. Howard), New York: Hill & Wang.

Bronfen, Elisabeth (1992), *Over Her Dead Body: Death, Femininity and the Aesthetic*, New York: Routledge.

Cleland, John (1888), *A Directory for the Dissection of the Human Body*, 3rd ed., London: Smith, Elder, & Co.

Cleveland, Emeline Horton (1858), *Introductory Lecture on Behalf of the Faculty to the Class of the Female Medical College of Pennsylvania for the Session of 1858–59*, Philadelphia: Merrihew & Thompson, Printers.

Daston, Lorraine and Galison, Peter (2007), *Objectivity*, New York: Zone Books.

Dwight, Thomas (1896), 'Our contribution to civilization and to science', *Science*, 3, pp. 75–7.

Ellis, George Viner and Ford, George Henry (1882), *Illustrations of Dissections in a Series of Original Colored Plates the Size of Life Representing the Dissection of the Human Body*, 2nd ed., New York: William Wood & Company.

Hunter, Mary (2015), 'Intern, orderly, artist, corpse: Emerging masculinities in Henri Gervex's *Autopsy at Hôtel-Dieu*', *Oxford Art Journal*, 38:3, pp. 405–26.

Hurren, Elizabeth (2012), *Dying for Victorian Medicine: English Anatomy and its Trade in the Dead Poor, c. 1834–1929*, Basingstoke: Palgrave Macmillan.

Jordanova, Ludmilla (1989), *Sexual Visions: Images of Gender in Science and Medicine between the Eighteenth and Twentieth Centuries*, Madison: University of Wisconsin Press.

Kaiser, Robert M., Chaff, Sandra L. and Peitzman, Steven J. (1984), 'Notes and documents: a Philadelphia medical student of the 1890s: the diary of Mary Theodora McGavran', *The Pennsylvania Magazine of History and Biography*, 108:2, pp. 217–36.

MacDonald, Helen (2006), *Human Remains: Dissection and its Histories*, New Haven: Yale University Press.

McGavran, Mary Theodora (n.d.), 'Life and Work of Mary T. McGavran', MS ACC-169, Philadelphia: Drexel University School of Medicine Legacy Center, Mary Theodora McGavran, M.D. Papers.

Park, Katharine (2010), *Secrets of Women: Gender, Generation, and the Origins of Human Dissection*, New York: Zone Books.

Ponce, Rachel N. (2013), '"They increase in beauty and elegance": Transforming cadavers and the epistemology of dissection in early nineteenth-century American medical education', *Journal of the History of Medicine and Allied Sciences*, 68:3, pp. 331–76.

Richardson, Ruth (1987), *Death, Dissection, and the Destitute*, London: Routledge & Kegan Paul.

Sappol, Michael (2002), *A Traffic of Dead Bodies: Anatomy and Embodied Social Identity in Nineteenth-Century America*, Princeton and Oxford: Princeton University Press.

Ware, John (1850), *Success in the Medical Profession: An Introductory Lecture Delivered at the Massachusetts Medical College, November 6, 1850*, Boston: David Clapp, Printer.

Warner, John Harley (2009), 'Witnessing dissection: photography, medicine, and American culture', in J. H. Warner and J. M. Edmonson (eds), *Dissection: Photographs of a Rite of Passage in American Medicine 1880–1930*, New York: Blast Books, pp. 6–29.

Warner, John Harley and Edmonson, James M. (eds) (2009), *Dissection: Photographs of a Rite of Passage in American Medicine 1880–1930*, New York: Blast Books.

Warner, John Harley and Rizzolo, Lawrence J. (2006), 'Anatomical instruction and training for professionalism from the 19th to the 21st centuries', *Clinical Anatomy*, 19, pp. 403–14.

Wells, Susan (2001), *Out of the Dead House: Nineteenth-Century Women Physicians and the Writing of Medicine*, Madison: University of Wisconsin Press.

FILM

'SEE FOR YOURSELF': AUTOPSY FILM AS AUDIO-VISUAL MEDIATION OF LEARNING EXPERIENCES, c.1928–62

Christian Bonah and Joël Danet

I n the office of a grey-haired professor of pathology at the medical faculty in Strasbourg, France, an almost forgotten, yet still treasured, silver metal can sit on a remote corner of a shelf. The professor says it contains a film strip. He keeps it as a silent witness of the foregone tenure of his predecessor, Professor Louis Frühling (1916–62) (Philippe 2001; Olivier-Utard 2009). He has not watched the 35mm movie since his days as a young assistant, as the institute no longer has a projector. Projected on a silver screen, the film turns out to be a challenging viewing experience. The 101-minute work, entitled *Techniques Anatomopathologiques de l'Autopsie, Cours Cinématographique du Dr. Frühling* (Vierny et al. 1962), is a filmed autopsy lesson produced in 1962 by Alain Resnais's Parisian production crew and was not commercially distributed. The movie is not an isolated, idiosyncratic curiosity. A similar production is listed in the catalogue of France's Centre National de la Cinématographie, under the title *Techniques des Autopsies* (Benoit-Lévy 1928).[1] These two autopsy films bookmark a period of medical education (1920s–60s) when instructional movies were used for producing and transmitting medical knowledge in autopsy practice. Seen today, these spectacular, transitional and ambivalent works appear as tokens of a century-long didactic effort to use the motion picture in medical education, and material traces of the agency of that era's modern communication technologies in medical knowledge production and transmission (Orgeron et al. 2012; Elsaesser 2009; Bonah and Laukötter 2009).

What does autopsy do to educational motion pictures and what do they do to autopsy? This chapter examines the influence of educational motion pictures on autopsy practices and, conversely, the influence of these practices on the medium. Working through the two films mentioned above, Jean Benoit-Lévy's 1928 teaching film *Technique des Autopsies* and Louis Frühling's 1962 *Cours Cinématographique*, we will use the cinematographic concept of the *frame* as a central analytical category. According to French film critic and theorist André Bazin, one of the first to have theorised the specificities of the cinematic language, *le cadre est un cache*, framing means hiding (Dudley 1978; Bazin 2018). The film theorist Jean-Louis Comolli elaborates:

> Framing in film is about making things fit into a frame, adapting to the frame: placing the sky, the sea, the landscape, the body, the thing in a more or less extended rectangle, one that cuts out a visible portion of the shot and forces what is being filmed to fit within these bounds or to remain outside of them. (Commoli and Sorel 2015: 106, author's translation)

In autopsy film, we argue, framing the corpse, 'which before it is filmed, is obviously not framed', consists in 'making it enter a frame, and therefore subjugating it, disciplining it, regulating it' (Commoli and Sorel 2015: 106). In this sense, autopsy film reproduces what autopsy and its method themselves are already doing: framing, and therefore rendering visible, making students see (Fleck 1986: 129). An autopsy is not the random cutting and slicing of corpses, but a highly regulated exercise. The ordered, standardised procedure, which pathologists call their 'method', is itself a procedural frame for containing the exercise and its inherent violence. Autopsy film adds a visual frame to the procedural frame, a practice called *surcadrage* in film theory, a frame within a frame. This practice also acutely raises the question of the place of the spectator, since the cameraman makes the spectator an accomplice in the way he looks at the corpse. It orients the gaze and frames the emotions of student spectators. And it reveals a homogeneity and filmic tradition of surgical and pathology filming since cinema's earliest days. Our central concept suggests three functions. First, autopsy film as teaching material mechanically reproduces views of a real autopsy frame after frame: the scenes can be copied and projected again and again. Second, it adds the camera's frame to the procedural frame; third, framing directs spectators' emotions.

Autopsy films will be analysed as pedagogical tools along three lines. First of all, films and their specificities are presented from a didactic perspective, considering why films joined the ranks of books, blackboards and autopsy theatres as learning tools and how the mechanical, frame-by-frame reproduction autopsies worked for larger audiences. Second, filmic choices of clarity and soberness will be analysed in light of the frame in a frame, considering how the production and reproduction of medical knowledge are shown, and how movies were thought to prepare and extend the practice of autopsies as learning experiences, raising the question of the statuses of patient and corpse in these movies. Third, filmic choices aimed at toning down sensory knowledge and the emotions of the autopsy will shed light into the role of film technique in the respectful treatment of corpses and in the anonymisation and control of emotions – framing for the purpose of transmitting. Lastly, we will examine the influence of filming techniques on autopsy knowledge, the opening of corpses and the emotions and feelings it triggers, pointing to the importance of their management in the secular history of the autopsy. Often requested, difficult to evaluate historically, we lack information on how students received these films: did they feel that the film was a substitute for this experience, did they see the film as a complementary pedagogical tool, did they find in the film treatment a different, and perhaps disturbing, embodiment of this motif of the open and examined body? Without student notes or interviews of the time, we suggest to take reception into account indirectly through an approach based in particular on film theory of spectator experience.

Reproducing the frame

Since the beginning of the nineteenth century, the autopsy has become one of the key practices through which medical students learn to correlate clinical observation with post-mortem pathological findings. The advent of the autopsy, which in Greek literally means 'seeing by your own eyes', has been described by Michel Foucault as the very moment when humankind transformed itself into an object of scientific inquiry and as the medical practice that grounded the 'birth of the clinic' (Foucault 1975). In different cultural settings, including in German-speaking countries, the practice is called 'opening corpses' (*Leicheneröffnung*), which describes the post-mortem practice more than the gaze. During the nineteenth and twentieth centuries, autopsies were performed by the thousands in teaching hospitals for medical education. They gave crucial momentum to biomedical, evidence-based medical practice (Bonah 2008). By the late nineteenth century, the autopsy had its material culture in form of dissection theatres, rooms, tables and tools (Filliquet and Bonah 2008) (see Figure 7.1).

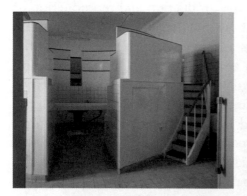 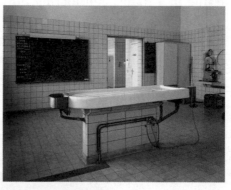

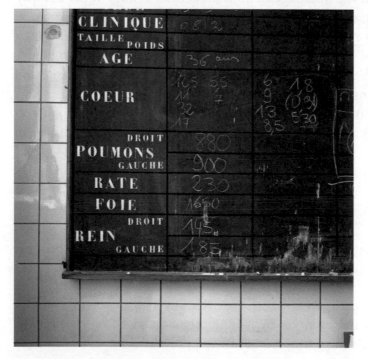

Figures 7.1: Views of the autopsy rooms, tables and theatre at the medical faculty in Strasbourg built in 1878. Photographs by the artist Pierre Filliquet. Filliquet and Bonah (2008).

How did autopsy film complement this material culture that had existed since the 1920s and what does it add to the existing teaching media combination of blackboard or printed drawings, textbooks, and dissection facilities, allowing for a hands-on experience? First, it is worth recalling that since the beginning of the twentieth-century scientists invested in the educational film, and valued it as an extremely useful tool for teaching. The film makes it possible to highlight details and make them visible to an entire class. A lecture in cinematic form can be replayed countless times, allowing for the mechanical reproduction of proper technique (Bonah 2012). *Technique des Autopsies* and *Cours Cinématographique* are two examples of such a use of film for teaching purposes, applied to autopsy. Their vocation is didactic: in this sense, the films are about autopsy methods rather than a particular autopsy per se. They belong to the instruction and utility film genre. Although over twenty years elapsed between the two, their approaches and treatments are similar, reflective of a form or sub-genre of teaching film. Both showcase a particular form of transmission of a tried and tested method. Both enlist a physician who is actively involved in teaching his art. Both involve recognised documentary film technicians, and both resonate with the history and newest developments of *film d'enseignement*, film as a teaching aid (Porcile 1965: 235). Here, their comparison evidences a shared effort to adapt a medical textbook to the screen as a complement to written learning material and as a preparation for hands-on learning. Additionally, the contexts of production of both films – respectively the international structuring of the medical film field in the 1930s and the significant post-Second World War growth of utility film – reflect the credit and scientific interest such films garnered, far beyond the confines of the medical departments where they were shot (Bonah and Laukötter 2009).

A textbook turned into a movie

In content and structure, *Technique des Autopsies* consists of the partial adaptation of the eponymous textbook by Gustave Roussy and Pierre Ameuille (1910), respectively, head practitioner and assistant at the pathological anatomy lab of the Paris Faculty of Medicine. The textbook was geared towards students--'non-residents who are eager to learn but deprived of appropriate guidance', states the preface penned by Professor

Pierre Marie (1910: vi) – as well as anatomical pathologist colleagues. It drew not only on the authors' theoretical knowledge but also on their personal experience as practitioners. Its aim was to guide the person in charge of 'examining and opening the corpse for the purpose of identifying as thoroughly as possible the traces left by various medical conditions in the form of anatomical lesions' (Roussy et al. 1910: 2). The textbook contrasts the 'unicist' or French method, wherein the same clinician who treated the patient performs the autopsy, with the 'dualist' or German method, wherein the autopsy is assigned to a specialist in pathology (Roussy et al. 1910: 6–7). Although essentially literary in form, alongside reproductions of pieces like the autopsy protocol (Roussy et al. 1910: 36–38), it contains images, specifically drawings based on 'snapshots taken specially for each stage' (Marie 1910: vi). These images punctuate the demonstration, beginning in the chapter on 'the autopsy of nerve centres' (Roussy et al. 1910: 64), serving as visual aids for understanding the explanations provided in the text. Likewise, *Technique des autopsies* presents itself as an on-screen lecture, as if it were updating the treaty's effort to visualise the content through drawings, by moving from a static to a dynamic approach.

The production of *Technique des autopsies* was closely monitored by medical educationists who believed in the educational value of the film. Gustave Roussy, whose film promoted the autopsy method he had developed with Pierre Ameuille, was in 1930 appointed as the head of the Comité Français d'Etudes Médico-Chirurgicale par le Cinématographe (French Committee for Medical and Surgical Studies through Film), an organisation operating under the supervision of the ministries of education and foreign affairs. Dr. Roger Leroux, head practitioner in anatomical pathology at the Paris Faculty of Medicine, is shown in action in the film. He would later contribute to the promotion of surgical film by giving a lecture on 'medical and surgical teaching through film' at the international teaching and educational film conference (Vignaux 2004). Lastly, Jean Benoit-Lévy, the film's director, worked both to further the techniques of surgical films and to expand their diffusion. Alongside the operator Edmond Floury, he made a series of six surgical films, including *Technique des Autopsies*, produced by the aforementioned Comité Français d'Etudes Médico-Chirurgicale par le Cinématographe, of which he then became the secretary. The goal was ultimately to create an Encyclopaedia of medical and surgical films (Benoit-Lévy 1945).[2] When he committed to this project as director and coordinator, Benoit-Lévy was well aware that surgical film already had its milestones and key figures. In a 1926 conference, he gave at the *Foyer Civil* (a venue for the promotion of secular social work) in Châlons-sur-Marne, he discussed the legacy of Dr. Doyen, the surgeon who pioneered surgical film, who 'in 1898, had himself filmed during one of his operations for his own edification and that of his students' (Vignaux 2004: 2). Edmond Floury also combined directorial and producing duties. This led him to create a company in his name, which began producing a series of surgical films in 1946.

A lecture in image and sound

Shot in 1962, as scientific film flourished against the backdrop of a global surge in documentary production, the *Cours Cinématographique du Dr. Frühling* embraced and updated the approach initiated by Benoit-Lévy and Floury. Like *Technique des Autopsies*, the film is based on a specific written teaching content – albeit not a textbook, but a university lecture. Its title, which translates as 'Dr. Frühling's filmic lecture', defines it as the image-and-sound equivalent to a lecture conceived and taught by the physician himself. As is specified in the end credits, Dr. Frühling was at the time the 'Director of the Institute of anatomical pathology at the Strasbourg Faculty of Medicine'. Ever since he had taken up that position in 1953, he had taught intensively and strived to modernise his laboratory's equipment as much as possible (Philippe 2001). Frühling used the income from the medical tests performed at his institute to fund equipment purchases. For instance, in 1957, he had Strasbourg's second electronic microscope delivered to the institute. He used the same funding to hire Alain Resnais' film crew to produce his film in 1962. The impetus behind the film was to preserve and showcase the art of a recognised educator and pathologist who has developed his own protocol for performing the autopsy. Considering their growing numbers, it also aimed at making the professor available to more students. Frühling envisioned screening it to third-year medical students, and to distribute copies to faculties of medicine all over France (Philippe 2001).

Like *Technique des Autopsies*, Frühling's film brought first-rate filmmakers into the field of utilitarian film. In the 1950s, the genre gained a new momentum, thanks first to public investments in communication on the progress of post-war economic reconstruction, and second to the emergence of multiple production initiatives by firms and researchers

(Bonah 2020). This favourable economic context gave room for young talents to take the opportunity to experiment and make a name for themselves. Most of the names listed in the credits of Frühling's film are associated with that emerging post-war generation whose films were valued to such an extent that the period was called a golden age of documentary film (Odin 1998). Take, for instance Sacha Vierny, one of the three camera operators listed as *cinéastes* (literally filmmakers or directors) in Frühling's film. Sacha Vierny was a director of photography for such luminaries as Alain Resnais (*Nuit et Brouillard*, 1954; *Le Chant du Styrène*, 1957), Agnès Varda (*Opéra Mouffe*, 1957) and Robert Menegoz (*Seul le Brouillard est Gris*, 1965), which drew praise for its 'highly innovative camera work' (Dériaz 2010: 69).

The film and the experience

The two films we discuss in this chapter are teaching films. As their titles indicate, they transmit a method, a savoir-faire. The use of the filmic medium is intended to best prepare and perfect the students' skills of observation in anticipation of hands-on autopsy exercises. As a 1923 article on teaching the experimental method in physiology explains:

> Only experience counts. Let that be clear. But to what extent can students be made to take part? What benefit will they be able to derive from what we will show them? What will they be able to see? What will they be able to understand? This is what we shall have to discuss.
> (Richet 1923: 386, translation authors' own)

This discussion was made all the more urgent by the fivefold increase in the number of medical students between 1870 and 1918, growth that continued exponentially between 1918 and the 1960s. The filmic lecture thus served as an intermediary in this strained ecosystem of medical training. At a first level, motion pictures which demonstrate a method allow for the transmission of detailed knowledge to an entire class, and help to prepare successful individual hands-on autopsy exams (see American Medical Association 1962). They become an additional link in a chain of transmission. At a second level, autopsy motion pictures enhance visual learning experiences. They can provide close-ups when viewing is difficult, use slow motion and symbols and diagrams to orient the spectator. Most of all, as mechanical reproductions, they can be re-played as often as desired or required. At a third level, since the early surgical films of Eugen Doyen, motion pictures by physicians have always served as a form of self-promotion as well. They spotlight the physician and co-author and promote a name.

Autopsy yields visual proof (*prevue*), and it is a difficult experience, an ordeal. The systematic practice of autopsy is a core feature of evidence-based medicine. It embodies medical knowledge, initially in research producing pathological knowledge, later as a fundamental learning experience. At a time when student populations were growing, *Technique des Autopsies* and *Cours Cinématographique* presented themselves as credible, large-scale learning tools. The methods they depicted were sufficiently recognised to warrant an ambitious direction and diffusion, beyond strictly internal use. They were conceived with specialised physicians and directed by skilled documentary filmmakers who used their talents for teaching purposes. In the age of the mechanical reproduction of images and medical films, the lived experience of autopsy became, in certain instances, audio-visually mediated in a didactic media alliance which included books, drawings, photographs and *in presentia* autopsies: filmed autopsies became additional links in an expanding transmission chain. *Technique des Autopsies* as well as *Cours Cinématographique* were not substitutes for *in presentia* autopsies. They are audio–visual moving image guidelines for students to follow before they perform the actual procedure. They provided background information, presented details to entire classes of increasingly numerous students and displayed the proper techniques to adopt for a successful post mortem examination.

A frame within a frame

Medical instructional films emerged at the very beginning of motion picture production, in the late 1890s (Nichtenhauser n.d.). Surgical films figured prominently in turn-of-the century cinema, as part of what Tom Gunning has called 'the cinema of attractions' (1990: 56). Initially a mix of instruction and entertainment, surgical films became full-fledged educational tools by the 1920s.[3] In the age of mechanical reproduction, they offered access to larger audiences, the possibility of including animated diagrams, verbal and visual learning tools in the place of static illustrations. Our autopsy films connect seamlessly to this traditional strand of scientific filmmaking (Lefebvre 2004; Strauven 2006; Curtis 2015).

Autopsies are individual experiences of medical education. The opening of corpses gives insight into bodily transformations scrutinised indirectly, in the form of external traces, during clinical exams. Autopsies are also spectacular procedures, and separating the spectacular from the didactic was an essential goal of the burgeoning field of scientific teaching film in the 1920s.

The autopsy may have a potential for spectacle and a transgressive essence, but its performance has always been framed by a strict methodology. Autopsy textbooks are not only technical guides but they also serve to order and contain the experience. The autopsy films we analyse follow that line, and in filming the experience they add the camera frame to the procedural frame: a frame in a frame. *Technique des Autopsies* and *Cours Cinématographique* respectively originate in a textbook and in a lecture: this difference in source teaching material creates a distinct relationship to space in each of the films. Imitating the principle of theoretical writing, Benoit-Lévy's film is presented as a succession of actions on a corpse, it limits itself to showing a succession of operations on a body, without matching it with a related action or seeking to contextualise it: no settings, no anecdote. As it comes from a lecture, which is by nature embodied in a real-life setting, the *Cours Cinématographique* has a broader scope, and shows events connected to the autopsy, taking place both before and after the procedure. It opens with a handwashing scene and ends with the examination of removed organs, two situations in which the corpse is not present. Conversely, in *Technique des Autopsies*, the camera remains pointed at the dissection table throughout (see Figure 7.2), for technical reasons (the cameras were not very mobile at the end of the 1920s) as well as in order to concentrate the point of view.

Frühling's film ends with a shot of a laboratory and this comment: 'From the shock of pathological morphology and pathological physiology, an understanding of disease will emerge' (*Cours Cinématographique*, 1:29:59). This is a reference to the chain of tasks in which autopsy is a link, whereas in Benoit-Lévy's film, the autopsy is depicted as a standalone process. Still, while they each follow their own logic, both films exemplify film teaching applied to surgery and its efforts to distance learning from the spectacle. Their *mise-en-scène* reflects a constant effort to take the viewer's hand, to never leave them behind as the procedure unfolds, by addressing them and by filming the corpse in a sober and straightforward manner. These framing and narration choices are where the line is drawn with entertainment films, in which surprise and suspense are part of plot construction. In addition to their different approaches to space, what sets both films apart lie mostly in their respective uses of the technical resources offered by the production and of the innovations of their time.

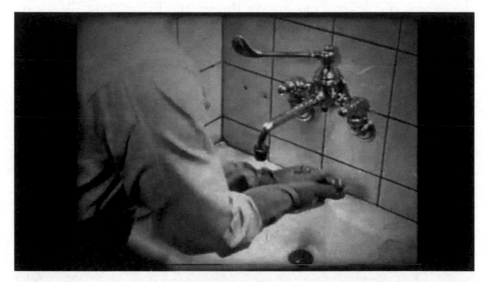

Figure 7.2: Practicing pathologist handwashing scene, Sacha Vierny et al. (1962). France © DHVS. 00:01.

Devices to draw the viewer's attention and to derealise the situation

In *Technique des Autopsies*, Benoit-Lévy made use of the tried and tested methods of film didacticism applied to surgery. The corpse is a field of intervention on which tool-equipped hands act; this field of intervention defines the scope of the shot, and the gestures made during the intervention are the subject of each shot. As recommended in the 1920s by German physician Alexander von Rotha, Benoit-Lévy did not seek to personalise the surgeon by including shots of his face; he is embodied only by his hands moving into the frame above the corpse (Nichtenhauser n.d.). Like Professor Charles Claoué, who began filming his own plastic surgery operations in 1924, Benoit-Lévy steered clear of long shots, which were perceived as too anecdotal and too far removed from the subject to be adequately informational (Thévenard and Tassel 1948). *Technique des Autopsies* is characterised by an effort to emphasise educational value over all other filmic considerations throughout. It uses two devices to neutralise the reality effect inherent in shooting a surgery in real time. First, each time the surgeon picks up a new tool, he presents it to the camera. Such shots punctuate the film (see Figure 7.3), echoing the figures in chapter 2 of Gustave Roussy and Pierre Ameuille's textbook, which are entirely dedicated to the description of the necessary tools (Roussy and Ameuille 1910).

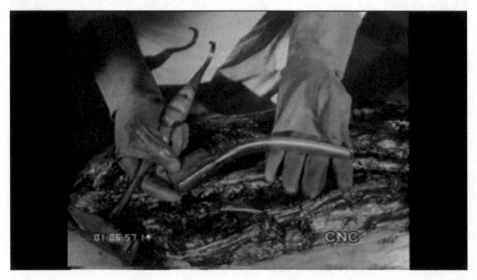

Figure 7.3: Pathologist picking up a tool, Jean Benoit-Lévy (1928). France © Jean Benoit-Lévy family, 06:58.

Second, Benoit-Lévy shoots cardboard cards that are inserted into the frame to call attention to an important anatomical detail. When, for instance, the optic nerve or brain swelling need to be shown, an assistant's hand enters the frame to place a label indicating the anatomical feature in question. This curious device, which replaces the insertion of an animated diagram, adds a strictly theoretical element to the shot. This intrusion forces the viewer to derealise the situation, to no longer take it as a moment seized in its integrity, by shifting his or her attention to the new object. The method being demonstrated prevails over the situation created by the demonstration.

For the most part, *Cours Cinématographique* employs the same narrative outline and visualisation methods as *Technique des Autopsies*. For

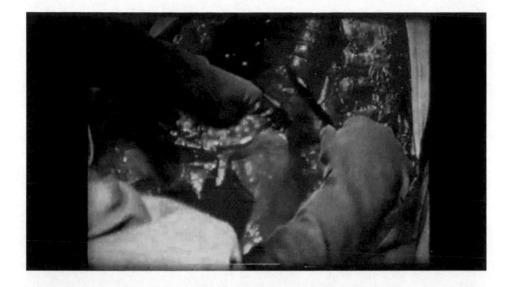

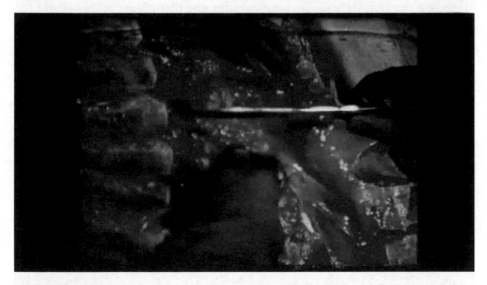

Figure 7.4: Technical autopsy scenes with off-voice comment, Sacha Vierny et al. (1962). France © DHVS, 06:32 and 33:32.

similar purposes, the director takes advantage of the new filmic techniques that have been introduced in the meantime. Since the film is no longer silent, a voiceover replaces intertitles to provide explanations. Although the person speaking is not visible on screen (see Figure 7.4), he directly addresses, calls out to the viewer: 'make sure the incision is deep enough to reach the bones!' (Vierny et al. 1962: 44:36). As a device, these addresses to the viewer, resembling a teacher's address to a class or student, can be seen as equivalent to the cards inserted by Benoit-Lévy. A monotonous, almost liturgical tone is adopted to recite what pathologists consider to be the 'catechism' of the autopsy. This verbal addition to the camera's framing keeps the viewer's attention focused.

Likewise, the introduction of colour and improved lighting lend the images greater legibility. The dark blue gloves covering the hands that cut the corpse contrast sharply with the bright red of the organs (also mirrored on the wide surface of the scalpel). It is easier for the viewer to make out the different parts of the body and events such as blood flow during the incision here than in Benoit-Lévy's grainy black-and-white images.

Filming an open corpse

Based on the template of the surgical film, the directing choices made for both two films were intended to help the viewer follow the succession of steps in the autopsy without disruption. Unlike in a fiction film, the goal is to avoid surprise and dramatisation. This applies both to narrativisation and to how the corpse is filmed: the idea is to tone down dramatic elements. In *Technique des Autopsies*, explanatory intertitles precede the shots, so that the viewers are filled in by the time the shot actually comes, and hence remain one step ahead of the filmic narrative (see Figure 7.5).

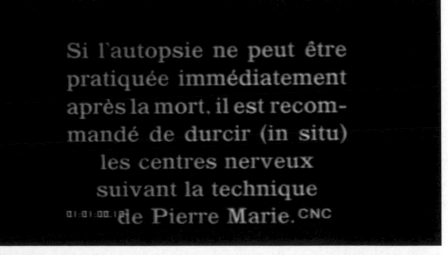

Figure 7.5: Explanatory intertitles preceding autopsy shots, Jean Benoit-Lévy (1928). France © Jean Benoit-Lévy family, 01:36.

As Bernadette Nguyen and Emmanuel Nuss (2020) point out on the film's page in the Medfilm database, only two shot scales are used for the film's two main sections: medium shots to show the beginning of the autopsy, focusing on the spinal cord, and close-ups to show subsequent acts performed on the brain and cerebellum. Directorial choices are sometimes not as pertinent as they should be, however. In the scene that displays the skin incision along the spinal line, the camera operator Edmond Floury opted for repeated lateral tracking shots that follows the cut from the neck down to the buttocks, then back up again to show the disinsertion of muscles and grooves, and so on. To avoid sweeping back and forth over the field of intervention, which destabilises the gaze, he would have had to stick to a long, high-angle shot capturing the entire subject. This is what is done in the film by Vierny, Penzer and Brun; this choice allows them to introduce understated pan shots to follow the surgeon's gestures. *Cours Cinématographique* films the corpse along a vertical axis, whereas Benoit-Lévy favoured a longitudinal view (see Figure 7.6).

While this choice was probably designed to limit variations in shot scales, the change of angle curiously mirrors the one that occurred between Rembrandt's depictions of two anatomy lessons, in a shared 'migration of images' from painting to film (Aumont 2005: 56). Whereas *The Anatomy Lesson of Dr. Tulp* (1632) places the corpse in a similarly longitudinal position, *The Anatomy Lesson of Dr. Joan Deijman* (1656) has it 'stretched out before the surgeon in much the same abrupt foreshortening as Mantegna's *Dead Christ*', in the words of Otto Benesch, who argues that this is a 'clearly developed' example of 'the compositional principles of Rembrandt's late style' (Benesch 1990: 105). Likewise, from one autopsy film to the other, the change of angle results in a more remarkably stripped down filmmaking style.

In both films, the framing of the autopsied corpse consists in 'making it enter a frame, and therefore subjugating it, disciplining it, regulating it' (Commoli and Sorel 2015: 106). Adding their visual frame to the procedural frame, our autopsy films double and reinforce the regulation of spectator gaze. In doing so, they embrace the essence of the autopsy experience as a learning exercise and they fully testify to the specificities of instructional motion pictures as a genre, marked by their dedramatising soberness, and an effort to convey information and a method, as opposed to emotions.

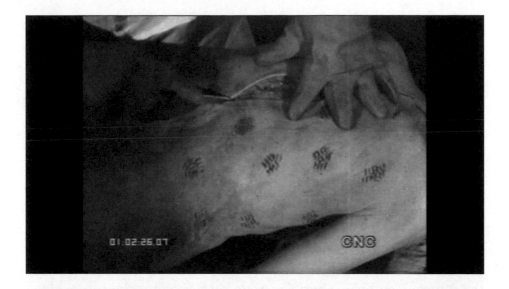

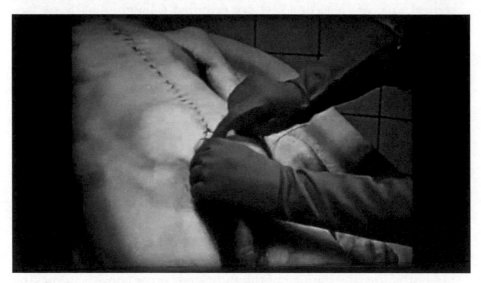

Figure 7.6: (a) Initial skin incision technique, Jean Benoit-Lévy (1928). France © Jean Benoit-Lévy family, 02:27. (b) Initial skin incision technique, Sacha Vierny et al. (1962). France © DHVS, 89:35.

Framing emotions

Autopsy not only provides visual proof embodying medical knowledge but also at the same time, as Harley Warner has demonstrated, for western medical students, it has been for two centuries an ordeal, in the sense that it is a difficult experience and a rite of passage to become a physician

(Warner 2009). The autopsy is a face-to-face existential and personal experience with an emotional impact. When they were introduced in the 1920s, autopsy films carried an inherent contradiction in the sense that they staged and mediated what had been in essence since the beginning conceived as a live, direct sensory experience accompanied by the foul odour of the formalin used to preserve the bodies and the dissection tools that spoke to the violence of the act: a sensory encounter with death. As such, a first hypothesis is that the motion picture introduced distance, annihilated odour, sanitised the exercise. As described above, this sober framing not only provided guidance and dedramatised the exercise but also contained its emotional impact.

Since the mid-nineteenth century and Claude Bernard's canonisation of the experimental method in his *Introduction to Experimental Medicine* for physicians, scientists have suggested that 'fruitful and enlightening generalisations on vital phenomena will never be achieved for as long as we have not ourselves experienced and moved about the foul and pulsating terrain of life, in the hospital, the amphitheatre or the laboratory' (Bernard 1865: 28). Autopsy exercises are indeed emotional, foul and thrilling experiences, despite the containment strategies and the framing to which they are subjected. The two films can be seen as the filmic transposition of the precautions taken to anticipate emotional reactions to facing this reality. In addition to an effort to show and explain, there is an emotional (and ethical) factor involved in filming a corpse that the autopsy will require opening and prying into under the spectator's gaze. *Technique des Autopsies*, for instance, may be aimed at an audience of future doctors and specialists, but it still has to show as much respect to the autopsied subject and to the viewers' emotions as possible by adopting a restrained approach. A practitioner does not have the same relationship to reality when they are actually doing the job as when they watching the job being done in a film where the job is framed and edited, shown in a certain light and in an expanded scope. In doing so, the two autopsy films transpose and transform the autopsy ordeal and its emotional management (Sadoul 1960). This is where the power of film comes in: it lends an aura to the objects it depicts. According to the painter Francis Bacon, the filmic depiction of an object transforms the feeling it inspires:

> One's sense of appearance is assaulted all the time by photography and by the film. So that, when one looks at something, one's not only look-

ing at it directly but one's also looking at it through the assault that has already been made on one by photography and film [...] it's the slight remove from fact, which returns me onto the fact more violently. (Sylvester 1987: 30)

For Bacon, in the film the dematerialisation of a situation, which is screened and not experienced in the flesh, adds violence and emotion rather than subtracting it. The camera's gaze draws viewers in more than it creates a sense of detachment. It's framing further subjugates the corpse subjected to autopsy. Bacon's reflections, not incidentally, were nourished by his fascination for scientific photographs, such as Eadweard Muybridge's chronophotographic series and the photographs depicting positions for radiographers in K. C. Clark's 1939 book *Positioning Radiography*.

Bacon describes the effect of the image as a filter on the subject that is being tackled, which as it is 'assaulted' in turn assaults whoever is looking at it. The risk of filming the process of cutting the corpse into pieces is that it could intensify the assault to the extent of making the autopsy lesson unwatchable. In a sense, through the aura of the image, the autopsied dead body might lose its status as an object of knowledge and, covering the dimension of mystical horror that has been lent to him, revert to 'something that has no name in any language', in the words of Tertullian as quoted by Jacques-Bénigne Bossuet in his *Sermon on Death* (Bossuet 1926). The directorial choices made in *Technique des Autopsies* precisely appear to reflect a concern with appealing to the spectator's emotion as little as possible. Whereas the drawings in Roussy and Ameuille's textbook show the face of the corpse on numerous occasions, Benoit-Lévy stops at the neck or looks at the back of the head during the part on the brain and cerebellum. The longer and more detailed *Cours Cinématographique* does include a passage where the face is visible, as an incision is made from the chin to the lower lip. However, the very tight close-up used for that scene de-personalises the corpse. Additionally, Frühling's film includes a long sequence on the extraction and examination of pelvic organs that presents the respective techniques appropriate for male and female bodies, requiring the presence of an additional female corpse in the scene (Vierny et al. 1962: 54:35–1:08:03). By adding this second corpse, the film again de-personalises the viewer's relationship to the autopsied subject. Here, anonymising the corpse becomes the ultimate way of framing the student spectator's emotions.

Conclusion

A motion picture is a series of individual frames being produced and reproduced. The film itself can be copied and reproduced, and projection reproduces viewing experiences. Autopsy films are thus a mechanical multiplier of the essence of autopsy, which is to see for yourself. Autopsy films are in this sense a pedagogical adaptation to the considerable increase in the number of students and a complementary teaching aid. Indeed, mechanical visual reproduction was partly used to make up for teaching staff shortages.

This involves a particular use of the filmic image, which consists in an attempt to reduce it to a generic representation of the reality it depicts, much like a textbook does in textual form. Thus, when an intertitle in *Technique des Autopsies* or the voiceover in *Cours Cinématographique* mentions a limb or organ subsequently shown on the corresponding image, the spectator is expected to consider what is shown in the shot as their strict translations. Yet, and this is where the limitation of using film as an instrument of basic knowledge arguably comes in, filmic expression based on live-action shots do not operate following the same principle of semantic symbolisation as textual expression.

Likewise, in an autopsy film, the image of the corpse refers to no other corpse, which crucially restrains its theoretical reach and introduces a contradiction with its intention to stick to fundamental knowledge. The film's contents constantly tend to seep out of the frame where the director intended to box them, precisely because they are individuated, especially when it comes to a corpse.

With *Cours Cinématographique*, and its shots depicting what happens before and after the autopsy, we are closer to the experience. Still, the direction also seeks to abstract the sensations inevitably associated with it. As Claude Bernard pointed out, though, the intimate experience of these sensations should be part of the lesson. As they neglect this initiatory dimension of autopsy teaching, both *Cours Cinématographique* and *Technique des Autopsies* remain incomplete learning tools. These two teaching films can be usefully compared to the journalistic treatment in public French television channel Antenne 2's 1986 'Autopsie' report, broadcast in the programme *Moi Je*, dedicated to investigation in secret areas of society, particularly in various professional fields. Seen through the eyes of the reporter, Eliette Leriche, the programme tackles the physical and psychological experience of autopsy head-on. The director introduces subjective shots (allowing us to look as if we were the surgeon) and counter shots (showing the faces of the surgical team members), which would have been unthinkable for Benoit-Lévy and the filmmakers enlisted by Frühling. To shed light on the emotional charge of the images, excerpts from an interview with the autopsy practitioner have been inserted: 'the corpses we autopsy are always cold' he says. 'If a sufficient period of time has elapsed since the death, they are inert, unresponsive; it is entirely different, how you approach them, the physical contact is very different from what it is with a living person, even if they are asleep' ('Autopsie' 1986: 05:54). Later, the same doctor discusses his post-autopsy routine, but not in connection to the laboratory examination of removed organs, focusing instead on the moment when he comes back home to his wife and children: 'I can perfectly kiss my wife or children as usual after a day performing autopsy; I just make sure I don't smell and I've washed my hands' ('Autopsie' 1986: 09:10). The physician repeatedly mentions that smell, which might result in social awkwardness if it lingers on the hands. This precision on the olfactory dimension of the autopsy reminds us that the two films we studied, *Cours Cinématographique* and *Technique des Autopsies* are devoid of any attempt to restore such sensory experience: the students who see them are not facing the ordinary, peculiar smell of formaldehyde. Both in form and content, the 1986 report provides additional information on the reality of autopsy as an experience that is repeatedly lived over the course of a pathologist's lifetime. The report has a complementary teaching value in that it embraces the sensory and affect-laden dimension of the autopsy, and acknowledges the fact of individual learning by experience.

The cinematographic reproduction of an autopsy is *transitional* in the sense that this analogue copy makes an initial move towards digital dematerialised teaching methods while producing its own material culture, namely the film strip in its can. By the early 2000s, the number of routinely performed autopsies attended by medical students every year in large teaching hospitals, previously in the thousands, had dwindled to almost zero. Autopsy rooms and theatres are closed. What remains are visual motion picture traces, reused in digital teaching and learning. Interestingly, this dematerialisation and distanced learning does not necessarily imply that the images circulated are any less violent or emotionally charged – quite the opposite, in fact. Much could be learned from the film directors of autopsy films, who struggled with framing that subject for half a century between the 1920s and 1960s.

Acknowledgments

This research received funding from the European Research Council's 'The Healthy Self as Body Capital' (BodyCapital) Project under the European Union's Horizon 2020 research and innovation programme (Grant agreement no. 694817).

Endnotes

1. Further mentions of filmed autopsy lessons are mentioned in the American Medical Association (1962) film *The Motion Picture in Medical Education*.Intended to stimulate greater use of film in teaching, includes a cranial autopsy scene among its filmic examples.
2. The other films were *L'Obstétricie Opératoire* (1927), *L'Appendicectomie* (1932), *La Bronchoscopie* (1932), *La Biopsie* (1933) and *Opération du Cancer du Sein* (1933).
3. The well-documented case of Eugène Doyen's surgical films (produced from 1898 onwards) illustrates the point. To counteract accusations of self-publicity, the surgeon filed a legal suit against his camera operator, Parnaland, for screening these motion pictures at fairs.

References

American Medical Association (1962), *The Motion Picture in Medical Education*, USA: Sturgis-Grant Productions Inc. [https://medfilm.unistra.fr/wiki/The_motion_picture_in_medical_education. Accessed 19 November 2021.].

Aumont, Jacques (2005), 'Migrations' ou le spectre de la peinture', *Matière d'images*, Paris: Images Modernes, pp. 41–83

'Autopsie' (1986), Eliette Leriche (dir.), *Moi je* (5 February, France: Antenne 2) [https://medfilm.unistra.fr/wiki/Autopsie. Accessed 19 November 2021.].

Bazin, André (2018), *André Bazin: Écrits Complets*, 2 vol., Paris: Macula.

Benesch, Otto (1990), *Rembrandt*, New York: Rizzoli.

Benoit-Lévy, Jean (1928), *Techniques des Autopsies*, France: Edition Française Cinématographique for Faculté de médecine de Paris [https://medfilm.unistra.fr/wiki/Technique_des_autopsies. Accessed 19 November 2021.].

Benoit-Lévy, Jean (1945), *Les Grandes Missions du Cinéma*, Montréal: Parizeau.

Bernard, Claude (1865), *Introduction à la Médecine Expérimentale*, Paris: Baillière.

Bonah, Christian (2008), 'Autopsy ordeals', in P. Filliquet and C. Bonah (eds), *Autopsies*, Paris: Monografik-editions, pp. 125–32.

Bonah, Christian (2012), 'Une introduction à l'étude de la médecine expérimentale à l'ère de la reproduction mécanique: Un legs de Claude Bernard et / ou d'Etienne Jules Marey?', in B. Jean-Gaël Barbara and P. Corvol (eds), *Les élèves de Claude Bernard: Les nouvelles disciplines physiologiques en France au tournant du XXe siècle*, Paris: Hermann, pp. 151–72.

Bonah, Christian (2020), '"Réservé strictement au corps medical": Les sociétés de production audiovisuelles d'Eric Duvivier, l'industrie pharmaceutique et leurs stratégies de co-production de films médicaux industriels, 1950–1980', *Cahiers d'histoire du CNAM: Le cinématographe pour l'industrie et dans les entreprises (1890–1970): histoire, acteurs, usages et configurations*, 12:12, pp. 135–59.

Bonah, Christian and Laukötter, Anja (2009), 'Moving pictures and medicine in the first half of the 20th century: Some notes on international historical developments and the potential of medical film research', *Gesnerus*, 66:1, pp. 121–45.

Bossuet, Jacques-Bénigne (1926), *Sermon on Death* (trans. C. O. Blum, from Œuvres oratoires), IV, Paris: Desclée.

Commoli, Jean-Louis and Sorel, Vincent (2015), *Cinéma, mode d'emploi: De l'argentique au numérique*, Paris: Verdier.

Curtis, Scott (2015), *The Shape of Spectatorship: Art, Science and Early Cinema in Germany*, New York: Columbia University Press.

Dériaz, Philipe (2010), 'Grandeur et servitudes du cinéma industriel', in N. Schmidt and P. Dériaz (eds), *Du film Scientifique et Technique*, Condé-sur-Noirau: Corlet.

Dudley, Andrew (1978), *André Bazin*, New York: Oxford University Press.

Elsaesser, Thomas (2009), 'Archives and archaeologies: The place of non-fiction film in contemporary media', in V. Hediger and P. Vonderau (eds), *Films that Work. Industrial Film and the Productivity of Media*, Amsterdam: Amsterdam University Press, pp. 19–34.

Filliquet, Pierre and Bonah, Christian (2008), *Autopsies*, Paris: Monografik-editions.

Fleck, Ludwik (1986), 'To look, to see, to know', in R. S. Cohen and T. Schnelle (eds), *Cognition and Fact: Materials on Ludwik Fleck*, Dordrecht: Reidel, pp. 129–51.

Foucault, Michel (1975), *The Birth of the Clinic: An Archeology of Medical Perception*, New York: Vintage Books.

Gunning, Tom (1990), 'The cinema of attractions: Early film, its spectator and the avant-garde', in T. Elsaesser and A. Barker (eds), *Early Cinema. Space, Frame, Narrative*, London: BFI Publications, pp. 56–63.

Lefebvre, Thierry (2004), *La Chair et le Celluloïd: Le Cinéma Chirurgical du Docteur Doyen*, Brionne: Jean Doyen Editeur.

Marie, Pierre (1910), 'Préface', in G. Roussy and P. Ameuille (eds), *Technique des autopsies et des recherches anatomo-pathologiques à l'amphithéâtre*, Paris: Doin, p. vi.

Nguyen, Bernadette and Nuss, Emmanuel (2020), 'Techniques of autopsy', *MedFilm*, April, https://medfilm. unistra.fr/wiki/Technique_des_autopsies#tab=Contexte_2. Accessed 19 November 2021.

Nichtenhauser, Adolf (n.d.), *A History of Motion Pictures in Medicine* (unpublished book MS, *c.*1950), Adolf Nichtenhauser History of Motion Pictures in Medicine Collection, MS C 380, Maryland: Archives and Modern Manuscripts Program, History of Medicine Division, National Library of Medicine, Bethesda.

Odin, Roger (ed.) (1998), *L'âge d'or du documentaire – Europe: Années Cinquante*, Paris: L'Harmattan.

Olivier-Utard, Françoise (2009), 'Frühling, Louis Armand. Pseudonyme dans la Résistance: "Commandant Gérard"', in J. Maitron (ed.), *Le Dictionnaire Biographique du Mouvement Ouvrier et Social*, 25 February, https://maitron.fr/spip.php?article24719. Accessed 20 March 2020.

Orgeron, Devin, Orgeron, Marsha and Streible, Dan (eds) (2012), *Learning with the Lights Off: Educational Film in the United States*, New York: Oxford University Press.

Philippe, Muriel (2001), *Louis Frühling (1916–1962) et la Méthode Anatomo-Clinique*, Thèse de Médecine, Strasbourg: Université Strasbourg.

Porcile, François (1965), *Défense du Court Métrage Français*, Paris: Cerf.

Richet, Charles (1923), 'L'enseignement de la physiologie', *Revue des Deux Mondes*, 18:2, , pp. 365–94.

Roussy, Gustave and Ameuille, Pierre (1910), *Technique des Autopsies et des Recherches Anatomo-Pathologiques à l'Amphithéâtre*, Paris: Doin.

Sadoul, Georges (1960), *Conquête du Cinéma*, Paris: Gedalge.

Strauven, Wanda (ed.) (2006), *The Cinema of Attractions Reloaded*, Amsterdam: Amsterdam University Press.

Sylvester, David (1987), *The Brutality of Fact: Interviews with Francis Bacon*, London: Thames and Hudson Ltd.

Thévenard, Pierre and Tassel, Guy (1948), *Le cinéma scientifique français*, Paris: La Jeune Parque.

Valérie Vignaux (2004), 'Contribution à une histoire de l'emploi du cinéma dans l'enseignement de la chirurgie', *1895, revue d'histoire du cinéma*, 44, pp. 73–86.

Vierny, Sacha, Jean Pezner and Philippe Brun (1962), *Techniques Anatomopathologiques de l'Autopsie: Cours Cinématographique du Dr. Frühling*, France: Institut d'Anatomie pathologique de Strasbourg.

Warner, John Harley (2009), 'Witnessing dissection: Photography, medicine and american culture', in J. H. Warner and J. M. Edmonson (eds), *Dissection: Photographs of a Rite of Passage in American Medicine 1880–1930*, New York: Blast Books, pp. 7–29.

FILM

'NOW WE ARE GOING TO LOOK AT A PIECE OF FILM': PROJECTING MEDICINE IN TWENTIETH-CENTURY MEDICAL EDUCATION

Angela Saward

Lurking in medical museum archives and libraries, unseen for near-ly half a century, are a multitude of audio-visual treasures. They are not feature films distributed to cinemas and watched eagerly by a global audience of millions. The films focused on in this chapter are those created and seen by a limited number of professional medical audiences. This chapter argues that medical films made in the twen-tieth century are a 'hidden cinema'; those films made for and shared only amongst the medical professions in their often-cloistered worlds, but which are now accessible to wider audiences, thanks to digitisation. As a curator of historical medical film, video and audio material, I find these films fascinating in their use of the idiom of film which makes medical film education distinct from other pedagogical media. This gen-re of filmmaking was bound by intra-professional conduct, pre-dating patient-centred medicine, and the written record is sparse on their au-diences' reception. However, these historical films can tell us something about the way medical knowledge was perceived, how it was learned and reproduced in the past. The continued existence of these films is due to individuals and institutions who have carefully sequestered this material for over a century in the hope that historians of the future would be in-terested in them (see Figure 8.1). As film projectors have gathered dust in storerooms, films not viewed for decades can now be rediscovered, with many titles, especially those with perceived historical value, gaining diverse and exponentially larger audiences, something inconceivable to the original producers.

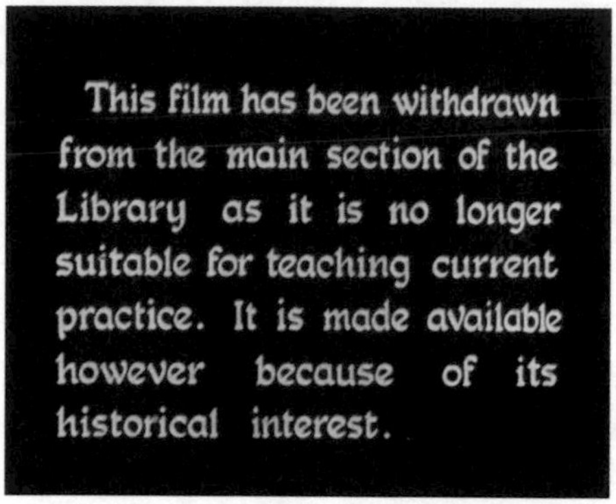

This film has been withdrawn from the main section of the Library as it is no longer suitable for teaching current practice. It is made available however because of its historical interest.

Figure 8.1: Film still, opening intertitle, *Coal Gas Poisoning and Resuscitation*, Sir Joseph Barcroft (writer), 1935. UK. Public Domain.

This chapter explores some of the contradictory views which prevailed in the medical profession about the role of film in teaching and learning and its rocky path to respectability, focusing on the mid-twentieth century film. Through a curatorial journey, looking at the provenance of two films held by Wellcome Collection in London, UK – a museum and library dedicated to challenging how we all think and feel about health – some of the issues around medical filmmaking, its educational value and the transnational historiography of film collecting are explored, while also considering its transnational nature.

Understanding aggression

The training and recruitment film, *Understanding Aggression* (Thomson 1960), is the first of two films I focus on in this chapter. *Understanding Aggression* was made for trainee nurses and produced by the Central Office of Information for the Ministry of Health, a government department in the United Kingdom. It illustrates one example of how the presentation of a film was managed in a medical educational setting. Embedded into its narrative, medical students settle into their seats, the lights are dimmed, and the lecture begins – an occurrence repeated many times in medical schools over the twentieth century, until the demise of the film projector in the 1980s. This film also shows how medical films evolved to resemble mainstream cinema. In previous years, before film had become a respectable and integral part of the teaching and learning experience, the act of watching film within medical educational settings had been thoroughly scrutinised by the profession. This film arguably represents a watershed moment in the maturation of the medium.

Understanding Aggression (see Figure 8.2) begins with Nurse Joan, who is running late for a lecture on aggression, the subject of the film. She is late due to an 'upset' on the ward, in what we discover is a mental hospital of the time. This hospital is one which has enlightened practices and asks the staff to engage in the idea of the hospital as a 'social laboratory' where the emotions of its staff are just as much under review as those of the troubled and sometimes difficult patients. In the opening sequence, in order to introduce the topic of aggression, the viewer is invited to follow Nurse Joan into a classroom where the lecture has already begun. This sudden immersion into the drama assumes a sophisticated level of cinematic viewership by the audience, one that is already habituated to learning using film and familiar with this setting. Later, we understand alongside Joan that her actions have inadvertently caused a mental crisis in a patient, Susan Morris. We are then invited to imagine Susan's complex thought processes and understand the roots of her anxiety.

In parallel, a male patient, Andrew Lewis, who has aggressive behavioural traits and demonstrates a cynical and manipulative side, proves troublesome for a male nurse, Nurse Ferguson. A romantic *frisson* between colleagues (Nurses Ferguson and Joan) creates jealousy between the staff and the patient (Andrew). Another feature of the film is its depiction of the emerging diaspora of people within the National Health Service from Britain's former colonies providing a rich contextual backdrop to the film and situating it in the early 1960s when immigration to supplement labour shortages was supported by the governments of the time. The aim of the film, understanding aggression, is achieved by a series of events, culminating in a fractious cricket match between the staff and the patients: patient Andrew, when batting, is caught out by a fielder, when he becomes angry and argumentative he is then ordered back to the ward. Afterwards, the staff have cause to reflect on their own behaviour and the existential nature of mental illness – thereby achieving the aim of the film by understanding aggression in practice.

Understanding Aggression draws upon reality, with footage of children displaying normal aggressive behaviour and hurting each other in normal play settings screened to the students within the film. The footage is

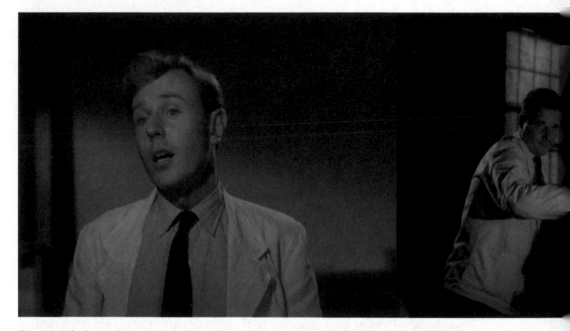

Figure 8.2: Left to right, composite of three film stills; lecturer, projectionist, film-within-the film of children playing, *Understanding Aggression*, Margaret Thomson (writer and director), 1960. UK. Crown copyright. Courtesy of the BFI National Archive.

framed in the film by the teacher–trainer and this layering of the 'film-within-the-film', a meta-cinematic device, is a way of introducing the purpose of the film:

> Part of the business in growing up is to learn how to direct it in useful channels. Now we are going to look at a piece of film, which shows some scenes of young children before they have learnt to control their aggressive urges. What children want at this age they want with the whole of them. They haven't learnt yet that other people have needs and wishes just as urgent as theirs. And because we humans are social animals, we want to be liked by other people and to like them in return. We want to work and play together. (*Understanding Aggression* 1960: commentary at 00:00:56)

Understanding Aggression has a clarity of purpose; a sound understanding of the audience (hence the inclusion of seemingly extraneous content, such as the romantic backstory); a well-scripted narrative; and then a well-chosen milieu in which to place these elements. This contributes to one of the ways in which films created within the medical sphere still

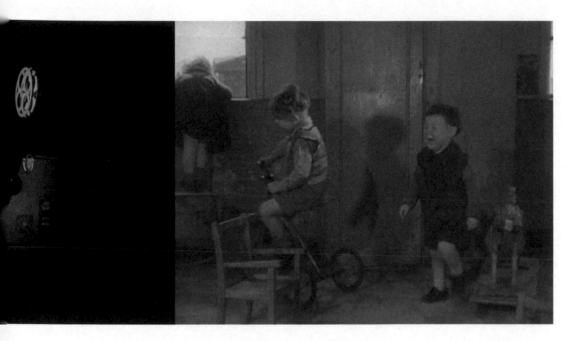

have enduring appeal: the learner–trainer in the film explains how the enacted scenarios contribute to empathetic understanding by the 'gift' of imagination. Films with a psychiatric focus were the hallmark of the writer–director, Margaret Thomson, whose directorial style was to mix drama and realism: one factor in illustrating how film can reflect psychological 'realism' and therefore provide 'humane staff education' (Russell 2018), perhaps film's richest contribution to medical education.

The medical motion picture

In terms of a starting point for understanding the role of medical film in education, an earlier film, *The Medical Motion Picture* (Creer 1947), also made for medical professionals, is an example of a film about the history of early medical filmmaking; these insights were used to inform and then shape the creation of new films. Made on the occasion of the 100th anniversary of the American Medical Association (AMA), its purpose was celebratory, presenting important examples of medical filmmaking. The first twenty minutes of the film comprise of a compilation of

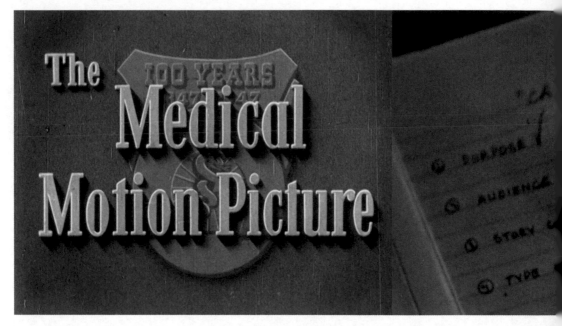

Figure 8.3: Film stills, left to right, composite of the opening intertitle, elements of a successful film, projecting the finished film, *The Medical Motion Picture*, Ralph P. Creer (technical adviser), 1947. USA. Public Domain.

the most scientifically interesting and medically significant films made in the United States to date, with commentary about why filmmaking techniques improved alongside improvements in film stocks and technological innovations in the laboratory and clinic. Thereafter, the film looks at how to make a new medical film, entitled *Management of a case of Thyroid Cancer*, from concept to delivery, with a focus on the intended audience and the final purpose of the film. Behind the scenes, the production process is demystified, showing the creation of animations, the patient being filmed, and then the final film assembled for screening. This sequence codified how to create a 'good' medical motion picture through the enacting of this 'film-within-a-film', thereby underlining the growing professionalisation in the sector. The enactment is a mode of meta-cinema that testifies to what degree the genre was evolving.

Globally, films have been exchanged, hired, and sold over time, including those catering specifically for the medical professions and as a result of these transnational exchanges, a sixteen millimetre copy of *The Medical Motion Picture* was donated by the AMA to its British professional equivalent, the British Medical Association (BMA) (Anon. 1957a: 195). The film's technical adviser, Ralph P. Creer, may have been

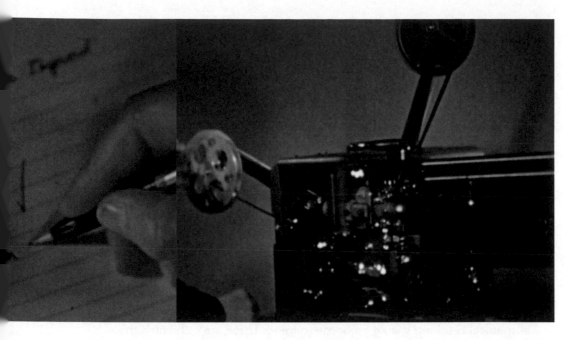

party to this donation as he travelled to the United Kingdom to participate in the World Congress on Medical Education (Anon. 1953: 560).
Creer's life and career (1909–2000) spanned the evolution of medical
illustration from pencil and paper to photography and then onto film.
He was a technician with a passion for film and a desire to promote
excellence in the field. In his role as Senior Clinical Photographer in
the Photographic Department of Yale Medical School, he wrote to the
AMA lobbying for the production of better-quality medical photography and a framework for excellence (Creer 1934: 1325–26). Motivated
by the coexistence of photography and film in clinical work, Creer's expertise led him to become Secretary of the AMA Committee on Medical Motion Pictures in 1950.

On both sides of the Atlantic, film reviews were systematically included in the journals of both the AMA and BMA, reflecting the growing professional interest in medical films. In America, the AMA was
more advanced in its promotion of film as a pedagogical medium, perhaps spurred by Creer's influence. This is evident in the film title which
followed *The Medical Motion Picture*, *The Motion Picture in Medical Education* (1962), made to promote the AMA's expanding library with a

department dedicated to the operation of the acquisition and loan of medical films. This later film is 25 minutes in duration and comprises a survey of films made since 1947 which the AMA deemed excellent, after which it briefly looks at their film library. A nod to Creer's legacy is made in the final sequence, showing a library record card for a film about the medical value of a film on obstetrics, annotated in Creer's handwriting; that it was 'a good case presentation' (*The Motion Picture in Medical Education* 1962: onscreen at 00:24:41).

In 1938, in Britain, mirroring Creer's initiative in the United States, the BMA had also received a recommendation by its Council to establish a film library, but thwarted by the war, it only started collecting films in 1946. A Film Committee to explore 'The Scope and Use of Medical Film in Education' was set up in 1947 and reported on the pros and cons of film in education:

> In considering the scope of films in medical education the broad aims of medical teaching should be borne in mind. These are to furnish the requisite knowledge, develop judgment and skill, cultivate the right attitude towards patients and give opportunities for experience, and to encourage students to think for themselves.

However, somewhat contradictorily,

> Only knowledge and understanding can be imparted by means of the film in education. To a lesser degree the student's attitude to medicine and its various branches can be moulded by the film, but his experience, skill, and judgment cannot be materially influenced by means of the motion picture. (Anon. 1947a: 141)

The view expressed by the BMA (in the first comment) was directed at the objective quality of individual films, thereby narrowing the film's potential role aesthetically and emotionally in teaching. In 1949, the organisation inaugurated a film competition to attract medical films of merit for its library, graded by a panel of experts. Submissions were solicited from members and non-members alike, with calls placed in the organisation's journal (and no doubt elsewhere). Medals were awarded to films from different categories – originally just two, commercial and non-commercial film (Anon. 1957a: 195), rising to four by 1971 – reflecting the development of the genre over time. Winners went on to form the basis of a growing film library available to its members. 'Amateur' films (those not made by professional film units in hospitals or sponsored by pharmaceutical companies) had always been welcome and received awards. A point made in 1947, something of an afterthought in the report but demonstrating some foresight, was that there may be historical interest in such a collection of films in the future: indeed when the BMA donated its film library to Wellcome Collection, London, in 2006, *The Medical Motion Picture*, amongst a thousand other titles, formed part of the collection of films transferred featuring all aspects of medicine. Subsequently, these films have become accessible worldwide and once digitised can be easily consulted by researchers. Through this acquisition, the films moved from the realm of the medical profession into that of the broader research community; Creer had foreseen this possibility many decades before – that there would be historical value in these films (see Figure 8.4).

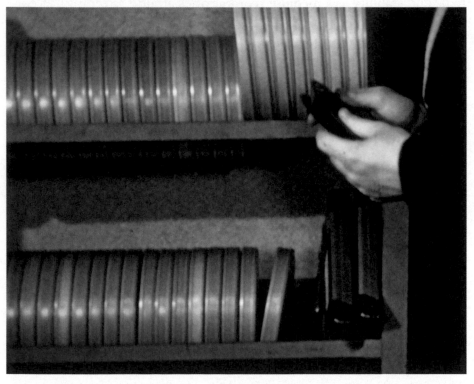

Figure 8.4: Film still, 'Many excellent reels are added to the growing film libraries' [commentary], *The Medical Motion Picture*, Ralph P. Creer (technical adviser), 1947. USA. Public Domain.

Film's 'peculiarity'

The 'peculiar advantages' of the medical film genre within medical education had already been noted in an anonymous review of Creer's film (Anon. 1947b: 903). In the opening commentary on the film's soundtrack, it is stated that the film aims to be 'a valuable adjunct to teaching' (*The Medical Motion Picture* 1947: commentary at 00:00:24). The reviewer of the film scoffed at this laudable aim; 'The film demonstrates applications for medical films: it neither asserts nor denies that a film can shake a thermometer, but it does prove that a film could show how a thermometer is shaken' (Anon. 1947b: 903). This written comment is indicative of the crossroads that medical films had reached in terms of educational credibility; films were readily available but not considered mainstream educationally for reasons relating to their reliability (variability in content) and stability as a medium (complexities around screening). A consensus had started to emerge that the educational benefit of film related to viewership; the 'presumption of mimesis' and 'kinesthetic empathy' in the transferral of skill from the practitioner to the audience (Curtis 2012: 162). The image was considered physical and immediate whereas the word was seen as intellectual. The reviewer of the film sought a more assertive role for the genre because the film did not explicitly identify when or how films could be used most effectively.

By the 1940s, cinema was an established leisure pastime, but there was a dissatisfaction with spectatorship versus viewership within medical education. Naysayers pointed to uncertainty surrounding the educational merit of the medical film, leading to robust debate within the profession: one evening's screening convened by the BMA for its members with a mixed programme of (unspecified) medical films was criticised as potentially causing 'acute fatigue and confusion' in the audience, with the risk of luring medical students away from 'the straight and narrow way' (Anon. 1945: 87). The experience was described as approximating entertainment for the 'penny-gaff state of mind' (a derogatory reference to an end of the pier show, often lewd, available for a penny in the early years of cinema) (Anon. 1945: 87). In fact, these somewhat spiky comments were designed to invite a more considered blend of 'modern' teaching methods into the medical training curriculum with the film being augmented with discussion. It acknowledged that the time-honoured model of the apprentice-medical student learning in the shadow of a master–teacher ('the straight and narrow way') could be disrupted by the advent of film, although anecdotally, the majority of educators were unable to successfully unlock its potential through inexperience or indifference.

During the World Congress on Medical Education in 1953, Creer had this to say about the value of film to his peers at the BMA:

> Educational psychologists were of the opinion that the rate of learning was based on experience; therefore one of the most effective methods of teaching was to provide direct experience or an adequate substitute. That was where the use of the motion picture came in, for many types of previously unobtainable experiences were now only as far away as the motion picture projector. (Anon. 1953: 560)

Film used in medicine was, however, considered to not be without limitation; he concurred that its effectiveness was contingent on the skill of the teacher; the level of preparation and what he called a 'new method of teaching'.

The experience of reading a textbook versus watching a film differs in many respects: film is a time-based medium and so instead of words as units, these units are images. If an image is equivalent to a word, then an animation sequence is equivalent to a sentence; a procedure, a paragraph; a chapter, a case study (Anon. 1947a: 141). This suggests that films could have the potential to replace textbooks, although the challenge for teachers was to find and evaluate film material to fulfil this aim; both the AMA, in its film library, and the BMA, with its film competition, endeavoured to grade titles objectively by the usefulness of the films' content to reduce the effort required in finding a suitable film. The ease of using a textbook was in contrast to the difficulty in not only finding a 'perfect time' to show films (presumably due to the planning required in securing the right equipment and perhaps also a technician to set up and run the film) but also due to a visceral dislike of the distractions of running film; 'the darkening of the room, all the paraphernalia of shutters, the squeaking of the roller screen, the focusing of the picture' (Anon. 1947a: 141). The view expressed by the BMA Film Committee was that this should be a routine activity managed smoothly by the teacher or it would interrupt the receipt of knowledge.

The historiography of medical film

An early film portrayed in *The Medical Motion Picture* demonstrated the challenges in capturing the body true to life. The cumbersome nature of 35mm film cameras and the film stocks available in the 1910s and 1920s mitigated against the filmic representation of the human body with a high degree of fidelity. Film is a photochemical medium and footage shot in black and white, on film stock insensitive to reds, makes blood indistinguishable from the iodine which is liberally applied to the surgical area (both are uniformly black; *The Medical Motion Picture* 1947: commentary at 00:01:13–00:01:30). Not only is the colour field flattened but also the 'definite texture', the viscosity, of blood is absent (*The Medical Motion Picture* 1947: commentary at 00:06:58). An example of orthochromatic versus panchromatic film is contrasted using the technique of split screen with two black and white caesarean section film sequences shown side-by-side. The introduction of colour film stock led to better representation of bodily structures. Although the following film still, showing a split screen image (see Figure 8.5), scarcely does justice to the point being made in the film, that these 'structures' (presumably the patient, the baby) are better differentiated three-dimensionally. In the film, both film loops are running simultaneously (see Figure 8.6), although contemporary eyes still struggle to discern exactly what is depicted.

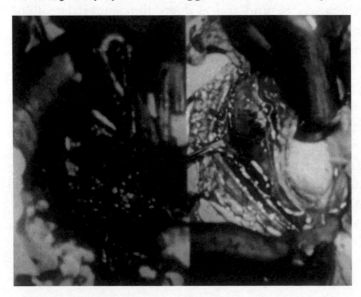

Figure 8.5: Film Still, split screen; left to right, a caesarean section at point of entry shot with orthochromatic film and panchromatic film, *The Medical Motion Picture*, Ralph P. Creer (technical adviser), 1947. USA. Public Domain.

Filmmaking techniques developed in the clinic, such as endoscopy, provided an opportunity for physiological phenomena to be captured more systematically, creating more research 'data' in the form of film. This gave clinicians ample opportunity to show normal versus abnormal physiologies, although early examples of filmmaking illustrated in the film are 'unusual cases' (Oppenheimer's Disease, an uncommon neuro-logical condition indicated by extreme floppiness in the new-born) and rare phenomena (in the case of the young woman with myasthenia gravis, whose speech improves after treatment in a 'before and after' sequence). Silent and sound cinema, animation and the use of medical illustrations are all considered in turn in *The Medical Motion Picture*. These carefully curated milestones illustrate how technology, in the development of film stocks or innovative cinematographic 'devices' (which enable laryngos-copy, cine-microscopy and cineradiography) could provide an experien-tial understanding of the body.

Bringing the clinic to the classroom became achievable both behind the camera, with the availability and relative ease of handling sixteen millimetre film cameras by amateurs and professionals alike, and then with the ubiquity of projector equipment across the sector in classrooms (as in *Understanding Aggression*) and lecture-theatres. From the 1930s onwards, sixteen millimetre gauge filmmaking became the norm: many physicians obtained cameras for their own personal use as well as utilis-ing them in their laboratories, clinics and surgeries (and no doubt lead-ing to the charges of filmmaking as a 'distraction' or hobby). It is not inconceivable that, as more clinicians made or had direct influence over the films they needed for their medical speciality, acceptance grew. Trade in film supplies, such as projector equipment aimed at teaching hospi-tals as well as general practitioners, developed in parallel, indicating the breadth of the film market amongst the medical professions, something evidenced in two advertisements in a catalogue of medical films, see Fig-ures 8.7 and 8.8. The adoption of sixteen millimetre as a distribution format also greatly added to its transnationality.

Medical etiquette

Looking at the impact of these films beyond the medical profession, why were these medical films not more widely known? 'Medical eti-quette' governed who watched them: one organisation, Kodak, known

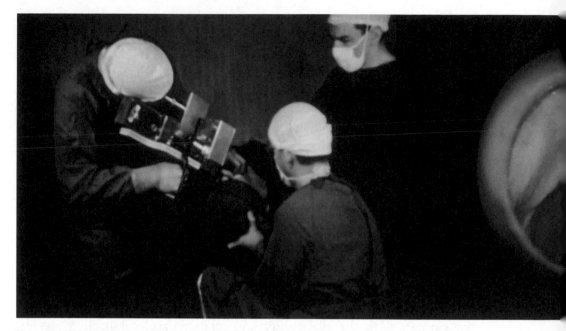

Figure 8.6: Film stills, left to right, composite of three frame grabs of clinicians using a laryngoscope, healthy larynx, unhealthy larynx with papilloma of both portions of anterior vocal cords, *The Medical Motion Picture*, Ralph P. Creer (technical adviser), 1947. USA. Public Domain.

for its production of cameras and film to consumers and professionals, also managed a commercial library of medical films. In the preface to a catalogue published in the United Kingdom, it warned that,

> The Kodak Medical Film Library is intended only for circulation within the limits of the Medical Profession [...] they will not be exhibited to any persons other than qualified medical men and registered medical students [...]. Non-compliance with this stipulation will be regarded as a serious breach of medical etiquette. (Kodak Ltd c.1939: n.pag.)

'Medical Etiquette' was an unwritten code of conduct between medical professionals and although on the surface the objective was laudable (to avoid the prurient gaze and prevent harm, to avoid anxiety or fear in the patient), in actuality it had more to do with mitigating against professional disagreements with colleagues. It is indicative of how medicine had become a bounded disciplinary domain with the siloing of medical specialities with language unfamiliar to the public (one such example is the word 'neoplasm', a medical term for a tumour in cancer diagnosis, widely in use in medical educational materials throughout

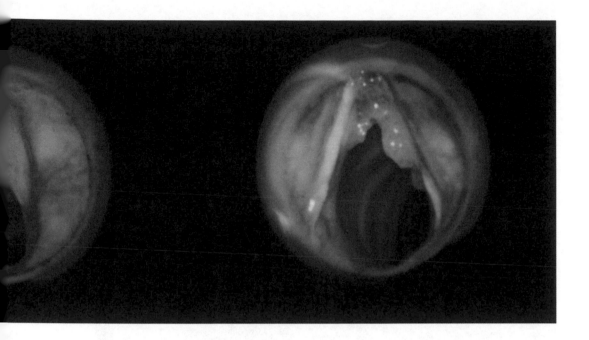

the twentieth century, but still liable to confuse the unwary cataloguer who has not encountered this before). The construction of these codes of etiquette relate to policing the boundaries of medical knowledge and practice (indeed, the right to hire further films is mentioned as a specific sanction). These strictures can be viewed as an attempt to control how much the public could see of medical practice in case it undermined the authority of the practitioner. However, by digitising these historical medical films for audiences beyond medicine – even though they are outdated, and sometimes visceral in content – museums, archives and libraries have disrupted the notion of 'medical etiquette', leading to the visibility of this 'hidden cinema'. A recent example, during the global COVID-19 pandemic, illustrates how historical medical film has travelled beyond academic research, and has allowed for the rediscovery of medical technology in respiratory medicine; shortages in the supply of medical equipment have resulted in clinicians looking to the internet for historical references to help in the reconstruction of medical equipment, which was in short supply.

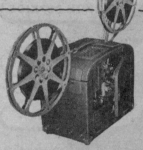

Figure 8.7: Trade advertisement by G. B. – Bell & Howell (Scientific Film Association 1952: 9). England. Copyright of Bell and Howell. Image source: Wellcome Collection.

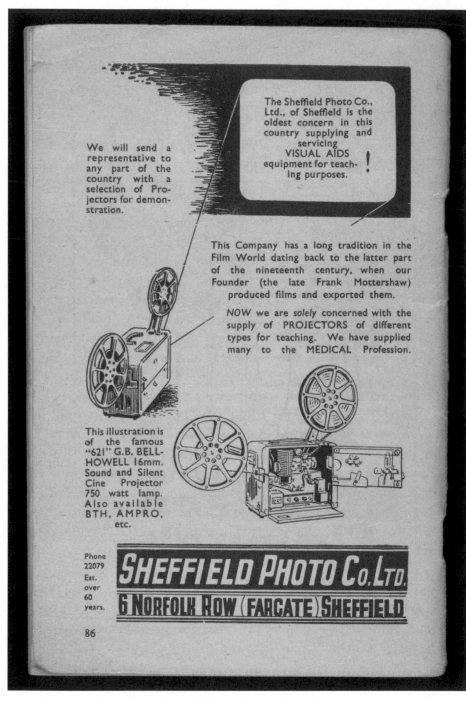

86

Figure 8.8: Trade advertisement by Sheffield Photo Co. Ltd (Scientific Film Association 1952: 86). England. Copyright of Sheffield Photo Co. Ltd. Image source: Wellcome Collection.

Conclusion

Medical films have borne witness to considerable technological innovation during the mid-twentieth century with film brokering new understandings of the working of the body by bridging the gap between the laboratory, clinic and education. It has proved a robust, enduring and transnational medium within the medical professions. Film's physical materiality (the film stock, the equipment for creating moving images, processing and then screening it) appealed to many medical practitioners, particularly those embedded in technical disciplines such as Ralph P. Creer, who became one of the leading international authorities and historians of medical motion pictures (Gibson 1981: 30). Often film's staunchest advocates were clinician–filmmakers themselves.

Over the course of the second half of the twentieth-century, educational audiences themselves shifted in their reception, understanding and appreciation of the moving image. Film was designed for re-use, providing repeatable content over time, although there has been surprisingly little research into the effect of film on its audiences. The dissenting voices discouraging the use of film in medical education ebbed away over time. Evidence of a shift in the acceptance of film is hinted at in a British Government report published in 1965 by Brynmor Jones, Vice-Chancellor of the University of Hull. The report included the findings of a 1963–64 survey on the audio–visual educational landscape around the world. It outlined differences in the adoption of audio-visual aids in higher scientific education (not just the 'ambient' use of film in teaching to 'pad out' the lecture). It made a powerful case that media literacy would grow and that students would become 'picturate' and more receptive to images versus text:

> The view of the controlled and disciplined utterances of film and television may lead to the realisation that these media have a significance for us comparable with that of El Greco, Titian and Michael Angelo in a less literate world. (Jones 1965: 2–3)

This comment was prescient, media 'literacy' has indeed grown exponentially over the course of half a century; *Understanding Aggression* illustrates this shift in audience behaviour.

In reconstructing history, the care taken in the selection of the case studies outlined in *The Medical Motion Picture*, a film about filmmaking, belies the considerable cinematographic (and medical) knowledge required. The earliest examples of surgery, as articulated in the film, were created as 'films of record' from the nineteen-teens, capturing important medical moments, and noted as being made within living memory. Yet even in 1947, many of these 'excellent reels' had not survived due to damage or loss, a situation consistent across the film sector throughout the twentieth century. Then, once the films no longer represented current practice, they become inactive agents in film libraries, and this rich heritage was forgotten.

The medical film deserves fresh eyes. The film, as an educational genre, was an important step in the historical evolution of medical imaging of the body from illustration, through to photography, and onwards to 3D imaging. Film as a distribution medium lasted as long as film reels were in circulation and as long as technology supported screening in the classroom or lecture theatre. For medical audiences, this was a shared, but hidden, cinematic experience, replicated across the medical professions for much of the second half of the twentieth century. Digitisation has proved to be transformative; watching medical film is no longer site nor specialism specific; medical knowledge can now freely circulate, unimpeded by the medical profession itself.

Acknowledgements

With thanks to Michael Brown (*Performing Medicine: Medical Culture and Identity in Provincial England, c.1760–1850*, Manchester: Manchester University Press, 2011) for help in understanding medical etiquette from a pre-cinema perspective.

References

American Medical Association (1962), *The Motion Picture in Medical Education*, USA: Sturgis-Grant Productions Inc. [https://medfilm.unistra.fr/wiki/The_motion_picture_in_medical_education. Accessed 28 August 2020.].

Anon. (1945), 'The medical film', *British Medical Journal*, 1:4385, p. 87, https://doi.org/10.1136/bmj.1.4385.87. Accessed 24 April 2020.

Anon. (1947a), 'Appendix II, the scope and the use of the film in medical education, preliminary [Committee] report', *British Medical Journal*, 1:4511, S127, pp. 140–8. https://10.1136/bmj.1.4511.S127. Accessed 24 April 2020.

Anon. (1947b), 'Medical motion pictures: Film reviews, the medical motion picture – It's development and present application', *Journal of the American Medical Association*, 137:10, p. 903.

Anon. (1953), 'Section C: Techniques and methods of medical education: The moving picture in medical education', *British Medical Journal*, 2:4835, p. 560.

Anon. (1957), 'Annual report to council: Medical films', *British Medical Journal*, 1:5023, S161, p. 195. https://10.1136/bmj.1.5023.S161. Accessed 24 April 2020.

Creer, Ralph P. (1934), 'Correspondence: Photographic illustration in medicine', *Journal of the American Medical Association*, 103:17, pp. 1325–26.

Creer, Ralph P. (1947), *The Medical Motion Picture*, USA: Audio Productions, Inc. https://wellcomecollection.org/works/bs44aq39. Accessed 27 July 2021.

Curtis, Scott (2012), 'Dissecting the medical training film', in M. Braun, C. Keil, R. King, P. Moore and L. Pelletier (eds), *Beyond the Screen: Institutions, Networks and Publics of Early Cinema*, Eastleigh and Bloomington: John Libbey/Indiana University Press, pp. 161–67.

Jones, Brynmor (1965), *Audio-Visual Aids in Higher Scientific Education; Report of the Committee Appointed by the University Grants Committee, the Department of Education and Science and the Scottish Education Department in February, 1963*, London: Her Majesty's Stationery Office, pp. 2–3.

Kodak Ltd (*c*.1939), *Catalogue of Kodak Medical Film Library*, London: Kodak Ltd.

Gibson, Henry Lou [Louis] (*c*.1981), 'The Biological Photographic Association, Its Half Century', USA: Biological Photographic Association: https://bca.org/about/BPA50th.pdf. Accessed 29 August 2020.

Russell, Patrick (2018), 'The NHS on film', *The National Archives*, 6 July, https://blog.nationalarchives.gov.uk/the-nhs-on-film/. Accessed 29 April 2020.

Scientific Film Association (1952), *Catalogue of Medical Films: A Revised Edition of the Catalogue of Medical Films Published in 1948 for the Royal Society of Medicine and Scientific Film*, London: Royal Society of Medicine.

Thomson, Margaret (1960), *Understanding Aggression*, UK: Ronald H. Riley (RHR Productions), in association with the Film Producers Guild, https://wellcomecollection.org/works/dpys458f. Accessed 29 April 2020.

GARDENS

GROUNDWORK FOR PLANETARY HEALTH: REIMAGINING GARDENS IN MEDICAL EDUCATION

Stacey Langwick and Mary Mosha

The dual environmental and health crises that have shaped the opening decades of the twenty-first century raise challenging questions for medicine, including the content of medical education. Some medical schools are responding by developing curricula to train 'climate aware' physicians, by supporting research that tracks how ecologies will alter the distribution and longevity of disease, and/or by planning for the new level of emergency response required to address climate events (Howard 2019; Maxwell and Blashki 2016; Lemery et al. 2021; Philipsborn et al. 2021). While important steps, these initiatives stop short of reckoning with the ways in which biomedicine is entangled with, and complicit in, climate change (Whitmee et al. 2015).[1] Few acknowledge that biomedicine shares many of the epistemic commitments that have shaped anthropogenic impact on the planet. By limiting concerns to the consequences of toxic pollution, warming atmospheres, rising seas, unpredictable weather events and expanded ecological zones for known vectors of disease on human health, even progressive initiatives in medical schools continue to hold nature and the (human) body as ontologically separate. In this chapter, we share the experimental beginnings of a project that strives to cultivate a space to ask questions about medicine's obligations to planetary health and reimagine medicine's epistemic objects in the face of climate change. We suggest that new ground – literally and figuratively – is needed to envision interdisciplinary projects that work to both rethink and restage healing on, *and of*, the planet.

In 2017, a group of scholars, public health specialists, clinicians and community leaders from Tanzania and the United States came together over a shared desire to think more deeply about the relationship between healing and environment, and the kind of medical education needed today. We recognised the need for a creative, multidisciplinary space – one that would join the classroom, the laboratory and the clinic – in order to hold out the possibility of epistemic emergences that might interrupt the ecological and health emergencies that increasingly defining our historical moment. We built on members' shared experience in designing and teaching in a global health exchange programme between Kilimanjaro Christian Medical Center (KCMC) and Cornell University. Each year since 2008, we had worked together with groups of Tanzanian and American students from the summer policy course, who had developed elaborate case studies that elucidated the ways that geopolitical histories and social inequalities resulted in uneven distribution of the health impacts. In coming together as the Uzima Collective, we were committed to exploring the forms of knowledge needed to mobilise healing as a mode of justice, simultaneously medical, ecological and social.

In 2015, a Rockefeller Foundation-Lancet Commission called for a programme on Planetary Health, that would address the ways that human impacts on the earths system have created health challenges for (and between) human and natural systems. Research on planetary health strives to consider how widespread environmental change shapes not only human health but the landscapes in which health is possible. This work pushes against the academic siloing of concerns into either 'nutrition' or 'environmental health'. Yet, such research, even as it expands conversations in medicine, often remains tied to Euro-American historical notions of what Donna Haraway has called natures/cultures and their conceptions of humans. As the Uzima Collective came together, we were challenged by the long histories of public healing in Tanzania, and elsewhere in Africa, that intervened in the dynamic social and material worlds through which the capacities of individual and collective bodies become possible. We also were inspired by local engagements with global ecological movements and the Tanzanians who work across multiple scales to nourish plants, soils, communities and economies in the name of health. We wanted to garden together.

The name Uzima holds us accountable to these alternative histories and attuned to the current innovations that bring them to bear on everyday life and assessments of strength, vitality, and health in Tanzania. In Swahili, '*uzima*' connotes the qualities of having transitioned to fullness, maturity, wholeness, wellness, of embodying a vitality that both are life and extends beyond individual embodiments of life. It gestures to an understanding of health that is more-than-human and more-than-a-right. Gardening offered an embodied practice through which to think with plants and landscapes about how ecological entanglements shape contemporary notions of the 'therapeutic', and provincialise 'planetary health'.

What sort of knowledge is therapeutic in response to the ecological and social threats shaping this century? What material conditions might cultivate the practices of noticing, the kinds of awareness and the modes of perception that will not only innovate medical technologies but also generate the healing of ecologies, bodies, communities and economies? The consequences of climate change not only challenge technological innovation but also challenge the matters through which medicine is taught, healing conceptualised, and health evaluated. The Uzima Garden is a space in which to explore the sorts of epistemological projects and methodological collaborations that these alternatives might offer, as well as their potential for an alter-politics (Hage 2015). This project does not focus on finding a single answer to the question: what must medicine do to address the impacts of climate change on human health? Rather the collective strives to create spaces for the learning, questioning and healing that is needed for medicine to begin to rethink itself in the face of climate change.

Our vision continues to be inspired by contemporary grassroots efforts in Tanzania, to redefine healing at the intersection of medicine and agriculture. One of us (Langwick) has conducted extensive fieldwork on such work, focusing on the rise of a new configuration of plant-based healing in Tanzania. *Dawa lishe* (nutritious medicine) heals by feeding, nourishing, strengthening and maturing. The efficaciousness of interventions rests in their cultivation of the forms of strength that make places, times and bodies livable again (and again). Treatments attend not only to individual bodies, but also to relations between people, plants and soil. Some of the most provocative work catalyses healing through the extensions of gardens, lush spaces full of therapeutic foods and herbal medicine. These biodiverse gardens are cultivated without synthetic chemical pesticides or fertilisers. Flora is chosen for the ways that species interact and support each other's maturation and fertility as well as its nourishment of humans. Plantings make affordances for some species to self-propagate, and to surprise their human companions. Gardeners attend to these surprises as well as to compost and other liveliness generated by the impermanence of life and the shifting shapes in which it instantiates itself. These *dawa lishe* gardens align themselves with food sovereignty movements, rather than with projects to expand access to medicine or initiatives to develop new drugs (Langwick 2018). In so doing, they strive to locate the therapeutic in efforts to re-imagine the forms of sovereignty possible in Africa today. The Uzima Project draws strength from this innovative work.

Gardens in medicine are not new. Modern medicine and medical education emerged with, and through, the botanic garden. Yet the *dawa lishe* gardens, even as they are explicitly therapeutic, and often include signage and labels, stand in sharp contrast to botanic gardens. What kind of garden would foster the evaluations of the efficacy of medicine and medical knowledge based on whether it was nourishing to both soil and body? In the emergent design and hands-on work, taking place in a plot at the entrance to a major teaching and research hospital in the foothills of Mount Kilimanjaro, Uzima is reimaging the garden as an epistemic object in medicine.

Gardens

The science of botany, and with it, institutional botanic gardens and herbaria, arose in the 1500s (Egerton 2003). A request by the medical school of the University of Padua in 1545 resulted in The Botanical Garden of Padua, which is now celebrated on the UNESCO World Heritage list as the 'original of all botanical gardens throughout the world' (Hallett 2006: 177). Botanic gardens labour to turn plants into academic objects, breaking explicitly from the relations between plants and people that shaped diverse histories of herbalism and delineating an evolution from medieval 'physic gardens' often attached to monasteries (Doyle 2008). The sixteenth and seventeenth centuries saw botanic gardens spread from northern Italy to other parts of Europe as medical schools began to appoint professors of botany. These university-run medicinal gardens both produced plant-based remedies and trained students how to attend to plants as medical objects (Olszewski 2011). They became key sites to structure physicians' epistemic commitments to the natural world, as context and resource, and to human bodies as the focus of therapeutic intervention.

In the eighteenth and nineteenth centuries, botanic gardens expanded with the goals of empire (Batsaki et al. 2016; Tchikine 2016). Directors of gardens in Europe and the fledging United States sought out plants from Asia, South and North America, and Africa, designing gardens that manifested dreams of geopolitical dominance (Brockway 2002). Plants like cinchona from the Andes came to be seen explicitly as a 'tool of imperialism' (Headrick 1979). The antimalarial quinine in its bark became critical to the survival of Europeans in the tropics and plantations remaking the landscapes of colonies in the tropics (Roy 2017). Shaped by the epistemologies and ontologies of colonialism, botanic gardens moved beyond the purview of medical schools and focused more broadly on commercially viable plants: plants for agriculture and building joined those medicine in collections. Britain, France, Germany and the Netherlands all established botanic gardens in their colonial territories. Botanic gardens, such as the Amani Research Station in Tanzania, organised colonial flora into sites that could generate scientific knowledge (Tilley 2011). In the process, they initiated the movement of plant materials along routes that established colonial centres and peripheries.[2]

Colonisation is an important part of the story which saw botany develop into a weighty academic science outside of medical schools. Ethnobotanical studies contributed to the organisation of the botanic gardens in the metropoles and the territories, mapping plants and their usage. Once removed from the contexts in which they had dwelled, plants used to heal could be articulated into pharmacopeias, which were comparable, combinable and researchable. Mastery over the pharmacopeias which had located the authority of the doctors came to shape the relations between biomedical doctors and biological sciences. The pull of such gardens continues, inside and outside of medicine, often mediating the boundary between traditional and modern medicine. In postcolonial Tanzania, efforts to mine indigenous plants for pharmaceutical research, as well as for the production of herbal remedies, motivated the Institute for Traditional Medicine to cultivate a garden of indigenous therapeutic plants (Langwick 2015, 2021).

In an effort to grapple with the epistemological traditions that inhere in these gardens, Nancy Scheper-Hughes and Margaret Lock (1987) turned to culturally distinct styles of noticing plants and producing knowledge at a key point in their classic essay on the 'Mindful Body'. They compared 'non-western' traditions to illustrate that a variety of 'holistic' conceptions of the body have emerged from diverse ways of articulating humans' relations with nature, and they contrast them with 'western' ways of apprehending nature. Scheper-Hughes and Lock justified their deconstruction of the biomedical body by illustrating how it limits both clinical knowledge and health care delivery.

Byron Good (1994) and Annemarie Mol (2003) extend these epistemological concerns by describing the specific clinical practices through which the body is enacted, and how it then comes to organise medical work. Good's ethnography of an American medical school highlights the role of medical education in the emergence of the biomedical body as a distinctive form of reality. He examines how medical students learn the micropractices of seeing, writing and speaking that formulate the objects – the bodies and diseases – to which clinicians attend. While anthropologists have long drawn attention to work 'beyond the body proper' (Lock and Farquhar 2002), the formative processes Good describes still guide medical education.

Today, small gardens affiliated with some medical schools in Europe and the United States celebrate medicine's roots in ethnobotany, phytochemistry and pharmacology: be they designed to recognise herbs that have been used medicinally in the past, or poisonous plants that have long histories in the imperial pharmakon, or spaces that hold out 'nature' as an antidote to the harms of modern life. These little green spaces for students or medical professions to take a break or eat lunch on sunny days are traces of the history in which the garden served as a key epistemic object in the development of modern medicine.

Bodying forth

Over the past three decades, infectious disease researchers and public health scholars have promoted analytical frameworks that locate biomedical concerns in the context of human–animal–environment relations.[3] Approaches, such as Planetary Health and One Health, have supported multidisciplinary work, expanded the objects to which medicine proper attends and highlighted more complex conceptualisations of disease and fields of intervention. Initiatives foreground the complex dynamics among humans and nonhumans, between life and its environs. The conceptual structure of these multidisciplinary initiatives, however, continue to mobilise health as an achievement of individuals (human or animal). Broad epistemic agreement across disciplines has maintained the dualisms that organise Euro-American philosophical traditions – such as body/environment, human/nonhuman, life/nonlife, inside/outside (Lerner and Berg 2017). Offering moments of encounter as the ground for transactional exchange (e.g. parasites moving from animal host to water to human host), centres descriptions around discrete, even if porous entities. Narratives hold distinct form (bodies) and context (environments).

Ed Cohen (2011) sketches a position from which to undo these dualisms when he suggests how viruses might inspire a refocusing of accounts away from tracing the trajectories of entities and towards narratives of those forces that animate life and nonlife. Drawing inspiration from virology, Cohen focuses attention on the capacities that enable viruses to move DNA through bodies, across populations, over time shaping and reshaping that which is brought into being – bodied forth. His proposal undoes the subjects and objects of public health accounts; that is, body and environment (form and context) constantly emerge and re-emerge through each other. Cohen's work exemplifies the kind of humanities scholarship that Wolf (2014) argues is important to dislodging assumptions, seen in many public health and environmental initiatives, of a discrete body that grounds individual being (and rights) (see also Cohen 2008, 2020).

Julie Livingston (2019) continues to extend this effort in her latest book, *Self-Devouring Growth*. In drawing on histories of rainmaking, animal cohabitation, and transportation in southern Africa, she de-naturalises contemporary ways of apprehending the forces that body both 'us' and 'the planet' forth and suggests a re-mapping of the relations that are at stake. Livingston argues that the health, environmental and social crises we face in the twenty-first century are rooted in a world propelled by devasting, 'self-devouring', forms of growth. Her planetary parable seeks to unlock 'our collective imagination' (Livingston 2019: 9), opening up new ways that public health might conceive of, no less intervene in, ecological and bodily capacities, debilities and relations through which particular forms of life, growth and health – as well as death, decay and disease – manifest.[4]

How might rethinking what sort of garden is at the heart of medicine – and therefore the relations between people and plants that inhere in its design – provide a space to cultivate alternative notions of growth? What sort of garden might create epistemic engagements that articulate the therapeutic in the forces that body us – humans and nonhumans – forth? The Uzima Collective began gardening together in an effort to imagine an educational and therapeutic space that would hold open the question of what sort of knowledge would help health professionals generate new modes of attention and new possibilities for intervening in the entanglements of ecological and bodily capacities.

The *dawa lishe* gardens that extend through non-governmental projects, such as support groups for people with AIDS, people with disabilities, and vulnerable children, as well as outreach efforts around nutrition, inspire us. These plant–human projects re-articulate human health within the dynamic set of relations that animate planetary 'ongoingness' (Haraway 2016; see also Weston 2017). They challenge the economies and efficacies that frame biomedical articulations of health by demanding that therapies be nourishing to humans and their environments. They are not, however, epistemic projects. Uzima was forged in the friction between these activist efforts and the demands of educating future health practitioners. Our experiment is a collaboration dedicated to cultivating pedagogical innovations that animate a notion of therapeutic sovereignty *within* medicine.

Uzima project

The Uzima Garden is in its early stages. In 2018, the Kilimanjaro Christian Medical Center (KCMC) dedicated two and a half acres of land along the entrance to the college–hospital–research complex to our project. The site is ideal as it abuts the Nutritional Rehabilitation Unit (NURU), highlighting the historical shifts in the forms of agriculture developed as solutions to nutritional problems, and in biomedical interventions into hunger.

In the early 1970s, KCMC – similar to other major hospitals in newly independent Anglophone African countries – instituted a NURU programme.[5] High rates of severe malnutrition driven by drought as well as fluctuations in the world economy, ecological stresses, demographic pressures and the effects of class formation marked these first years of independence. The medical community identified women and children to be at particularly high risk for malnutrition, yet the effect of treatments available to clinicians on the ward when patients presented as severely malnourished were limited. While a critical piece of comprehensive programming to fight malnutrition, hospital-based intensive nutritional therapies then, as now, were not deemed sufficient for generating long-term change. Nutritional Rehabilitation Units were farms with residential programmes within hospitals. A patient whose condition was diagnosed as primarily one of malnourishment could be prescribed a residency on the farm. These patients were invited to live on the farm, work in the fields learning new agricultural techniques and eat the food produced. Then, after several months, when the mother and child had recovered, they returned home healthier and equipped with new agricultural knowledge and techniques for food preparation.

KCMC initiated NURU during an era in which national and international health goals focused on primary health care. In the mid to late 1980s, as Structural Adjustment Programs altered the political frame through which medicine functioned, such primary-care-oriented, social interventions began to decline. Through the 1990s and 2000s, with the re-configurations of health care driven by the rise of global health, the political economy of nutrition changed and the priorities of the KCMC leadership changed with it (for more on the political economy of postcolonial nutrition, see Nott 2018; Redfield 2012; Scott-Smith 2014). NURU came to embody a different set of commitments. Patients at KCMC were no longer prescribed a residency on the farm. The goals of the unit turned to agricultural production. For two decades, the fields were primarily planted with maize, mono-cropped for ease of mechanised harvests, as well as with a couple of smaller plots for the cultivation of bananas, green vegetables and beans. The harvests supplied the Kitchen Department of the hospital and contributed to programmes focused on admitted patients. In the past year, a new venture is emerging. KCMC has started renting the land to a company interested in the commercial production of vanilla. The goals of NURU then are continuing to change, as the land is now imagined as a resource for entrepreneurial agricultural production, and the shared profits as going to partially fund food for hospitalised patients.

As the goals enacted through NURU evolved over the past five decades, the maintenance of the NURU buildings has been inconsistent. Currently, they contrast sharply with a new, bright white structure surrounded by gates and protected by an armed guard that sits on the adjacent plot of the biotechnology research centre. This new building houses the laboratory guinea pigs bred for pharmaceutical research. The visual contrast evokes the concerns of many public health scholars and medical practitioners: global health initiatives have shifted attention away from primary health care and toward a pharmaceuticalisation of health (Biehl 2007; Nguyen 2010).

Not only institutions but also the disciplinary focus of nutritional science has shifted globally, as social priorities and political will turned away from primary health care and towards acute (secondary and tertiary) care, emphasising pharmaceutical intervention. The layered challenges of malnutrition and metabolic disorders however suggest the limits of pharmaceuticals, supplements and ready-to-use therapeutic foods (RUTFs) in the face of the nutritional challenges that Tanzania faces today. The Uzima Project emerged from a shared analysis that the changes in the burden of disease in Tanzania calls for a rethinking of the role of nutrition in health care and a corresponding update to the concept of the NURU. It is an argument that twenty-first-century nutrition must exceed the critical crisis-oriented responses to caloric insufficiencies and micronutrient deficiencies. Members of the collective are interested in cultivating enduring interventions into the environments of health. The Uzima Project poses these questions through a process-based design of a therapeutic and educational space, a garden. A garden in which the very philosophical assumptions about humans' relation with nature, assumptions that underlie biomedicine and constitute the specific version of the body to which clinicians attend, might be explored and re-invented.

Uzima garden

These dreams are big. But the work is concrete. The work is the everyday work of cultivating the relations of a team that cannot only hold the idea of a garden as pedagogical object, but be willing to engage in the constant intellectual upheaval of trying to reinvent the garden that has been central to the production of modern medical knowledge. It is bringing a biocultural collections expert with experience working with Native American groups in the United States, who have explicitly articulated their plant collections as a materialisation of sovereignty, to lead a workshop in the Tanzanian medical school. It is listening to those on the mountain who farm with the land and continually learn from the plants. It is studying with elders about the plants with which they have healed themselves and their families. It is about engaging with entomologists who can teach us how the termites that are thriving on these two and a half acres can be engaged as co-gardeners. It is about seed exchanges with the community groups that inspire us, and about cultivating alternative economies of health. It is about testing the soils for toxicity, given that the area is potentially exposed to run-off from the gas station, NURU, and the large biotech research complex that borders it. In addition, at different times in the recent past, the plot has been farmed with chemical fertilisers and pesticides and used as a place to dump and/or burn garbage. With that information we must decide on remediation strategies that will enable the soil to regenerate a vitality that has been taken from it. It is debating how these micro-decisions can be brought to medical students, within and beyond their required modules in the Community Health Department, and opened up to the KCMC public in ways that generate conversation about how we live in and through toxicity. It is about composting (see Figure 9.1) and composting more, as we work together for new ways to articulate biomedicine's obligations to the waste it produces.

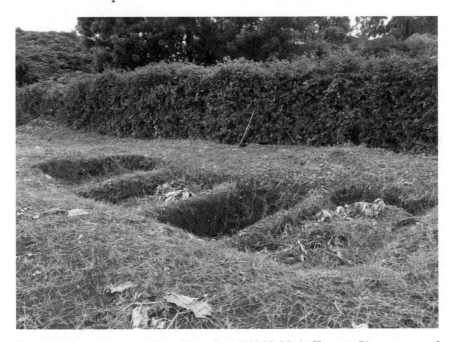

Figure 9.1: First compost pits when clearing land, KCMC, Moshi, Tanzania. Photo courtesy of Sabina Mtweve, 2020.

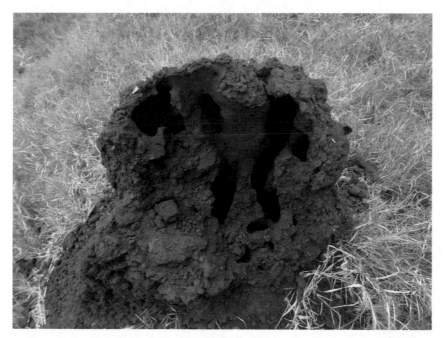

Figure 9.2: Mounds of termites who, in moving leaf litter, contribute to the distribution of nutrients throughout the plot, KCMC, Moshi, Tanzania. Photo courtesy of Mary Mosha, 2020.

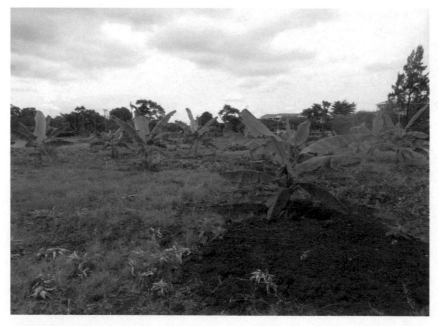

Figure 9.3: Planting the first banana trees in kihamba, KCMC, Moshi, Tanzania. Photo courtesy of Mary Mosha, 2020.

It is about working with medical students to design research projects that will draw out the sorts of stories and processes of storying (seeing, writing and speaking) that could stimulate this process; about finding and working with landscape architects who are excavating forms of process-based design knowledge that have been marginalised over time. It is about sharing the harvests from the first cover crops with others. It is about having the patience to not just create a garden design, but to hold the space for the iterative work through which the project team, medical school staff and students, community members, termites, rains, plants, soils, waters, histories and curriculums might engage over time, bodying forth a new kind of garden with a new kind of learning, new kinds of perception, and medical objects that can meet the demands of the twenty-first century. It is about generating ethical subjects who can meet the demands for healing to be fundamentally about justice.

At each turn, we grapple with how this work can be integrated into medical curriculums at both KCMC and Cornell. We refer to the first (and ongoing) phase of the Uzima Project as 'Health from the Soil Up.' This work expanded the literature critical to cultivating the space as therapeutic. Medical faculty not only engaged in soil toxicity tests but also thought about the histories of development on land bordering the plot (biotechnology buildings, NURU, a petrol station). Uzima holds a space for reflecting on the forms of growth and health that have given rise to that which borders our place and asks how that stands in relation to those form of health and growth that give rise to *dawa lishe* gardens. When wondering about the role of the termites that had colonised the field, the Uzima Collective enlisted public health students at KCMC to observed the termites and others at Cornell to reach out to entomologists in their institution. These students shared observations, photos and entomological studies in order to discern the species, as well as their lifestyles and gardening styles (see Figure 9.2). The way the creatures dwelling with us laboured became critical to how the collective imagined engaging (and eventually working) with them in redistributing plant debris and nourishing the soil. Global health students in the United States have conducted literature reviews, developed working bibliographies, and archived collections of relevant literature to assist students design policy case studies in the KCMC-Cornell Global Health summer course, as well as to overcome barriers to access teaching in both institutions.[6] They began writing a story of our soil as 'a story of gathering community and giving to the systems that sustain our health' (Maurer 2020: n.pag.).

Students at KCMC have designed a poster to communicate the relations they see in the garden, and built a labyrinth to draw others to move through the space, to invite them to be part of the garden and to contribute to envisioning it from there.

Epistemic decisions are also materialised in the nitty-gritty decisions in the care for soil and plants, and the non-human others welcomed into the space. When the Uzima Collective faced a decision about crop cover, we debated whether soy beans would be a plant that supported and extend Uzima's notion of the relations that constitute therapeutic space. They are nitrogen fixing, however they also participate in the dispossession of indigenous and small-scale farmers (particularly in the genetically modified versions that circulate so readily in South America and Africa) (Hetherington 2013). Our collective strove to understand the materiality of beans, together with their political–economic collaborations, as critical to the constitution of our space and an object for medical training. We turned to our community collaborators for recommendations – choosing to cultivate different relations through our cover crops, ones that supported the seed sharing work of local NGOs and international connections between environmental organisations and the food sovereignty movement. As the eagerness to plant drove some of us forward more quickly than others, we realised the need for a Living Collections Policy to help guide our reflection on and labour over plant selection. Not only did 'Beans, Bananas and Other Biodiverse Foods of Tanzania' emerge as one of our collections, but the process of articulating the Collective's shared values and the goals of the project through the themes around which we would gather plants and people, as well as naming the collections themselves, pushed against the epistemological boundaries of botanic gardens. The themes that energise our attention; the plants gathered into the space; the forms of care brought to soils, flora, fauna, and the people who enter; and our collective design work and outreach in specific classes are all guided by collective reflection on the garden as an epistemic object. At each turn, the seven members of the Uzima Collective ask themselves, as well as students and collaborators working with them, to explicitly articulate the relations through which they are conferring therapeutic value on plants, and to make clear how they see those relations work toward holding medical practice and knowledge accountable to being 'nourishing'. For example, how do they work against logics of extraction? How do they disrupt analytical frames that render medical waste invisible? What assumptions to do they make about bodies and ecologies? What kinds of labour do they require from plants and people?

As The Living Collection Policy guides our planting, it describes some of the concrete actions through which Uzima is striving to experiment with the cultivation of this new epistemic space. The first efforts started in mid 2020 with the design and planting of a *kihamba* (Kichagga, singular) in one section of the garden: a style of intensive planting dominated by banana that has given rise to homesteads in the Kilimanjaro region over the past several hundred years (see Figure 9.3). *Vihamba* (plural) enact a method of planting and dwelling that enables the farmer to continue production over time without purchasing extensive external inputs (Fernandes et al. 1984). Research on the slopes of Kilimanjaro has found that *vihamba* maintains 'about 520 vascular plant species including 400 non-cultivated species' and exemplifies a way for densely populated areas to be managed for human and nonhuman life (Hemp 2006: 1). The modes of production and habitation that constitute *vihamba* manifest a distinctive formulation of reality, of dwelling. They are spaces fed, energised and activated by the transfer and transformation of 'life force' or 'bodily power' among humans, animals and crops (Myhre 2018). Elders are buried in their *kihamba* and it holds those living to be accountable to many different human and ecological pasts. *Vihamba* attune our philosophies and our activism to bodies as effects of activities that channel the capacity for life (human and nonhuman, individual and collective). In addition to drawing on a regionally unique manifestation of plant and human relations, and capturing a wide range of plants used to nourish, heal and sustain liveliness for people and animals, as well as linages and lands over time, the *kihamba* opens up a space to elaborates on two central themes in the Living Collections Policy: 'Plants are Always More than Resources' and 'Working Against Historical Forms of Dispossession'. The collective is exploring, in very concrete ways, how a *kihamba* might be cultivated and sustained in the garden. After all, these are lineage formations and not public gardens. Questions of whether a *kihamba* can even be cultivated as an epistemic object in a public garden are complex. We remain present to these questions as we engage in this space with medical and public health students. More broadly, *vihamba* offer medical students an opportunity to reflect on the times and spaces of medicine, as well as the political, economic, cultural and ecological values that structure interventions deemed therapeutic. More concretely, for example, *vihamba* have long relations to fields, and attending to these relations could expand the ways that health development experts engage in food security debates that often pit small scale farming against larger scale initiatives.

Vihamba stand in contrast to the botanic gardens that have grounded the relations between plants and humans at the heart of medicine. They draw attention to the ways that humans, plants, animals and soil are 'bodied forth' together, through collective human and nonhuman work. In this space, Uzima invites students and staff to develop ethical, technical, and aesthetic projects that explore healing as a way of approaching the contingent liveliness of bodies and ecologies as they work through and within each other. Plants co-create a space for dwelling: cultivating the capacities of bodies and place and the relations through which lineages might extend over time and place. From within a *kihamba*, assessments of the therapeutic value of plants cut across medicine and agriculture; they open up new questions about the relations that must be supported and nurtured in service to our vital interests; and they insist that therapeutic efficacy be grounded in notions of nourishment beyond the individualised human bodies. The frictions between *vihamba* and the gardens that render plants as resources for extraction – from botanic gardens to the NURU fields that border our project – are providing a fruitful catalyst for the conversations and projects through which the Uzima Garden will continue to emerge. Drawing on the *vihamba* as a pedagogical space renders concrete the political, economic, social and ecological values that inform the medicine into which students are being disciplined.

Conclusion

In the beginning of the twenty-first century, as experts speculate on the likelihood that we are entering an era characterised by zoonotic pandemics, and as the publics witness the ways that COVID-19 exploits the fault lines of our social and material worlds, the urgency of experimenting with the matters of medicine is palpable. Medical schools strive to conceptualise how the field might evolve to address climate change. Many are increasingly interested in how medical schools might train doctors and others to manage the effects of environmental crises on human health and the impacts of what Julie Livingston has called 'self-devouring growth' on human life. Without acknowledging biomedicine's epistemic commitments to the extractive logics that articulate plants and people as resources, and to the analytical practices that hold bodies and ecologies as ontologically distinct, these efforts remain reactive. They stop short of reimagining medicine and healing. The Uzima Garden is an experiment rendering the epistemic boundaries that define medicine visible and as sites of experimentation. The project seeks ways to innovate how the medicine might more effectively apprehend the many complex, scalar relations that make up bodies and ecologies. Rather than medicalising human-environment relations, the Uzima Collective strives to reimagine pedagogical investments in health and medicine. We strive to expand attention beyond biomedical bodies and the ways that their environments impact them, and toward the 'possibilities [that] might enable us to body forth and flesh out new ways of living together with more equity, more justice, more compassion and more grace' (Cohen 2008: 122).

This effort, we suggest, demands the remaking of the relations of plants and humans at the heart of medicine, a reworlding that will challenge agriculture and drug development, as it reimagines the garden through which medicine has long structured its answer to the questions: what are plants? What counts as knowledge of them? What confers their therapeutic value? For the Uzima Collective, gardening has become a practice through which to explore new modes of attention and labour in medical education. Our garden, as a pedagogical space, reorients teaching and invites students to locate challenges to bodily and national sovereignty in the actions of plant collection, soil cultivation, planting strategies, harvesting and sharing food and herbs. It invites those who work in the garden to attend to links between health and governance, as these links are formulated in the practices through which plants are rendered therapeutic. In classes, internships and cross-cultural projects, Uzima supports the innovation of therapeutic objects of intervention that insist on thinking of bodies and land as instantiations of relations, and of immune systems and ecologies as ways of describing the affordances that shape their production as particular instances. This process holds space for medical students, professors, doctors, researchers, patients, artists and community members to debate what sort of medicine is needed in the face of climate change and what sort of garden can cultivate understandings of the 'body' and 'planet' that socialises and politicises (rather than individualising) disease.

Acknowledgements

The thinking in, and the work discussed through, this essay is a product of the joint effort of all those in the Uzima Collective, including Gloria Damion, Rhoda Maurer, Rehema Mavura, Jeanne Moseley and Florida Muro. Thank you to the student at KCMC and Cornell who have contributed to the project. Our appreciation for The Qualities of Life working group through which the initial discussion that led us to these issues developed and the Mario Einaudi International Studies Center that not only supported this working group but also provided seed funding for the Uzima Project. Special gratitude to Helen Nguya and Rose Machange who inspired the vision of this garden and continue to advise, share materials and collaborate with our experiments into the spaces that might both provide healing and generate healing knowledge. We would also like to thank the Kilimanjaro Christian Medical Center for their openness and support. KCMC has donated the use of two and a half acres of prime land along the entry way to the medical complex for the Uzima Project. They have also supported the ongoing KCMC-Cornell global health exchange programme, through which some of the most hands-on pedagogical innovations are taking shape.

Endnotes

1. The Rockefeller Foundation-Lancet Commission on Planetary Health in 2015 began to open up a space to ask some of these questions in that it draws attention to the political, economic and social systems that govern the effects of environmental change on human health.

2. Latour (1987) in *Science in Action* offered European botanic gardens as a prime example of his concept of 'centers of calculation'; that is, those places that came to define the production of modern knowledge through forms of accumulation driven by colonialism and racialised capitalism.

3. Journals supporting research in that elaborates this framework, include: *Infection Ecology and Epidemiology*; *One Health*; *Veterinary Sciences*; *International Journal of One Health*; *Journal of Animal Genetics*; *Transgenesis and Zoonoses*. See also call for One Health collaboration in response to COVID-19 (Amuasi et al. 2020)

4. Both Cohen's and Livingtson's accounts could be mobilised as a call for medicine to attend to questions of 'spatial justice', a concept that previously has been the reserve of geographers and the provocation of landscape architects, urban planners and conservationists (Harvey 1973; Soja 2010).

5. For an account of the NURU unit at KCMC, see Howard and Millard (1997). For a broader historical analysis of severe malnutrition in Africa and global interventions into it, see Tappan (2017).

6. Thank you to Nico Modest for a bibliography and collection of literature on 'The Connection Between Biodiversity and Human Health', to Ronald Nemac on 'Environmental Change and History of North Tanzania' and to Desiree Wright on 'The Intersection of Soil Health and Human Health'.

References

Amuasi, John H., Walzer, Christian, Heymann, David, Carabin, Hélène, Huong, Le Thi, Haines, Andrew and Winkler, Andrea S. (2020), 'Calling for a COVID-19 One Health research coalition', *The Lancet Healthy Longevity*, 395:10236, pp. 1543–44.

Batsaki, Yota, Cahalan, Sarah Burke and Tchikine, Anatole (2016), *The Botany of Empire in the Long Eighteenth Century*, Washington, DC: Dumbarton Oaks Sumposia and Colloquia.

Biehl, João Guilherme (2007), 'Pharmaceuticalization: AIDS treatment and global health politics', *Anthropological Quarterly*, 80:4, pp. 1083–126.

Brockway, Lucile H. (2002), *Science and Colonial Expansion: The Role of the British Royal Botanical Gardens*, New Haven: Yale University Press.

Cohen, Ed (2008), 'A body worth having?: Or, a system of natural governance ', *Theory, Culture & Society*, 25:3, pp. 103–29.

Cohen, Ed (2011), 'The paradoxical politics of viral containment; or, how scale undoes us one and all', *Social Text*, 29:1, pp. 15–35.

Cohen, Ed (2020), 'A cure of Covid-19 will take more than personal immunity', Behavior and Society, *Scientific American*, 7 August, https://www.scientificamerican.com/article/a-cure-for-covid-19-will-take-more-than-personal-immunity/. Accessed 30 September 2020.

Doyle, D. (2008), 'Edinburgh doctors and the physics gardens', *Royal College of Physicians of Edinburgh*, 38, pp. 361–67.

Egerton, Frank N. (2003), 'A history of the ecological sciences. Part 10: Botany during the Italian renaissance and beginnings of the scientific revolution', *Bulletin of the Ecological Society of America*, 84:3, pp. 130–7.

Fernandes, E. C. M., Oktingati, A. and Maghembe, J. (1984), 'The Chagga homegardens: A mulistoried agroforestry cropping system on Mt. Kilimanjaro (northern Tanzania)', *Agroforesty Systems*, 2:2, pp. 73–86.

Good, Bryon J. (1994), 'How medicine constructs its objects', in B. J. Good (ed.), *Medicine, Rationality and Experience: An Anthropological Perspective*, Cambridge: Cambridge University Press, pp. 65–87.

Hallett, Susan (2006), 'World's first botanical garden has roots in medicine', *Canadian Medical Association Journal*, 175:2, p. 177.

Harvey, David (1973), *Social Justice and the City*, Athens: University of Georgia Press.

Headrick, Daniel R. (1979), 'The tools of imperialism: Technology and the expansion of European colonial empires in the nineteenth century', *The Journal of Modern History*, 51:2, pp. 231–63

Hemp, Andreas (2006), 'The banana forests of Kilimanjaro: Biodiversity and conservation of the Chagga home gardens', *Biodiversity and Conservation*, 15:4, pp. 1193–217.

Hetherington, Kregg (2013), 'Beans before the law: Knowledge practices, responsibility, and the Paraguayan soy boom', *Cultural Anthropology*, 28:1, pp. 65–85.

Howard, Beth (2019), 'Climate change in the curriculum', *Association of America Medical Colleges (AAMC) News*, 10 October, https://www.aamc.org/news-insights/climate-change-curriculum. Accessed 9 September 2020.

Howard, Mary and Millard, Ann V. (1997), *Hunger and Shame: Child Malnutrition and Poverty on Mount Kilimanjaro*, New York: Routledge.

Langwick, Stacey (2015), 'Partial publics: The political promise of traditional medicine in Africa', *Current Anthropology*, 56:4, pp. 493–514.

Langwick, Stacey (2018), 'A politics of habitability: Plants, healing and sovereignty in a toxic world', *Cultural Anthropology*, 33:3, pp. 415–43.

Langwick, Stacey (2021), 'Properties of (dis)possession: Therapeutic plants, intellectual property, and questions of justice in Tanzania', in H. Tilly (ed.) Special Issue: 'Therapeutic Properties: Global Medical Cultures, Knowledge, and Law', *Osiris*, 36, pp. 284–305.

Latour, Bruno (1987), *Science in Action: How to Follow Scientists and Engineers Through Society*, Cambridge, MA: Harvard University Press.

Lemery, Jay, Linstadt, Hanna, Rochford, Rosemary and Sorensen, Cecilia (2021), 'We need to train climate doctors', *Science & Diplomacy*, 22 January, https://www.sciencediplomacy.org/article/2021/we-need-train-climate-doctors. Accessed 7 September 2021.

Lerner, Henrik and Berg, Charlotte (2017), 'A comparison of three holistic approaches to health: One Health, EcoHealth, and Planetary Health', *Frontiers in Veterinary Science*, 4:163, pp. 1–7.

Livingston, Julie (2019), *Self-Devouring Growth: A Planetary Parable as Told from Southern Africa*, Durham: Duke University.

Maurer, Rhoda (2020), personal communication, 13 August.

Maxwell, Janie and Blashki, Grant (2016), 'Teaching about climate change in medical education: An opportunity', *Journal of Public Health Research*, 5:1, pp. 14–20.

Mol, Annemarie (2003), *The Body Mulitple: Ontology in Medical Practice*, Durham: Duke University Press.

Myhre, Knut Christian (2018), 'Kaa: Historical transformations in production and habitation', in K. C. Myhre (ed.), *Returning Life: Language, Life Force, and History in Kilimanjaro*, New York and Oxford: Berghahn Books, pp. 31–62.

Nguyen, Vinh-Kim (2010), *The Republic of Therapy: Triage and Sovereignty in West Africa's Time of AIDS*, Durham: Duke University Press Books.

Nott, John (2018), '"How little progress"? A political economy of postcolonial nutrition', *Population and Development Review*, 44:4, pp. 771–91.

Olszewski, Margaret Maria (2011), 'Dr. Auzoux's botanical teaching models and medical education at the Universities of Glasgow and Aberdeen,' *Studies in History and Philosophy of Biological and Biomedial Science*, 42, pp. 285–96.

Philipsborn, Rebecca Pass, Sheffield, Perry, White, Andrew, Osta, Amanda, Anderson, Marsha S. and Bernstein, Aaron (2021), 'Climate change and the practice of medicine: Essentials for resident education', *Academic Medicine*, 96:3, pp. 355–67.

Redfield, Peter (2012), 'Bioexpectations: Life technologies as humanitarian goods', *Public Culture*, 24:1, pp. 157–84.

Roy, Rohan Deb (2017), *Subjects: Empire, Medicine, and Nonhumans in British India, 1820–1909*, Cambridge: Cambridge University Press.

Scheper-Hughes, Nancy and Lock, Margaret (1987), 'The mindful body: A prolegomenon to future world in medical anthropology', *Medical Anthropology Quarterly*, 1:1, pp. 6–41.

Scott-Smith, Tom (2014), 'Control and biopower in contemporary humanitiarian aid: The case of supplemental feeding', *Journal of Refugee Studies*, 28:1, pp. 1–17.

Soja, Edward W. (2010), *Seeking Spatial Justice*, Minneapolis: University of Minnesota Press.

Tappan, Jennifer (2017), *The Riddle of Malnutrition: The long arc of biomedical and Public Health Interventions in Uganda*, Athens: Ohio University Press.

Tchikine, Anatole (2016), 'The echos of empire: Redefining the botanical garden in eighteenth-century Tuscany', in Y. Batsaki, S. B. Cahalan and A. Tchikine (eds), *The Botany of Empire in the Long Eighteenth Century*, Washington, DC: Dumbarton Oaks Sumposia and Colloquia.

Tilley, Helen (2011), *Africa as a Living Laboratory: Empire, Development, and the Problem of Scientific Knowledge, 1870–1950*, Chicago: University of Chicago Press.

Weston, Kate (2017), *Animate Plant: Making Visceral Sense of Living in a High-Tech Ecologically Damaged World*, Durham: Duke University Press.

Whitmee, Sarah, Haines, Andy, Beyrer, Chris, Boltz, Frederick, Capon, Anthony G., Dias, Braulio Ferreira de Souza, Ezeh, Alex, Frumkin, Howard, Gong, Peng, Head, Peter, Horton, Richard, Mace, Georgina M., Marten, Robert, Myers, Samuel S., Nishtar, Sania, Osofsky, Steven A., Pattanayak, Subhrendu K., Pongsiri, Montira J., Romanelli, Cristina, Soucat, Agnes, Vega, Jeanette and Yach, Derek (2015), 'Safeguarding human health in the anthropocene epoch: Report of the Rockefeller Foundation–Lancet Commission on planetary health', *The Lancet*, 386:10007, pp. 1973–2028.

Wolf, Meike (2014), 'Is there really such a thing as "one health"? Thinking about a more than human world from the perspective of cultural anthropology', *Social Science and Medicine*, 129, pp. 5–11.

GLOVES

THE CONTEXT OF TOUCH: GLOVES AND THE PELVIC EXAM

Kelly Underman

It is Saturday morning and I am standing in a small examination room with three medical students. My co-worker reclines on the table, a drape sheet over her lap and her heels resting in the stirrups. Together we are teaching these medical students the communication and manual skills of the pelvic exam: I play the role of instructor and she allows the students to practice on her body as she gives feedback. We are both gynaecological teaching associates (GTAs), a group employed by over 72 per cent of medical schools in the United States who follow this model of pelvic exam instruction (Dugoff et al. 2016). While there are many aspects of this work that are unique to the US, GTAs are also common in Canada, Australia, the Netherlands and Scandinavian countries, and are becoming more common elsewhere, such as in Turkey, the United Kingdom (Janjua et al. 2017; Sarmasoglu et al. 2016; Smith et al. 2015).

GTAs have a partial origin in the Women's Health Movement of the 1970s and one aspect of this lineage is the emphasis on the patient perspective (Underman 2020). GTAs teach medical students how to perform a full pelvic exam in a sensitive and patient-friendly manner. While GTA sessions are a very small portion of an increasingly full curriculum, they are designed to help medical students adopt the norms and values of the medical profession. One such norm is the professionalisation of touch – which, as I demonstrate in this chapter, is facilitated by the materiality of gloves.

The room where I teach has a sink and a counter, on which sit the plastic specula that we will use, a tube of lubrication, and several boxes of non-latex gloves. I am about to teach the first part of the pelvic exam, which involves the external inspection of the genitalia, but first I have to put on gloves. I explain to the students that this is what we call 'clean gloving technique': while the pelvic exam is not a sterile exam, it does need to be done with awareness of hygiene. As GTAs, we teach hundreds of pelvic exams a year and thus have a much higher risk for problems caused by dust or viruses. HPV, for example, can live on surfaces for up to a week (Roden et al. 1997) and has been detected on many outpatient clinic surfaces as a potential non-sexual mode of transmission – including on the outside of glove boxes (Sabeena et al. 2017).

I demonstrate how to locate the very cuff of the glove in the box and how to pull it out quickly and carefully so as not to let the clean fingers touch anything else. My co-worker half-watches me; she trusts me, but part of the job is constant vigilance over your body and the bodies of others (Underman 2020). I show the students how to pull a pair of gloves on without touching anything. Then I pull a third glove over my right hand, which is for me my non-dominant hand. I hold my hands up in front of my body, mimicking surgeons, and hook the wheeled stool with my foot. I make a joke about this being the hardest part of the pelvic exam as I seat myself without touching anything – or falling off the stool. As the teaching session continues, it is my job in the instructor role to keep a close eye on the students' gloves. I help them put on gloves with clean technique and, when they inevitably touch their faces or the stool as they sit, I remind them about cleanliness and help them re-glove.

The role of gloves in the pelvic exam is an interesting one. Studies of HPV contamination in the outpatient clinic, as I referenced above, demonstrate that gloves per se do not protect against disease transmission if care is not taken to avoid cross-contamination (Sabeena et al. 2017). Thus, providers wear gloves not just to avoid disease transmission. Gloves also serve an important symbolic function: they make it allowable for strangers to violate bodily taboos and touch the genitals of a complete stranger (Henslin and Biggs 1971). Gloves, I argue, combine with other affective, cultural, and material aspects of the pelvic exam to render touch during it as distinctly *non-sexual*.

Much has been written about other material objects in the pelvic exam. The speculum, for example, has long been criticised by feminist scholars for its sexist and racist origins (Barker-Benfield 2004; Coopery

Owens 2017; Snorton 2017; Washington 2006). Ostensibly invented by a midwife in the early nineteenth century, the speculum gained notoriety among European physicians through its use in public exams of sex workers (Ricci 1949). In the United States, the forerunner of the bivalve speculum used today was developed by J. Marion Sims, the 'father' of gynaecology, through a series of brutal experiments on enslaved Black women (Cooper Owens 2017). Likewise, the lithotomy position favoured by US gynaecologists, which is reclining on the back with the legs separate and supported, has been criticised, as has the table and 'stirrups' used to maintain this position (Oakeshott and Hay 2006; Seehusen et al. 2006; Tillman 2016). The drape sheet – either cloth or disposable paper – is used to mark the 'regions' of the pelvic exam, separating the patient from pelvis (Henslin and Biggs 1971; Young 1997). Both speculum and table have undergone various feminist reclamations. Most notably, feminist self-help clinics reclaimed the speculum for self-exams (Kline 2010; Morgen 2002; Murphy 2012). As Donna Haraway describes, feminist iconography of the 1960s and 1970s depicts Wonder Woman holding a speculum and declaring her strength and readiness to fight the patriarchy (Haraway 1997). More recently, feminist designers have reworked the speculum to facilitate more patient-friendly examinations (Blei 2018; Pardes 2017).

Indeed, these material objects have received a great deal of commentary in the pelvic exam, but the role of gloves remains under-explored. There is a literature on strategies to desexualise the pelvic exam (Giuffre and Williams 2000) and another on the use of gloves in care work, which demonstrates that gloves form an important symbolic barrier that enables intimate contact between strangers (Twigg 2000). I want to build on this literature by exploring how the materiality of gloves enables these symbolic boundaries. How do gloves facilitate some forms of connection and disallow others?

The importance of gloves comes from the role of touch in clinical encounters (Harris 2016; Vinson and Underman 2020). More importantly, gloves are central to *professional* forms of touch. Physicians use their hands for many aspects of the medical exam, including palpation, which is medicalised touch that assesses the size, shape or texture of the body's parts and organs (Harris 2016; Underman 2020). Control of touch allows for a physician or other healthcare provider to shape the encounter: intimate touch is permissible so long as it has been desexualised (Emerson 1970; Giuffre and Williams 2000; Henslin and Biggs

1971). In the clinical encounter, touching a neutral part of the body (such as the elbow) is a way that medical students and physicians learn to express empathy (Vinson and Underman 2020). For the pelvic exam in particular, though, touching the genitals requires careful adherence to social scripting and, as I demonstrate here, the use of material objects.

Scholars have long commented on the symbolic role of the glove as a barrier. In their article on the dramaturgy of the pelvic exam, James M. Henslin and Mae A. Biggs (1971) note that intimate contact of the genitals by a strange man violates many deeply held taboos. Gloves are only one set of many 'props' used in the performance of the pelvic exam, joining other material objects like the magazines in the waiting room (to avoid eye contact with others) and the drape sheet (to separate the patient-as-person from the pelvis-as-object). Henslin and Biggs write, 'by using the glove he [the physician] is saying that he will not himself be actually touching the "private area" since the glove will serve as an insulator' (1971: 261). The glove thus serves an important role in desexualising the exam:

> Since the patient has essentially undergone a metamorphosis from a person to an object—having been objectified or depersonalized, the focus of the interaction is now on a specific part of her body [...] This [...] is an interesting and highly effective use of props and space. (Henslin and Biggs 1971: 261)

Thus, the glove as a material object has played a central role in the pelvic exam since the earliest sociological studies.

Studies of body labour focus as well on the role of gloves as a symbolic barrier in intimate contact (Gimlin 2007). In Twigg's work, 'Gloves were used by workers to protect themselves from the full intimacy of bathing work, and to put up a barrier of professionalism between the client and the worker' (Twigg 2000: 404). The materiality of gloves protected workers literally from the feel of their clients' aging skin, which was too intimate and personal, but also created a professional barrier to render their clients into a body that is to be 'handled' (Twigg 2000: 404). Gloves thus serve to symbolically bound emotions and bodies, containing what has been demeaned as culturally unacceptable as 'disgusting' or dirty. In a pelvic exam, this means the vagina – and all the ideas about disgust, degradation and impure sexuality they evoke (Underman 2020)

I observed this process in both my work as a GTA and in my interviews with GTAs, medical students, and medical faculty (Underman

2020). GTAs and medical students spoke of learning how to glove correctly, cleanly, in order to conduct the pelvic exam. Gloves were always mentioned in my interviews alongside the importance of hygiene. Medical students echoed GTAs: 'this isn't a sterile exam, but it is a *clean* exam'. In this way, gloves provide an important symbolic barrier, but they also make visible what is invisible in the exam: bacteria and viruses. Gloves stand in materially as a reminder of risk. The feel of gloves on yours hands, as a GTA or medical student, serves to reinforce that touch must be delimited: to the drape, the speculum, and the patient's body, as we used to teach in my programme. To touch otherwise means you must change your gloves.

Given the threat that the pelvic exam may be felt by its participants as overly sexual, and given longstanding associations of the vagina with disgust, desexualising the exam and rendering the vagina into just another body part in the eyes of the medical student is essential (Posner 2015). Medical students in my interviews spoke only in veiled ways about this issue; many talked of the exam as being unpleasant or anxiety-provoking. GTAs were more straightforward. A GTA that I call Anna spoke about the vagina as being an area of 'high privacy' in our culture. The use of distancing techniques such as gloves were essential, in her eyes and for other GTAs whom I interviewed, for helping medical students overcome their squeamishness about putting their hands inside a living person who is simultaneously teaching them about the pelvic exam. In this way, gloves symbolically separate a trainee from cultural taboos and demeaning affects that 'stick' to vaginas (Ahmed 2015).

Gloves thus also signal to patients in clinical practice that the provider is mindful of their health and well-being – and has no nefarious intentions. Countless guides for patients about their first pelvic exam state clearly that the provider will always be wearing gloves for genital examinations and that lack of gloves is a sign of lack of professionalism (e.g. see Shalby 2018). Here, gloves are a material representation of professional ethics and values that protect both patients and providers: patients can use gloves to assess whether the touch is medically necessary or not and providers can use gloves to demonstrate that their intimate contact is purely professional.

The materiality of gloves, however, introduces new sets of challenges into the encounter that a novice must learn to master. Medical students expressed many times that gloves reduce tactile sensation. In this way, gloves are a materially real barrier in skin-to-skin contact. Likewise, gloves cannot be taken by themselves to be clean – cross-contamination is just as possible when wearing gloves as not, hence my coworkers' and my vigilance. The feel of gloves on your hands as a trainee might in fact make you over-confident about your hygiene.

There is also something especially awkward and time-consuming about gloves. This hinges on how gloves combine with other material objects in the clinical space: water from washing your hands, sweat, powder on the inside of gloves, the quality of the glove material. Often times as GTAs we struggled to help a medical student put on new gloves because their previous, contaminated pair had made their hands sweat. We learned quickly to simply slide a new glove on the old, compounding the issues with tactile sensation. We knew as well which schools provided us with cheap gloves that were prone to rip when placed over one another. Some of us grew so frustrated by a new box of gloves, since locating a cuff among all the fingers was impossible, that we would pull them out in bunches and lay them on clean paper towels. This practice helped cut down on the students' discomfort. Instead of being forced to fumble with the box while their peers watched, they could easily pick up clean gloves.

My chapter thus demonstrates that the materiality of gloves gives touch its context: to wear gloves for a pelvic exam is to signal that you care about the health of your other participant and, more importantly, than you are a professional carrying out clinical work. Gloves, however, do nothing innately. Their meaning as material objects and the effects they can enact as a result depends upon other material, symbolic, and affective elements. Thus, in this way, the glove as a material object in the pelvic exam fosters some forms of connection (i.e. allowing the examination of the vagina, cervix, uterus and ovaries) and disallows others (i.e. emotional or sexual feelings, touching of other 'dirty' surfaces). This is most evident in how they render intimate touch nonsexual and distinctly professional.

Acknowledgements

Thank you to the Alice J. Dan Dissertation Research Award of the University of Illinois at Chicago for funding. Thank you to Danielle Giffort and Paige L. Sweet for comments on the draft.

References

Ahmed, Sara (2015), *The Cultural Politics of Emotion*, New York: Routledge.

Barker-Benfield, G. J. (2004), *The Horrors of the Half-known Life: Male Attitudes toward Women and Sexuality in 19th Century America*, New York: Routledge.

Blei, Daniela (2018), 'Women are reinventing the long-despised speculum', *The Atlantic*. 8 March, https://www.theatlantic.com/technology/archive/2018/03/women-redesigning-speculum/555167/. Accessed 24 November 2021.

Cooper Owens, Deirdre Benia (2017), *Medical Bondage: Race, Gender, and the Origins of American Gynecology*, Athens: University of Georgia Press.

Dugoff, Lorraine, Pradhan, Archana, Casey, Petra, Dalrymple, John L, Abbott, Jodi F., Buery-Joyner, Samantha D., Chuang, Alice, Cullimore, Amie J., Forstein, David A. and Hampton, Brittany S. (2016), 'Pelvic and breast examination skills curricula in United States medical schools: A survey of obstetrics and gynecology clerkship directors', *BMC Medical Education*, 16:314, pp. 1–7.

Emerson, Joan (1970), 'Behavior in private places: Sustaining definitions of reality in gynecological examinations', in Hans P. Dreitzel (ed.), *The Production of Reality: Essays and Readings on Social Interaction*, New York: Macmillan, pp. 74–96.

Gimlin, Debra (2007), 'What is "body work"? A review of the literature', *Sociology Compass*, 1:1, pp. 353–70.

Giuffre, Patti A., and Williams, Christine L. (2000), 'Not just bodies: Strategies for desexualizing the physical examination of patients', *Gender & Society*, 14:3, pp. 457–82.

Haraway, Donna J. (1997), 'The virtual speculum in the new world order', *Feminist Review*, 55:1, pp. 22–72.

Harris, Anna (2016), 'Listening-touch, affect and the crafting of medical bodies through percussion', *Body & Society*, 22:1, pp. 31–61.

Henslin, James M. and Biggs, Mae A. (1971), 'Dramaturgical desexualization: The sociology of the vaginal examination', in *Studies in the Sociology of Sex*, New York: Appleton-Century-Crofts, pp. 243–72.

Kline, Wendy (2010), *Bodies of Knowledge: Sexuality, Reproduction, and Women's Health in the Second Wave*, Chicago: University of Chicago Press.

Morgen, Sandra (2002), *Into Our Own Hands: The Women's Health Movement in the United States, 1969–1990*, Rutgers: Rutgers University Press.

Murphy, Michelle (2012), *Seizing the Means of Reproduction: Entanglements of Feminism, Health, and Technoscience*, Durham: Duke University Press.

Oakeshott, Pippa and Hay, Philip (2006), 'Commentary: Best practice in primary care', *BMJ*, 333, pp. 173–74.

Pardes, Arielle (2017), 'The speculum finally gets a modern redesign', *WIRED Magazine*, 5 October, https://www.wired.com/story/the-speculum-finally-gets-a-modern-redesign/. Accessed 24 November 2021.

Posner, Glenn D. (2015), 'The quandary of the sacred vagina: Exploring the value of gynaecological teaching associates', *Medical Education*, 49:12, pp. 1179–80.

Ricci, James Vincent (1949), *The Development of Gynaecological Surgery and Instruments*, Philadelphia: Blakiston.

Roden, Richard B. S. and Lowy, Douglas R. and Schiller, John T. (1997), 'Papillomavirus is resistant to desiccation', *Journal of Infectious Diseases*, 176:4, pp. 1076–79.

Sabeena, Sasidharanpillai, Bhat, Parvati, Kamath, Veena and Arunkumar, Govindakarnavar (2017), 'Possible non-sexual modes of transmission of human papilloma virus', *Journal of Obstetrics and Gynaecology Research*, 43:3, pp. 429–35.

Seehusen, Dean A., Johnson, Dawn R., Earwood, J. Scott, Sethuraman, Sankar N., Cornali, Jamie, Gillespie, Kelly, Doria, Maria, Farnell, Edwin and Lanham, Jason (2006), 'Improving women's experience during speculum examinations at routine gynaecological visits: Randomised clinical trial', *British Medical Journal*, 333:7560, p. 171.

Shalby, Colleen (2018), 'Is that normal? What to expect during a visit to the gynecologist', *Los Angeles Times*, 25 June, https://www.latimes.com/science/sciencenow/la-sci-sn-gynecologist-exam-basics-20180625-story.html. Accessed 17 May 2022.

Snorton, C. Riley (2017), *Black on Both Sides: A Racial History of Trans Identity*, Minneapolis: University of Minnesota Press.

Tillman, Stephanie (2016), 'Empowering gynecologic exams: Speculum care without stirrups', *Feminist Midwife*, 2 November, http://www.feministmidwife.com/2016/11/02/empowering-gynecologic-exams-speculum-care-without-stirrups/#.XrrAGURKiUk. Accessed 5 December 2020.

Twigg, Julia (2000), 'Carework as a form of bodywork', *Ageing & Society*, 20:4, pp. 389–411.

Underman, Kelly (2020), *Feeling Medicine: How the Pelvic Exam Shapes Medical Training*, New York: New York University Press.

Vinson, Alexandra H. and Underman, Kelly (2020), 'Clinical empathy as emotional labor in medical work', *Social Science and Medicine*, 251:112904, pp. 1–9,

Washington, Harriet A. (2006), *Medical Apartheid: The Dark History of Medical Experimentation on Black Americans from Colonial Times to the Present*, New York: Doubleday Books.

Young, Katharine Galloway (1997), *Presence in the Flesh: The Body in Medicine*, Cambridge: Harvard University Press.

HANDBOOKS

CHINESE MEDICAL ILLUSTRATIONS AND COMMUNIST MATERIALISM, 1950–66

Lan A. Li

Though medical canons often discussed the heart, liver, lungs, kidneys and spleen in classical Chinese sources like the *Huangdi Neijing* corpora and the *Shanghan Lun*, the same organs did not always take the same form across textual and graphic representations. Often, the heart and lungs sat in the chest; but there, they could swell or shrink on the page. The heart sometimes appeared slim, sometimes appeared bulbus. The lungs sometimes looked like large leaves, sometimes looked like thick thighs. Illustrators were less interested in realism – that was a concern for master artists. Instead, medical images were technical images that established particular rules within East Asian graphic genres (Bray et al. 2007). Technical images were meant to show less. Organs thus took the form of schematic drawings that presented an empty image to invite the imagination. While images in excessive detail seized the imagination, simple images liberated the mind.

The medical illustrator Wang Xuetai (1925–2008) understood the need for imagination. He had been commissioned to illustrate anatomical images for a textbook sponsored by Chinese Communist Party members in the 1950s. Yet Chinese medical anatomy, which included the heart, liver, lungs, kidneys and spleen, also included organs unknown in other medical fields, such as the triple burner, a membranous tissue that did not translate well (Lei 2012). These organs, both known and unknown, were connected to paths in the body known as *jingluo* 经络,

which have been translated as 'vessels', 'channels' and 'tracts'. These vessels were like cartographic meridians in that they guided physicians to locate therapeutic sites in the body. They resembled cartographic meridians in that they often moved depending on the time of day and one's physical orientation, both physical and ephemeral (Hsu 2010). Wang as an illustrator then needed to find the right kind of image – the right kind of body – to represent these flexible paths. He began by tracing the body of doughy Confucian scholars before creating his own template of muscular men, each version made in service of translating meridian paths to his readers.

Consider Wang's illustration of a muscular man in Figure 11.1. The man looked directly at the viewer and leaned to one side, his back leg supporting the weight of his body. He was in classic contrapposto. A single line stretched from the tip of his toe and moved up his leg. Small arrows on either side of the path directed it through a series of dots. The line continued along the man's calf, up to his thigh, and across his hip. The line then took a turn, dipping into the man's abdomen before moving back to the outer edge of the chest and into his throat. A profile view showed the path continuing up to his throat and ending at the tip of his tongue. This was the spleen meridian. Or, more literally translated, it was an image of the major-foot-Yin-spleen meridian or *zu taiyin pi jing*. Towards the end of the path, a target marked the centre of the man's abdomen with the character 脾 for 'spleen'.

Printed in 1966, the spleen meridian was one of 60 other images that appeared in a small handbook titled *Acupuncture Moxabustion Handbook*. The pocket-sized guide contained detailed instructions for preparing acupuncture needles, determining the appropriate angle for incision, and the procedure for condensing and burning dried mugwort (Wang 1966). Also known as moxabustion, cauterising the skin was another longstanding technique used alongside acupuncture. Wang's images identified the sites for applying acupuncture needles and burning moxa. They listed individual meridian paths with descriptions of their function that Wang collected from classical texts and empirical studies.

Wang's images were unusual. They were unusual in that his series of meridian men was one of the first to appear in this aesthetic form, with male bodies depicted in this way. For the first time, meridian men were muscular and lean. They took the form of dismembered Roman statues. Simple markings that articulated the knee, groin, chest and shoulders graphically associated these new meridian men with classical European

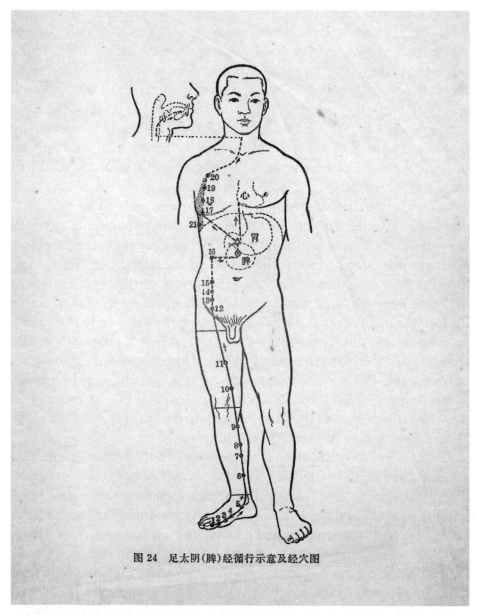

图 24　足太阴(脾)经循行示意及经穴图

Figure 11.1: Xuetai Wang, 'Diagram of the path and sequence of the major-foot Yin spleen meridian' (zu taiyin [pi] jing xun xing shiyi ji jing xue tu 足太阴 [脾] 经循行示意及经穴图), illustration for *Acupuncture and Moxabustion Handbook* (Wang 1966: 71).

graphic genres. These images invoked the spirit of Renaissance realism, which had characterised Andreas Vesalius's famous *De Humani Corporis Fabrica* (1543) and later Henry Gray's *Gray's Anatomy* (1859). Graphic details made the spleen meridian an anatomical figure. Although the man's skin did not peel away to reveal layers of tissue, the viewer could see into his body and appreciate the spleen, stomach and heart.

Wang Xuetai had presented these new versions of meridian men to translate meridians through classical European graphic realism. Schools of classical Chinese painting were also known for their detailed realism, but this impulse did not apply to technical drawings. Though Wang's technical images were not the first to take inspiration from European texts, he was one of the first to apply these graphic references to meridian men. It justified the inclusion of meridian men in Chinese anatomical education. It also represented Communist dialectical materialism, insofar as Communist dialectical materialism was related to Communist Chinese and Communist Soviet scientific discourse. The recent success of the China Communist Party in the late 1940s reinforced political alliances that dictated the terms of knowledge production and reproduction (Andrews 2015). Chinese scientists had turned to their Soviet counterparts in Russia for models of the material body, translating and printing tens of thousands of manuals on needling and heating techniques that resonated with a shared materialist – and uniquely Communist – ideology.

For instance, Wang and his contemporaries drew on the work of Ivan Pavlov (1849–1936), who investigated the material components of the mind and the soul. For Pavlov, the idiosyncratic body expressed itself through physiological responses – through conditional reflexes. These were basic reactions such as the excretion of gastric juices in response to external stimuli, including fragrances, buzzing sounds and electric shocks. While the elderly Pavlov began his work long before the formation of the Russian Communist Party, the Party had adopted Pavlovian research into a broader Communist–materialist ideology (Todes 2014). So, too, did Wang and his contemporaries build on Pavlov's work decades after his death.

Articulating the materiality of ephemeral connections in the body undergirded Communist materialist inquiry. Chinese Communist materialism, meanwhile, stood to maintain a cultural legacy of 'traditional' images from classical texts alongside new 'modern' ones. Illustrators then drew multiple versions of the body. To this end, Wang used his muscular meridian men to reconfigure Chinese medical bodies. It was not that classical Chinese medicine did not have anatomical figures. They did (Kuriyama 2002). The second century BCE corpus, known as the *Huangdi Neijing*, or *Yellow Emperor's Inner Canon* offered detailed descriptions of the body's inner organs and inner movements (Lo and Barrett 2018). Thousands of historical manuscripts contained images (Wang and Fuentes 2018). Medical treatises from the eleventh century made special reference to prints that displayed the oesophagus, lungs, heart, stomach, kidneys, liver, gallbladder, bladder and their surrounding membranes. Organs were organised based on a particular cosmology. Half of the major organs in the body were classified as Yang; the other half were classified as Yin. Half of the Yang organs were major; the other half were minor. Half of the Yin organs were major; the other half were minor. For instance, the *Inner Canon* explained that among the major Yin organs, the spleen was the most Yin of the Yin vessels (Unschuld 2016: 53).

As objects of history, meridians were illustrated on specific kinds of bodies. They portrayed scholars, sages, officials and monks who were standing, sitting or gesturing. These were not Greek gods. They were divine bodies of a different kind. A version of these classic meridian men appeared in Wang Xuetai's first rendition of the spleen meridian in 1950, seen in Figure 11.2. The block of characters above the image read, 'Diagram of the major-foot Yin spleen meridian' or *zu taiyang pi jing tu*. This man looked soft and round, with arms and legs slightly bent; his face turned towards the viewer. Wang had copied him from a version of the fourteenth-century classic, *Treatise of the Fourteen Meridians*, first published in the Ming dynasty (1368–1644). Among the fourteen men and the fourteen meridians from the fourteenth century text, this spleen man looked generically Chinese – a complex cultural identity, to be sure. He could have been a Confucian scholar with his hair secured in a tight bun and beard and moustache neatly groomed. The spleen meridian now started on the right foot. It again initiated from the tip of the toe, continued up the leg, and over the hip. Only this time, it made no detours and terminated under the armpit and not in the mouth.

Wang Xuetai traced this image shortly after he graduated from medical school. As a young physician, he was approached by the Vice Minister of Health for the Chinese Communist Party, Zhu Lian (1909–78), who herself was recently inspired by the therapeutic effects of acupuncture. Zhu had treated her own sciatica with surprising results before treating other top Communist cadres for fatigue and insomnia. Zhu developed

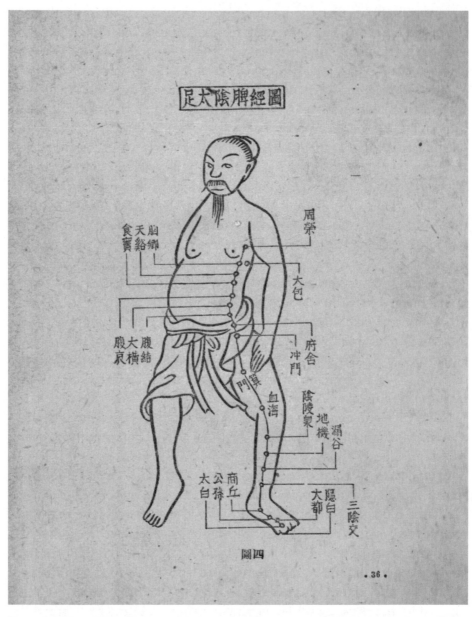

Figure 11.2: Xuetai Wang, 'Diagram of the major-foot Yin spleen meridian' (*zu taiyang pi jing tu* 足太阴脾经图), illustration for *New Approaches to Acupuncture Moxabustion* (Zhu 1950: 36).

a series of lecture notes, and her colleagues urged her to write a book. So, she did (Zhu 1950). She gathered a team of experts, including the young Wang Xuetai, who joined the team in 1948, to publish *New Approaches to Acupuncture Moxabustion* in 1950. Wang was the primary illustrator.

New Approaches to Acupuncture Moxabustion was not completely new. Revised manuals and books on acupuncture and moxabustion had appeared in the Republican period decades before, in the 1930s (Lei 2016). Despite this, Zhu Lian intended to make a pedagogical and political statement with *New Approaches*. It made the false claim that the Communist Party alone upheld China's cultural legacy, unlike its predecessors who had tried to eliminate it. Zhu Lian had taken her own call to action from a 1944 meeting in Yan'an, where regional government officials fashioned a slogan to render Chinese medicine 'scientific' and western medicine 'popular'. *New Approaches* aimed to do both (Taylor 2005).

Helping to sustain this narrative, Wang Xuetai studied and traced many images of early modern meridian men in addition to creating lithographs of écorché hands, heads and arms. These anatomical bodies made medical knowledge accessible. At least, it was made accessible based on the terms of the Communist Party that encouraged readers to recognise a text's content on the one hand and modernity's virtues on the other (Schmalzer 2016).

Zhu Lian and her team published a second edition of *New Approaches to Acupuncture Moxabustion* in 1954 (Zhu 1954). In this edition, Wang Xuetai produced a new set of images. Meridian men looked different. They appeared in colour. They had finer features. The major-foot-Yin-spleen meridian appeared on a man with red lips, seen in Figure 11.3. He had a blue handkerchief tied to his head and wore a blue patterned robe secured with a red sash. The spleen meridian, now red, began at the tip of the man's right toe, moved up his inner thigh, and passed his hips. In this version, the spleen meridian took a turn at the torso, folding into the belly before returning back to the edge of the torso, under the armpit, and up the neck. Zhu Lian claimed again that Wang had copied the image from the Ming dynasty classic, *Treatise of the Fourteen Meridians*. But it is more likely that Wang had found another version of the *Treatise of Fourteen Meridians* from the Qing dynasty (1636–1912). These versions showed the spleen meridian splintering in the centre of the abdomen, which more closely resembled other sets of meridian men printed in Japan during the Edo period (Huang 2003). It was this 1954 spleen meridian, its detour on the stomach and its lengthened path, that Wang

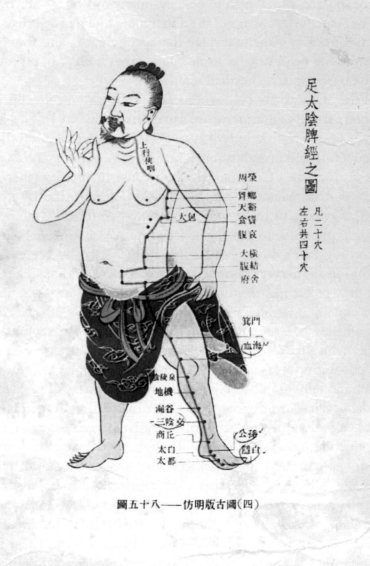

Figure 11.3: Xuetai Wang, 'Image of the major-foot Yin spleen meridian' (*zu taiyin pangguang jing zhi tu* 足太阳膀胱经之图), illustration to *New Approaches to Acupuncture Moxabustion* (Zhu 1954: 337–40).

used to create his own version of the image in 1966. As they continued to collaborate, Zhu began to edit out many of Wang's illustrations. She did not care for drawings of meridian men. She insisted that illustrators did not need to visually display therapeutic paths and sites (Ma 1952). Illustrations need not be so nostalgic. They need not reproduce paths from classical texts. They had science.

Like many of her colleagues in the 1950s, Zhu turned to her Soviet counterparts for alternative explanations (Fan 2013). She also leaned heavily on the translations of Ivan Pavlov's work to explain the effects of acupuncture and moxabustion. Zhu, like her contemporaries, announced that Pavlov was a Communist ally because his theory reflected the 'dialectical materialism' in nearly all fields of scientific practice (Zhang 2015). Pavlov and his many collaborators empirically interrogated observable phenomenon to speculate on unseen connections in the body. According to Pavlov, sensations were mediated by the excitation and inhibition of nerves. These connections were perhaps like attractions within a polarising magnetic field or more like a gravitational pull – each equally invisible, but understood through its effects. Zhu applied the same logic to acupuncture and moxabustion. She replaced meridians with Pavlovian descriptions of nervous function. In doing so, she denied the possibility of a classically Chinese epistemology in favour of this transnational Communist–materialist ideology. To Zhu, the unseen potential of nervous physiology was *more* material than meridians.

Wang disagreed. Images of meridians were essential to learning acupuncture and moxabustion. Though the therapeutic techniques of acu-moxa appeared unremarkable, the images of meridian men were uniquely 'Chinese'. Meridian men represented a broader cosmology. Meridian paths had specific names for specific orientations. The Yin meridians moved through the lungs, pericardium, heart, kidneys, liver and spleen. The Yang meridians moved through the small intestine, a membranous organ called the triple burner, large intestine, bladder, gallbladder and stomach. They started in the hands or the feet. The spleen meridian always began in the big toe. It always moved from the foot up through the leg. It was also always the most Yin of the Yin meridians. Wang Xuetai appreciated these longstanding descriptions of meridians. It was not that tradition was unchanging. Chinese medicine as a 'tradition' had been recently invented (Lei 2016). Still, meridian maps were ontological objects, epistemic guides. They defended a kind of cultural legacy and political imperative.

Despite their divergence, Zhu and Wang's modernist visions both represented different attempts to articulate physiology as anatomy that extended from a transnational Communist–materialist ideology. As Zhu Lian tried to emphasise the accuracy of lines as dots as nothing more than lines and dots, Wang relied on the material representation of meridians to explore its reach to other destinations that could never be drawn on the page. In other words, discourses of accuracy relied on rendering meridians as anatomical structures that invoked hundreds of invisible paths targeting many more unmarked destinations.

Wang Xuetai never signed his illustrations. No one did. Unlike paintings, technical diagrams were not scholarly work (Bray et al. 2007). These were works that belonged to the public. As Wang became independent of Zhu, he continued to compare, trace, and draw images. For Wang, the muscular template was another means for articulating meridian paths. In the *Acupuncture Moxabustion Handbook* (1966), he accompanied each muscular meridian man with a quote from a classical text. For the spleen meridian, he included a direct quote from a special section in the *Yellow Emperor's Inner Canon* that described the path moving from the toes, the legs, the hip, dispersing in the stomach, climbing up the diaphragm, reaching into the neck and ending in the tongue (Wang 1966). Drawing a new kind of body allowed Wang to superficially carve a new meridian path. In doing so, his images took on social and cultural currency that superficially supported discourses of Communist materialism.

Still, beneath that was a deeper tension. Wang's new images of meridian men both validated classical templates and rendered them obsolete. It was this paradox that continued to undergird debates on the role of meridians in Chinese medical anatomy. These tensions were made real in textbook images that reproduced muscular meridian men alongside bulbous ones; classical illustrations of spleens alongside biomedicalised structures. They continued to contribute to an orientalist tension between an imagined 'east' in antiquity and an imagined 'west' in modernity. In the 1950s, Communist discourses of dialectical materiality supported perspectives that both dismissed and reinforced 'traditional' anatomy. While Zhu Lian deferred to the invisibility of conditional reflexes, Wang Xuetai maintained the invisibility of *jingluo* 经络. Both Zhu and Wang justified their approaches as examples of dialectical materiality. They only diverged in their choice of invisible systems. But among these invisible systems, *jingluo* 经络 emerged as the only invisible structure that Wang continued to illustrate on paper. Whether on doughy Daoist bodies or muscular men, Wang's images communicated a kind of modernity that required conceptual negotiation between the invisible and the material, between the unseen and the illustrated.

References

Andrews, Bridie (2015), *The Making of Modern Chinese Medicine, 1850–1960*, Honolulu: University of Hawai'i Press.

Bray, Francesca, Dorofeeva-Lichtmann, Vera and Métailié, Georges (2007), *Graphics and Text in the Production of Technical Knowledge in China: The Warp and the Weft*, Leiden: Brill.

Fan, Ka Wai (2013), 'Pavlovian theory and the scientification of Acupuncture in 1950s China', in P. Cheng and K. W. Fan (eds), *New Perspectives on the Research of Chinese Culture*, Singapore: Springer, pp. 137–45.

Hsu, Elisabeth (2010), *Pulse Diagnosis in Early Chinese Medicine: The Telling Touch*, Cambridge: Cambridge University Press.

Huang, Longxiang (2003), *Atlases of Chinese Acupuncture Moxabustion History (Zhongguo Zhenjiu Shi Tujian)*, Qingdao: Qingdao Press.

Kuriyama, Shigehisa (2002), *The Expressiveness of the Body and the Divergence of Greek and Chinese Medicine*, New York: Zone Books.

Lei, Sean Hsiang-lin (2012), 'Qi-transformation and the steam engine: The incorporation of western anatomy and re-conceptualisation of the body in nineteenth-century Chinese medicine', *Asian Medicine*, 7:2, pp. 319–57.

Lei, Sean Hsiang-lin (2016), *Neither Donkey nor Horse: Medicine in the Struggle over China's Modernity*, Chicago: University of Chicago Press.

Lo, Vivienne and Barrett, Penelope (2018), *Imagining Chinese Medicine*, Leiden: Brill.

Ma, Jixing (1952), *Anatomical Cìjī Chart for Stimulating Acupuncture-Moxabustion Points (Zhēnjiǔ Zhìliáo Diǎn Jiěpōu Wèizhì Cānkǎo Tú)*, Beijing: Beijing College of Chinese Medicine and Technology at the People's Central Government Ministry of Health.

Schmalzer, Sigrid (2016), *Red Revolution, Green Revolution: Scientific Farming in Socialist China*, Chicago: University of Chicago Press.

Taylor, Kim (2005), *Chinese Medicine in Early Communist China, 1945–1963: A Medicine of Revolution*, New York: Routledge.

Todes, Daniel (2014), *Ivan Pavlov: A Russian Life in Science*, Oxford: Oxford University Press.

Unschuld, Paul (2016), *Nan Jing: The Classic of Difficult Issues*, Berkeley: University of California Press.

Wang, Shumin and Fuentes, Gabriel (2018), 'A survey of images from the Chinese medical classics', in F. Bray, V. Dorofeeva-Lichtmann and G. Métailié (eds), *Imagining Chinese Medicine*, Leiden: Brill, pp. 29–50.

Wang, Xuetai (1966), *Acupuncture-Moxibustion Handbook (Zhenjiu xue shouce)*, Beijing: People's Medical Publishing House.

Zhang, L., (2015), *Zhu Lian and Acupuncture Moxabustion (Zhulian yu zhenjiu)*, Beijing: People's Medical Publishing House.

Zhu, Lian (1950), *New Approaches to Studying Acupuncture-Moxabustion (Zhenjiu Xue)*, Beijing: People's Medical Publishing House.

Zhu, Lian (1954), *New Approaches to Studying Acupuncture-Moxabustion (Zhenjiu Xue)*, Beijing: People's Medical Publishing House.

HEARTS

THE HEART OF THE SIMULATED MATTER: INTERPROFESSIONAL TRAINING AND PRACTICES OF CLINICAL CARE

Ivana Guarrasi

This chapter is a critical reflection on the failing heart of a simulated patient. In a patient-actor's portrayal of a massive heart attack in the medical simulation laboratory, the simulated heart takes centre stage as a shared object of patient care around which medical, nursing and pharmacy students coordinate their interprofessional clinical skills training. This failing heart is not a bodily organ whose condition can be visually observed. Its elevated heart rate cannot be detected by palpating the wrist or carotid artery, and its abnormal sound cannot be auscultated with a stethoscope. Yet, this simulated heart is seriously ill and must be treated. By tracing the emergent and distributed materiality of the collective making of the simulated heart across both material objects and the coordination of skilled bodies, I show how biomedical knowledge and professional skills are reproduced through the dramaturgical organisation of clinical skills training. Breaking apart the fixity of professional scripts, participants in a simulation produce the existence of the same imagined heart through the joint coordination of different embodied performances of professional knowledge, role and vision, without collapsing into an indeterminate 'we'.

Using humans as patient surrogates in the training and standardised testing of clinical skills has become *de rigueur* over the past few decades in the United States, where my research is set, as well as other places around the world. Medical educators call a person, often an actor, trained to simulate a medical problem a 'standardised patient' (SP). Before interacting with students in a live simulation, SPs are carefully trained to perform disease processes and convey medical history, physical findings and emotional states in a consistent, repeatable manner for different students. They know how a doctor or nurse should talk to patients, how to touch their bodies, how to explain care, and what are the specific clinical skills medical, nursing, and pharmacy students are trained to master in each simulated scenario. Many SPs could give more compelling and expressive performances, but they are trained to hold back. Although students are asked to interact with SPs as if they were real patients, SP performers' acting skills are neither a priority for healthcare educators, nor part of the official SP training. Pointing to SPs actor's craft would delegitimise SP training methodology since medical education in the United States has relied increasingly upon methods of scientific management, standardisation procedures and measurable competencies.

My analysis here speaks to the limitations of such reductive practices. Exploring the complex and uncertain *simulated matter* of interprofessional expertise, I address the problem of how different healthcare professionals are trained to work, coordinate, and communicate in a team around a moment that is happening faster than any patient is prepared for. I show that in the context of Interprofessional Education (IPE) it is the SP's professional expertise that allows the student doctors, nurses and pharmacists to coordinate their dynamic moment-to-moment living through the unfolding activity of their interprofessional teamwork. By trivialising SP's actor's craft, and other resources that SP performers bring into simulations, the healthcare community might overlook what SP simulations can introduce into the training repertoire of a new generation of healthcare professionals. The imaginary heart of the SP does not simply simulate the anatomy and biomedical functioning of the heart; it simulates the practice of performing professional clinical skills on – and with – the body of the standardised patient.

I draw on the concept of 'professional vision' to develop a practice-based account of *interprofessional vision*. According to Charles Goodwin, the ability to see the things that matter in any profession is not a property of the eye or brain, but rather a property of 'systematic discursive practices, [such as] coding schemes, highlighting, and the articulation of material representations' (Goodwin 1994: 606), by which professionals demonstrate competence in their profession. He shows how the competent use of these discursive practices allows archaeologists, lawyers, and police officers to see – and help others see – the phenomenal objects of professional interest. I argue that interprofessional vision emerges when professional scripts, roles, and expertise, clash: it develops in the activity of making sensible the different professional perspectives as they intersect in one simulation to form a system of rearranged professional relations between students.

My argument develops an account of interprofessional vision as, first and foremost, bound up in the bodily interactions with others. The goal here is to identify the moments of the collective making of the imaginary heart – the moments of the heart's making as a living organ, grounded in the heart's biochemical, sociocultural and technological materiality, that makes itself known as a system of coordinated, constantly unfolding relations. An intersubjective mapping of the heart of an SP, that all participants inhabit during a simulation encounter, becomes a pathway for the re-ordering of their professional visions and embodied subjectivities. But this intersubjectivity is not only established by means of 'you' and 'I' engaging in co-existing relations but also through 'the public nature of perceptual objects', which are perceived by the self as well as other subjects, and thus they are 'intersubjectively accessible' (Zahavi 2001:155–56).

My analysis focuses upon the 'ethno' methods of an SP actor and students to reveal how they endogenously co-construct and understand their experiences of interprofessional vision. The basic premise of ethnomethodological method (Garfinkel 1988) postulates that there is an order in everyday activities, something which has already been organised by the participants following their 'common-sense' (Schuetz 1953) interpretations into procedures and forms of action.

Following a brief description of a clinical simulation script, the chapter is structured around a 'real time' description of participants' intersubjective encounters in simulation to emphasise the lived experiences of an SP actor and student teams. I first describe the intake in the clinic, and then the patient's transfer to the emergency department, where a second student team assumes care of the patient. My analysis of the video recorded simulation training is anchored in the perspective of the students from a post-simulation formative debriefing. The narrative is orchestrated as a performance of the script from the points of view of various professions: an actor performing the standardised patient, a medical student, a nursing student and a pharmacy student. These excerpts are interlaced with interpretative engagements of a social scientist, who is reading the script, viewing the video recordings, and conducting interviews to write this chapter.

Simulating heart attack

The nine-page-long training script for the SP actor includes a clinical case called 'Mark Reynolds'. Mark is a 49-year-old, former semi-pro golfer who presents to the clinic after experiencing two episodes of chest pain earlier in the day. He is 178 cm and weighs 82 kg. The clinical script includes a detailed description of Mark's family medical history, education, work, personal life, friends, what he eats, how much he drinks, and his exercise routine, even mentioning of his being 'Presbyterian… because I married one' – emphasising a close relationship with his wife. The most detailed section of the script is a step-by-step description of how the simulation scenario develops, first in a primary care clinic room and then in the Emergency Department (ED).

> Justin, an SP actor, reviews the script. I am meeting Justin for an interview on the university campus, as he had agreed to speak with me about his experiences.

> Justin: We go in like we are short of breath, and we have all this pale make-up and act like we cannot catch our breath. So the students are supposed to, like, do our blood pressure, listen to heart, lungs, and all of that. And they took us into the Emergency Room and they have actually, like, a fake arm set up, so they can do an IV, and there is actually fake blood in the arm, so, when they put the IV the blood came out… So it is pretty intense! They hooked me up to everything, so… I found it to be, as an actor, very emotional, because I immersed myself into that situation. It's like if, you know, if you think about the loved ones, you think about what you're doing, you think about – you know – 'Oh my gosh, I am having a heart attack, am I about to die!' You know, you start thinking about, 'Oh is this it?' It became very emotional! Plus we had to mimic, or, um, you know, create shortness of breath. So breathing like [forces his breath in and out repeatedly]. Where you get light-headed when you do that. But I was actually – tears veiled up my

eyes about three or four times during the event 'cuz, you know, I was into this guy who's got ready to check out, maybe. And he didn't know what's going on. It's pretty scary!

The SP's professional expertise

Although it has been recognised by the medical community that the cultural and social dimensions of medical simulation shape learning outcomes, healthcare simulations continue to be designed around psychometric research (i.e. Brennan and Johnson 1995) to evaluate the quality of clinical skills training and students' competence. Using assessment checklists and rating scales, simulation educators in the United States aim to scale human behaviour down to quantifiable and measurable units by reducing parameters of social behaviour that contribute to variation and contingency by defining them as biases. The work of medical anthropologist Janelle Taylor (2011) on SPs' performance of suffering is premised on a critique of simulation laboratories that are consciously discounting the actual experiences of real people, regarding them as distractions and obstacles to their educational goals. During the planning committee meeting, I attended before the IPE event, some of the healthcare educators expressed their concern that, in past years, SPs were 'being very different' in their portrayal of the selected patient case across groups of students, undermining the fairness of the teaching and assessment event.

For healthcare educators, the variability in SP performance is bias or lack of proper training, in life variability is essential to human behaviour. In his book, *Man's Rage for Chaos*, sociologist Morse Peckham (1967) uses the concept of dramatic metaphor to explain human behaviour. Ascribing to all human behaviour certain aspects of actor's behaviour, he states that the patterns of behaviour appropriate for specific social roles we play are organised around (dramaturgical) scripts for action. But, as he points out, even the most detailed script cannot account for all possible details of future actions. There is always a gap to be filled once individuals perform the script. When individuals learn to follow a pattern of behaviour, they in fact learn how to follow 'the range, the collection of bits which are socially acceptable in a given situation' (Peckham 1967: 58). Justin's account of his professional practice indicates that he needs to be aware and responsive to the always-changing interactional dynamic in the simulated encounter, deciding what behavioural patterns are called for by the clinical scenario script.

What educators deem the SPs' mistake of 'being different' across students is, in fact, the very professional SP quality upon which the teaching event depends. The sense of SP's ability to sustain and be responsive to a set of dynamically articulated social, embodied, and material relations, gives rise to a grounded professional epistemology. But this SP competence is not just the personal, individual experiences between students and the SP. It is 'a concrete expression of a given [socio-cultural] system', since the actors' creative work is not only social in nature but it also creates generally recognisable cultural forms (Vygotsky 1932: 237–41). As I will demonstrate through the case of the 'heart attack' simulation scenario in the next section, SP professional craft contributes the key element around which the student healthcare professionals organise their own in-role training.

Realtime description

On the day of the IPE event, the simulation starts with Justin performing as 'Mark Reynolds' to the 'primary care clinic' at the Medical School, complaining of chest pain. A team of medical personnel enters the room. The clinic team consists of two medical students, Doctor Lian and Doctor Riley; and a nurse, Nurse Jenny. While the students work with the SP in concert with one another for the first time, they are observed by three facilitators, each of whom represents one of the three participating professions – physician, nurse and pharmacist. I watch the clinic encounter unfold via video stream in the Monitoring Room. The laboratory is equipped with advanced simulation and information technology to record the simulation encounters.

> This morning, Mark had been playing golf with a client from a large VIP business account. The pain and pressure began in his chest.
>
> 'The pain was awful,' Mark says to the team in the clinic, grabbing at the center of is chest with his fist. 'I felt dizzy, like I was going to pass out. I had a hard time breathing and had to lay down on the greens.'
> The team performs the physical exam. Nurse Jenny measures his blood pressure. The blood pressure monitor is fixed to read high: 170/95. Doctor Lian performs a cardiac exam. She listens to the heart using

the ventriloscope, a simulation stethoscope modified to reproduce a patient's normal or abnormal auscultatory findings (heart and lung sounds), that can be used on healthy SP actors like Mark. She continues the exam by looking at the neck veins and feet for swelling and checks pulses in his hands and feet.

'I'm worried about your heart,' Doctor Lian says to Mark, and orders an EKG and X-ray. The EKG shows the patient having a serious type of heart attack, during which one of the arteries gets blocked. During the course of the visit, Mark develops a third round of chest pain, prompting the clinic team to arrange a transfer to the emergency department (ED).

'You may be having a heart attack,' Doctor Lian says, touching Mark's shoulder in a kind, empathic gesture, as Mark looks visibly shaken.

The 'Thingness' of the simulated heart

When I invoke caring for the fictionalised heart of the standardised patient, I am not referring to the staging of the heart attack as an illusion, or even to the staging of the laboratory encounter using advanced, high-fidelity simulation technology to achieve effective training. The rigged monitor showing high blood pressure, the ventriloscope for picking up abnormal heartbeats, the electrocardiogram (EKG) fabricated to support a diagnosis of a heart attack, the pale make up painted on the face of the SP, the fake arm allowing the nurse to administer the right dosage of heparin as IV bolus – they all contribute not to an illusion, but to the construction of the heart as simulated *matter* in the laboratory.

Literature in the cultural sociology of medical simulation (Guarrasi 2019; Johnson 2005, 2008; Underman 2015; Pelletier and Kneebone 2016) has established that it is fidelity to the culture of medical practice, discourse, and imaginary, and not the patient body, that makes immersive simulation a valid training tool. In my previous work (Guarrasi 2019), I examined how the standardised patient's body is transformed into an embodied map that systematises, organises, and classifies novices' knowledge into a unified system of clinical practice during the training of the standardised patient. For Ericka Johnson (2008), who studies practices of using high-fidelity pelvic simulators asserts, the high-fidelity simulator is a valid educational tool not because it realistically mimics the body of the patient, but because it authentically represents the body of the patient as experienced by the medical professional. These studies elaborate the epistemology that conceives the simulated body as an object that exceeds its 'objectness' by becoming a thing of simulated action.

The historian of science, Lorraine Daston (2004), asserts that objects are not equivalent to 'things'. She proposes a compelling epistemological framework that disrupts the traditional binary distinction between object and subject. In her view, the 'thing itself' produces different sets of relations in different domains of practice. Aligning my analysis with Daston's injunction to 'capture the thingness of things' (2004: 15), the collective caring for the simulated heart constitutes a new set of interprofessional relations that cohere with, but do not imitate, the established medical practices of treating disease and inhabiting professional identity in the clinic. Mark Reynold's heart functions as a shared cognitive and imaginative marker around which the collective making of the social reality of clinical practice becomes possible. A simulated heart is not an object of medical knowledge that students know from a textbook, but it interpellates their actions as a 'thing'. Tracing the coordination of professional practices of physicians, nurses and pharmacists, in the next section I make visible how the simulated heart lives through the orchestration of different lines of professional attention, skilled bodies, and the collective imagination of the participants.

Realtime description

In the Emergency Department, the second student team assumes care of the patient. The ED team includes Doctor Diane and Doctor Ben, both second-year medical students; Nurse Shelly is a third-year nursing student nearing graduation; Pharmacist Jasmine, a third-year student, has ample experience with simulation-based preparation at the School of Pharmacy. This is everyone's first interprofessional simulation experience. The expected ED treatment plan includes starting a heparin IV based on actual body weight of 180 lbs (82 kg). Heparin is a blood thinner, and the facilitators' guide says that students should administer it as 'IV bolus', meaning to rapidly inject a relatively high dosage of the medication for faster delivery. The infusion should be calculated based on the patient's actual body weight.

Ten minutes into the simulation Doctor Diane says, 'So his blood pressure is starting to look a lot better.'

Doctor Ben says, 'Should we give him heparin yet?'

'Yes!' Pharmacist Jasmine says, emphatically. 'We definitely want to give him heparin!' But she continues to study her medication administration notes with information about the dosage and administration procedures.

Nurse Shelly stands on one side of the bed, looking at the team, waiting.

'It will be a five ml dose of heparin, IV bolus,' Pharmacist Jasmine verbalizes out loud. She hands an IV bag to Nurse Shelly.

Nurse Shelly turns to Mark. 'What is your name and date of birth?'
'Mark Reynolds, May 12, 1971,' says Mark.

Nurse Shelly asks, 'How much heparin?'

Pharmacist Jasmine replies, 'Max 5000 units.'

'Over the first five minutes?' Nurse Shelly asks, attempting to confirm how rapidly she should 'push' the medication into the patient's bloodstream.

Pharmacist Jasmine pauses with a flustered look on her face and looks back down at her medication administration notes. 'I have converted the dosage, I just don't know for how long...' Both physicians join her next to the medication tray. They huddle together for several minutes. Doctor Diane reads the pharmacist's notes. 'It just says it's bolus.'
Nurse Shelly is holding a syringe, ready to inject the medication into Mark's simulated arm. 'Okay, so I am just confirming – I am giving 5,000 units over how much time?'
Everyone is looking at Pharmacist Jasmine. Pharmacist Jasmine is looking at her notes silently. Doctor Diane walks over to her and they are reviewing the notes together.

Doctor Ben turns to Nurse Shelly. 'Let's just hold off! Let's hold off.' For the next couple minutes, Nurse Shelly is standing next to the patient with the syringe ready in her right hand, waiting anxiously for the team to make a decision.

'I think we can go with one bolus,' Doctor Diane finally announces to everyone. 'It just says administer at once.'

'Okay, I just wanted to make sure,' says Nurse Shelly, and administers the shot.

At that point, the ED team students hear an announcement: 'Please proceed to your debriefing room to prepare your handoff and complete your team evaluation forms'. I am invited to join the students and facilitators who are sitting around a conference table in person. Debriefing is designed to deliver formative feedback to both student teams and reflect on the key takeaways from the event. These discussions make visible the markedly different professional visions that students had acquired as a part of their separate specialised educations. Once made visible in the performance of the script, it becomes possible to trace the ways in which their individual funds of knowledge clash with the demands of a real world interprofessional practice. It is in this process that they break away from the scripted versions of their intra-professional training to deal effectively with the controlled chaos of everyday practice.

Jasmine (ED 'pharmacist'): Having the med students come in and do the handoff so rapidly... you are not looking at your paper like when you are doing your usual training. But having to listen to everything and you don't have time to write things down. And then going from okay, do we give this? Did *they* [the clinic team] give this? What do we do next? Because *you have step-by-step in your mind*, but then you kind of have to figure out where to start. I went straight to my drug tray while I should have gone straight to the patient and started with that, or I should have gotten straight to the huddle and started with that. Because the way that we are taught, at least in pharmacy, first of all—*everybody is taught that they do everything by themselves.* So, immediately, me not talking to the patient and getting the entire history already turned me off, because it put me somewhere else in the line *where I'm supposed to be. And then on top of that you have an algorithm that you study in school, but it did not apply.*

The fact that the individual professional scripts available in an explicit form (e.g. as a written protocol of administering medication) that students are trained to follow 'do not fit' the simulated living practice illustrates distinction that Daston (2004) introduced with the notion of 'thingness'. As a physiological object, the student doctors, nurses and pharmacists share a wealth of common textbook knowledge about treating the heart. But seen as part of a culturally organised, scripted yet improvisational orchestration of professional roles, the heart reveals its fundamentally cultural and social nature and allows us to rethink its 'thingness'. The simulated, collectively imagined heart is located in the centre of the dynamic, collective effort to save the life of a whole human. Once the script (e.g. pharmacist's medication administration notes) is performed in coordinated action with the professional roles of others, it emerges in situation as a different 'thing'. As the students pointed out in the debriefing session, their conflicts – the moments of disruption and contested professional visions – as they worked together resulted in a paradigm shift, what Peckham calls the 'psychological insight' of the theater critic (1967: 57) – in how they thought about performing teamwork.

> Shelly (ED 'nurse'): For me it is understanding more the practicality—well—*the roles of each individual provider,* because, I am used to being in the clinic and doing everything on my own. But as Jasmine explained, how *she got the weight in pounds and you have to convert it to kilograms and then dose it out, and that whole thought process*—I would have never—we really don't know about that, and so understanding that, and then translating that into our actual work experience and kind of, like, of understanding why maybe some things take longer than we expect.

According to Jasmine and Shelly's reflection on their situational experience, the professional script they are following cannot be reduced to a list of clinical interventions; rather, in order to appropriately coordinate interprofessional work, the script must be interwoven into individual participants' active abilities to take on the other professions' perspectives and understand their professional roles. Looking at how an IPE simulation is organised and enacted 'as if it was in the theatre' rather than 'as if it was real' allows seeing how each profession conceives the clinical skills necessary to perform their professional role.

> Lian (clinic 'physician'): Hearing you guys dealing with the medications and what is going on in your mind helps me understand how I approach you and talk to you about the next step. *Getting that perspective of seeing the same case through someone else's eyes* is really useful to understand the same situation from a different perspective. So in the future when we work with them, we can think, 'that's why the nurse did that, or that is why the pharmacist did that because they are thinking of this.'

Using a sociocultural approach to learning and human development, Eugene Matusov (1996: 32) elaborates a participatory view of intersubjectivity by shifting the focus from individual action to individual contribution to joint activity at hand by making a distinction between 'having in common' versus 'coordination' of participants' subjectivities. In his view, [t]he metaphor of sharing as "having in common" implies intersubjectivity in a sociocultural activity as a process of unifying or standardising all the participants' contributions' (Matusov 1996: 27). In contrast, understanding the micro-development of intersubjectivity using the lens of 'coordination' allows understanding of interprofessional vision as lodged in the practices of each profession, each with their own optics, treating the heart according to their respective professional scripts and protocols. But these professional roles are not so much reduced representations of clinical skills as they are tools that mediate thinking and experiences in interprofessional activities.

Conclusion

The medical community recognises the importance as well as challenges of training interprofessional collaboration for the development of shared understanding and clarity regarding professional roles in healthcare (Hopwood et al. 2020). Medical, nursing and pharmacy schools have addressed this problem by starting to incorporate interprofessional training into the pre-licensure curriculum. But healthcare educators grapple with the question of how to create simulation training and assessment tools that are responsive to the complex nature of interprofessional skills and its assessment.

This chapter traced the multiple continuities of professional attention as they occur in performance-based simulation, so as to identify moments of the emergence of qualitatively different ways of knowing and doing that resist assessment by checklists that work to guarantee the gold standard of interprofessional teamwork in healthcare. The reproduction of medical knowledge in simulation requires productivities and interprofessional micro-negotiations that are often sidelined or invisible to the frameworks that dominate medical education. The dramaturgical analysis of social interactivity in clinical skills training I discussed here resists the acquisitive model of knowledge, characterised by measurable outcomes. It explored the social practice of engaging in interprofessional simulation as principally an intersubjective phenomenon.

By making the simulated heart of a healthy human actor the central object of my analysis, I evoked a particular form of knowing, and showed that the heart in the IPE simulation is not a mimetic copy of the physiological human heart. Rather, it is a collective, imaginative orienting that gives rise to a contingent, immersive, and distributed paradigm shift in interprofessional vision. It is the shift in the interstices of professionality that makes itself known in its unfolding against the background of other professional visions. Students learn how to remediate their professional skills, scripts, and roles – the institutionalised behaviours they inhabit when trained separately in their own professional silos – into a qualitatively new orchestration of moves. What the interprofessional training event allows each professional is to view the simulated heart as if through a kaleidoscope of joint activity.

Acknowledgements

I thank the organising committee members of the Interprofessional Education simulation event who generously offered their time and expertise during our collaboration. I not only empirically anchored this chapter but also provided invaluable insights on the topic of interprofessional healthcare training and enriched my identity as a scholar. I am indebted to Mike Cole for reading drafts of this chapter and providing me with invaluably sound advice.

References

Brennan, Robert L. and Johnson, Eugene G. (1995), 'Generalizability of performance assessments', *Educational Measurement: Issues and Practice*, 14:4, pp. 9–12.

Daston, Lorraine (2004), 'The glass flowers', in L. Daston (ed.), *Things that Talk: Object Lessons from Art and Science*, Brooklyn: Zone Books and The MIT Press.

Garfinkel, Harold (1988), 'Evidence for locally produced, naturally accountable phenomena of order, logic, reason, meaning, method, etc. in and as of the essential quiddity of immortal ordinary society (I of IV)', *An Announcement of Studies Sociological Theory*, 6, pp. 103–09.

Goodwin, Charles (1994), 'Professional vision', *American Anthropologist*, 96:3, pp. 606–33.

Guarrasi, Ivana (2019), 'Semiotic body of a standardized patient as a map of clinical practice', *Versus – Quadeni di studi semiotici*, 129:2, pp. 333–62.

Hopwood, Nick, Blomberg, Marie, Dahlberg, Johanna and Abrandt Dahlgren, Madeleine (2020), 'Three principles informing simulation-based continuing education to promote effective interprofessional collaboration: Reorganizing, reframing, and recontextualizing', *The Journal of Continuing Education in the Health Professions*, 40:3, pp. 81–88.

Johnson, Ericka (2005), 'The ghost of anatomies past: Simulating the one-sex body in modern medical training', *Feminist Theory*, 6:2, pp. 141–59.

Johnson, Ericka (2008), 'Simulating medical patients and practices: Bodies and the construction of valid medical simulators', *Body & Society*, 14:3, pp. 105–28.

Matusov, Eugene (1996), 'Intersubjectvity without agreement', *Mind, Culture, and Activity*, 3:1, pp. 25–45.

Peckham, Morse (1967), *Man's Rage for Chaos: Biology, Behavior, and the Arts*, New York: Schocken Books.

Pelletier, Caroline and Kneebone, Roger (2016), 'Playful simulations rather than serious games: Medical simulation as a cultural practice', *Games and Culture*, 11:4, pp. 365–89.

Schuetz, Alfred (1953), 'Common-sense and scientific interpretation of human action', *Philosophy and Phenomenological Research*, 14:1, pp. 1–38.

Taylor, Janelle S. (2011), 'The moral aesthetics of simulated suffering in standardized patient performances', *Culture, Medicine, and Psychiatry*, 35:2, pp. 134–62.

Underman, Kelly (2015), 'Playing doctor: Simulation in medical school as affective practice', *Social Science & Medicine*, 136–137, pp. 180–88.

Vygotsky, Lev (1932), 'On the problem of the psychology of the actor's creative work', *Collected Works of L. S. Vygotsky*, 6, pp. 237–44.

Zahavi, Dan (2001), 'Beyond empathy: Phenomenological approaches to intersubjectivity', *Journal of Consciousness Studies*, 8:5–7, pp. 151–67.

ILLUSTRATIONS

PERFORMED WITH CARE: ENACTING ACCURACY IN MEDICAL ILLUSTRATION

Drew Danielle Belsky

On a chilly afternoon in late September, I stand in a windowless and acrid cadaver lab in the basement of a brutish 1970s-era university medical building. A group of first-year biomedical communications students are sketching their most recent dissection from the morning's session. As they draw, the anatomy tutor asks about the drawings in relation to those in their textbook: 'So you scan the drawings and then the computer fills in the colours? How does it know where to put them?' The students laugh and patiently explain, 'It doesn't just do it automatically, we do it. A person colours it.' The anatomy tutor's expression conveys confused amazement, but for the students it is neither the first nor the last time they will need to explain that biomedical visualisations – from textbook drawings to 3D animations – are made by people.

A central paradox of biomedical illustration is that a well-crafted image is one that appears not to have been crafted at all. To understand the role of biomedical visualisations in medical education, one must understand the labour required to make images appear credible, natural and self-explanatory. In a literal sense, biomedical images play a key role in how medical personnel and laypeople alike learn to see bodies. However, the erasure of the material labour involved in the creation of such images leads to an understanding of medical images as unfiltered representations of the scientific truth of bodies. When particular kinds of bodies become naturalised as normal, others are marked as abnormal and in need of correction or elimination. Numerous scholars have argued that the construction of particular kinds of bodies as inherently pathological in medical visual culture results in serious health disparities for people of colour, women, trans and gender-variant people, and disabled people (Bauer et al. 2009; Massie et al. 2019; Parker 2016). Although many critical explorations of medical illustration begin with an image, it is crucial to resist reading images as detached from their making. The material and social practices through which an image comes into being as an object of knowledge are inextricable from its everyday circulation in education, medical and lay contexts. For this reason, my research centres on the human and non-human agencies through which biomedical visualisations are constructed.

My research draws on two years of participant observation and archival research in North American graduate programmes and professional gatherings for medical illustrators, as well as more than twenty interviews with students, faculty and practitioners. As a small, female-dominated profession whose knowledge practices are frequently illegible to outsiders, medical illustrators have struggled to gain recognition as active agents in the production of scientific and biomedical visuals. They distinguish their work from that of machines based on their ability to exercise judgement and selectivity. They emphasise their adherence to scientific values, as opposed to fanciful artistic flourishes, while at the same time differentiating their interpretive labour from what might be achieved mechanically. They substantiate the scientific and factual nature of their work by insisting upon their dedication to 'accuracy' while, at the same time, stressing the instrumental importance of their interpretive and aesthetic skills.

In this chapter, I focus on the social and material construction of 'accuracy' in biomedical visual communications. In order to understand the continued lack of bodily diversity in medical illustrations, I explore the material and social contexts within which medical illustrators create them. I examine the 'accuracy' not as a fixed, measurable attribute of images, but as a quality of human labour, enacted in and through social and material relations. I suggest that the relational practices of accuracy in medical illustration be cultivated as what Maria Puig de la Bellacasa has termed 'matters of care,' turning attention to the 'necessary yet mostly dismissed labours of everyday maintenance of life, an ethico-political commitment to neglected things, and the affective remaking of relationships with our objects' (2011: 100). Treating accuracy in medical education a matter of care may enable both medical illustrators and scholars to more substantively intervene in normative ways of seeing and understanding bodies.

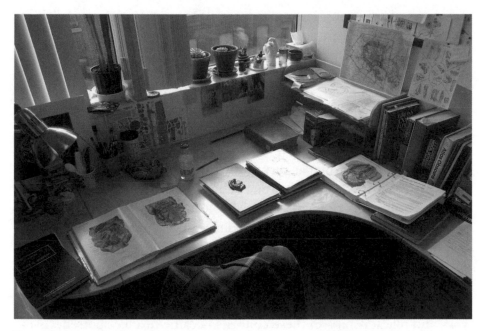

Figure 13.1: Personal workspace of a graduate medical illustration student. Shared computer labs, reference materials, and equipment are located in adjoining rooms within the department. Photo by the author (2017).

Crafting images

Medical illustrators produce images within a complex assemblage of material and social constraints. It is difficult to convey the breadth of practices that make up the field of biomedical communications and visualisation. The increasing technical and technological promiscuity of contemporary medical illustrators is clear in the range of their outputs. It is also tied to shifts in scientific research and inputs from which to draw. Although traditional work such as anatomical and surgical illustration still occurs, it is mainly accomplished using computer-assisted rendering tools and software. Growing demand for work at the molecular level entails frequent recourse to Protein Data Bank models and sophisticated representations of biochemical processes for medical and patient education, research publications, pharmaceutical advertising and science journalism. In addition to direct observation of objects and phenomena, medical illustrators use imaging technologies such as CT scans and MRIs, whose data can be extracted for 3D models. Such models can, in turn, be used to develop applications for learning anatomy, animations explaining surgical procedures, 3D printed surgical models, or even 2D printed illustrations.

Although mastery of the material practices of visualisation is integral to the profession (and comprise a large part of graduate training), shifts in outputs are not merely an effect of changing technologies. The markets and social economies of the work have also shifted. At the beginning of the twentieth century, the bulk of medical illustration work was the result of close, ongoing patronage-like relationships between the illustrator and particular surgeons or anatomists. The work consisted primarily in illustrating the patron's publications, including both articles and large long-term projects, such as book-length surgical and anatomical atlases. By the mid-century, as medical education and hospital medicine were expanding, hospitals and universities began to directly employ full or part-time medical illustrators in service to their medical staff and faculty. Several of these institutionally employed illustrators developed mentorship and training programmes for future medical illustrators. The work and relationships in these contexts became more dispersed, covering an ever-broader range of subjects and output formats. Budget cuts and administrative uncertainty in the 1970s and 1980s led to the decline of these more secure positions and a rise in freelancing and commercial work, which dried up again in the 1990s (Brierley 2013). Although the profession had long been a solitary and piecemeal one for those without a stable institutional position, the latter part of the century presented both greater precarity, as illustrators competed for contracts, and increasing autonomy, especially for those practitioners who were able to keep abreast (or ahead) of trends in graphic technologies.

Most contemporary medical illustrators accept these changes as inevitable, even positive, and understand the ability to assimilate new tools as an essential quality of any good practitioner. Although most cite technological developments as the greatest driver of change in their profession, they are rarely framed as a threat. They adapt to and exploit the affordances of graphical rendering tools rather than compete with them. However, the protean nature of their material practices continues to complicate the boundary-work of distinguishing their work as properly 'scientific', while managing professional boundaries against incursions from scientists, data specialists and non-medically trained artists and designers. Indeed, the most recognisable terms for what they do tend to elide the scope of labour and expertise involved in creating biomedical visualisations. As one practitioner explained:

I try to tell people I'm a medical illustrator cause I often think that that will be simple, but I realize very quickly it isn't cause nobody really knows what that is. [And] to clarify I say have you ever seen a textbook that shows drawings of anatomical specimens? And they'll say, yeah, yeah, yeah. And I'll say okay, well, you know, I do that, but I actually don't do a lot of that. I do something similar to that, so I might build software applications that incorporate visual elements or 3D representations of scientific or anatomical structures. (Respondent 05F)

It is easier to contextualise their work through a set of material practices and outputs than to describe a complex range of cognitive, perceptual and embodied skills. However, explanations based in technologies and artifacts obscure the human labour of their making. They do not convey the interpretive and craft skills that are particular to medical illustrators, making it difficult to articulate their expertise and to assert professional boundaries.

Medical illustrators are thus caught in a double bind. Making biomedical knowledge legible as 'fact' is understood to be the work of machines precisely because the expert labour of medical illustrators lies in naturalising their own artifacts. In the more contemporary context, Lucy Suchman argues that designers of autonomous technologies such as early forms of AI and interactive robots 'evidence a desire to naturalize them, to obscure their artifactuality' (2007: 214). Suchman's argument builds on Steven Shapin and Simon Schaffer's (1985) claim that '[t]he matter of fact can serve as the foundation of knowledge and secure assent insofar as it is not regarded as man-made' (Shapin and Schaffer cited in Suchman 2007: 214). Similarly, in order to 'achieve the appearance of matters of fact as given items' (Shapin 1984: 508), medical illustrations must not appear 'man-made'. As the anatomy tutor's comment demonstrates, the mythos of autonomous technology easily overtakes the messier material and social realities of agentive human medical illustrators. Because the structures and processes conveyed appear self-evident, medical illustrations must be naturally occurring or machine-made reflections of scientific truths, not human-made.

It is not an accident that a field dominated by women is also one where the agency of human practitioners is routinely effaced, their expertise overshadowed by visions of autonomous, value-neutral machines and artifacts which 'speak for themselves'. As historians of science have argued, the emergence of experimentalism in the seventeenth century entailed an emphasis on dispassionate rationality and 'gentlemanliness', casting suspicion on the embodied expertise of both artisans and women (Daston and Galison 2007; Schiebinger 1991; Shapin 1989; Shapin and Schaffer 2011; Smith 2012). The acceptance of biomedical images as objective representations of self-evident scientific truth depends upon this erasure of the human labour involved in their creation. Continued emphasis on the material technologies of making medical knowledge visible and teachable obscures the human agency and power relations invested in those renderings.

Crafting accuracy

For medical illustrators, accuracy is not a measurable quality or a fixed, value-neutral relation to truth but rather a product of human agency and the contexts of both production and reception. It includes not only thorough research and exactitude but also aesthetic, moral and pragmatic judgements emerging in the process of making. This complex process of decision-making must account not only for the fleshly organic matter of biomedicine and available scientific knowledge but also for the affordances of the materials used and the contexts where they will be deployed.

As a statistical concept, accuracy has a well-defined meaning which hinges on a knowable, verifiably 'true' value, or at least the assumption that such a value exists. Usually juxtaposed to 'precision', statistical 'accuracy' denotes a relationship between the measurement obtained and the 'true' value. Precision, on the other hand, refers to the degree of internal consistency between measurements. One is an ontological relationship which assumes a 'real' value (which may or may not be known/knowable), while the other is an epistemological one, intended to account for the variability inherent in the act of measurement itself. As Donald MacKenzie (1999) has explored in relation to nuclear missile testing, the concept of accuracy is subject to changing meanings in practice. Although the word suggests a relationship to truth, that relationship is dependent not only on the truth it purports to approach, but on the contexts of its enactment. According to McKenzie, the accuracy of nuclear missiles is constructed through a complex testing process, but 'whether the results of this process are facts' and whether those facts are transferrable to other contexts (such as from firing on a test range to firing on an enemy) have been repeated sites of controversy and uncertainty (1999: 346). In other words, accuracy is also an epistemological question.

During one interview, a faculty member in a medical illustration graduate programme described a recent encounter with a member of a review committee in the university, in which his data visualisation had been called into question:

> That assumption [that] as kind of visual arts-associated people, as communications people, we don't give a shit about truth and that we're likely to screw something up, that's kind of annoying. [...] That's probably the last thing you should accuse us of. You know, we're very concerned about accuracy and, you know, ultimate truth or whatever. I know, we could have philosophical discussions about whether those things actually exist but we're [...] but that's something we're obviously very concerned about and we're not about [...] you know, we're not about putting [...] lipstick on a pig or something. (Respondent 01F)

His impassioned outburst reflects the deep affective ties between medical illustrators and their work. It also conveys the complexity of accuracy as a concept both fundamental to their work and exceedingly difficult to explain or prove.

The social constraints within which medical illustrators work are deeply embedded in the concept of accuracy. Focusing on the pharmaceutical context, former medical illustrator Meaghan Brierly's (2013) dissertation explores the powerful role of economic and corporate power structures in producing images which illustrators can nevertheless evaluate as 'accurate'. She argues that 'accuracy is managed and entangled across aesthetic decisions, technological choices and the science narrative explained' (Brierly 2013: 175). Illustrations are deemed 'accurate' or 'legitimate' as a result of a lengthy process of negotiation between powerful pharma executives, researchers, art directors, and the illustrator herself. The social, political and cultural contexts of medical illustrators, including the temporal and economic realities of their employment *matter*.

However, accuracy is usually invoked by medical illustrators unproblematically. In their work and in interviews, they repeatedly stressed that 'accuracy is obviously super, super important' (Respondent 10F), with no further explanation. On the surface, the term seems to refer to scientific facticity: objective and legitimate knowledge, correctly obtained. Students, in particular, emphasised the amount of research necessary to be 'accurate'. Yet, when pressed, accuracy entailed far more than precise measurement or a relationship to legitimate knowledge and research:

Interviewer: When you say accuracy, what do you mean by accuracy?

Respondent 7S: Yeah, so that's a major thing that we focus on is accuracy. It's really what separates medical illustrators from just, you know, artists, fine artists. It's because of our accuracy in our work. I think the importance of that is to make sure that what we're conveying actually is beneficial and effective – I'll say effective, actually – because it can go as far as like, even causing maybe a surgeon or something like that to do a procedure wrong if we don't have accuracy in our anatomical illustrations correct. So, in that sense, like what we're doing, it has to be accurate because the way our work is used and what it's used for, for that understanding, really it shapes the outcome in people's lives and their health.

For this recent graduate, to meet moral and instrumental goals – to be 'beneficial and effective' – an illustration must be 'correct'. Tautologically, in order to be correct, it must be beneficial and effective.

Although aesthetic decisions are routinely figured as secondary or even opposed to correct scientific information, they are at the same time fundamental to the work of managing attention and interpretation. Which aspects are beautiful and why is bound up with both rendering skill and the purposiveness of the illustration as a source of reliable knowledge intended for a specific audience. On the one hand, 'there is value in aesthetic beauty. It attracts your eye to [...] the structures that you're meant to be looking at' (Respondent 04F); on the other, one might be obligated to 'eliminate these gorgeous aspects of an illustration in order to have the moment shine through that you're talking about' (Respondent 10F). The knowledge that viewers are expected to gain from the visualisation is a key factor in decision-making, governing both content and style of presentation. In this sense, accuracy is also a matter of negotiating interests and managing meanings toward a particular interpretive result.

Crafting care-full images

Feminist philosopher of science Letitia Meynell (2008) argues that interpretive flexibility is an inherent quality of pictures. She explains that 'there is a flexibility allowing imaginative differences within the constraints of the prescribed imaginings' (Meynell 2008: 17). 'Imaginings' in this context are how the viewer makes sense of marks on the page as standing in for objects or actions in the real world, to the point that they will refer to the image *as the thing* it represents, not as marks on a page (nor as an animation or a representation). The forms that such imaginings and interpretive actions may take are guided not only by the representational conventions which the illustrator chooses to follow or adapt but also by the viewer's prior knowledge and interests, including the representational norms with which the viewer is familiar. The medical illustrator's drive to understand 'the audience' is an attempt to maintain control over the potential imaginings a particular image makes possible.

Unlike many analysts of medical illustrations and visual culture, Meynell is careful to include the agency of illustrators and to account for elements, both social and material, which inform the process of bringing an illustration into being. Inclusion or exclusion of particular details and viewpoints come about through research, negotiation and aesthetic problem-solving, which constitute 'accuracy' for a medical illustrator. Taken as a whole, these inclusions and exclusions 'prescribe the imagined functioning of the system' (Meynell 2008: 23). She concludes that these contexts matter precisely because 'conceptual decisions about what is truly important inform the visual hierarchies that organise the depicted objects and their relations and provide a crucial point for the possible introduction of patriarchal norms' (Meynell 2008: 23). Thus, while the illustrator may intend accuracy when they omit or minimise the clitoris in conventional textbook illustrations of male and female genitalia, they suggest that it and its function are not relevant to reproductive processes. Moreover, these and other aesthetic decisions result in illustrations of male and female genitals which bear little resemblance to one another, obscuring the 'shared developmental history of the clitoris and the penis' and thus reinforcing the 'cultural unintelligibility' of intersexed bodies (Meynell 2008: 23).

As Meynell makes clear, the training of medical vision (and by extension the wider public) through medical illustrations constructs the intelligibility of particular kinds of bodies and relations as 'normal'.

Historians of science Lorraine Daston and Peter Galison (2007) have argued persuasively that medical image-making serves as a form of training the perceptual apparatus. The serious consequences of routinely privileging thin or athletic abled white male hetero- and cis-normative bodies as the standard in medical visuals are well documented (Bauer et al. 2009; Massie et al. 2019; Parker 2016; Schiebinger 1990). Yet despite ample documentation of the problem and its consequences over the last thirty years, little has changed (Parker 2016). The epistemic absences and normalisation of only a narrow (and idealised) set of bodies over all other bodies raise concerns both for longstanding critics and, increasingly, for medical practitioners and illustrators themselves.

Since 2016, the Association of Medical Illustrators (AMI) has undertaken various initiatives to redress the lack of racial diversity within the organisation as well as to address criticisms of medical illustrations themselves. Much of this work has focused on recruiting students from a wider variety of racial and ethnic backgrounds. Those involved with these efforts hypothesise that diversifying the profession will lead to greater diversity in their work. However, if the gender demographics of the field cannot guarantee a lack of sexism in the images they produce, it seems unlikely that a politics of inclusion will achieve substantive shifts in representational practices. As Sara Ahmed argues, the formation of 'diversity' committees and initiatives can 'function as a containment strategy' which ironically 'allow[s] organizations […] to conceal the operation of systematic inequalities' (2012: 53). Just as a predominantly female profession can still produce sexist images, racism in medical visuals will not disappear as a natural and logical result of expanding the racial make-up of the field. The conventions and norms of representation in medicine align a narrow set of athletic white, male bodies with normalcy and situate all others as deviant or problematic. These standards of practice are not only entrenched through long histories of colonialism and sexism but also through the continued organisation of social and material concerns that dictate which objects and relationships are 'truly important' and which are irrelevant or even distracting (Meynell 2008: 23).

When certain bodies are always presented as a neutral, anatomical baseline, then those that deviate become signifiers whose presence and unique characteristics are assumed to carry further meaning. Thus for many illustrators (and their employers), marking a body as female or of a particular ethnic group is understood to be inherently significant to the reading of the image. As one mid-career practitioner explained,

We don't want the person we chose in an illustration to stick out. We want the message to be in the organ that is being shown in the person or the molecule that's floating around their head. We don't want it to be noticeable, so we always pick a white man. You know? It's like, they blend into the background. They are human, you know. That represents all of humans. And the parts associated with women like breasts or the look of Africans, it like, I think as white people in medical illustration, we just think of it as distracting, automatically, you know?. (Respondent F10)

Enacted as a historical and disciplinary convention of representation and signification, the young, athletic white male anatomical body perpetuates and reproduces itself precisely by virtue of already being the standard. Nevertheless, as a 'beneficial and effective' representation of the range of human embodiments, this unmarked 'universal standard body' is quite simply inaccurate (Moore and Clarke 2001: 61).

How then can we account for the complex assemblages of material and social concerns that enable or discourage rendering practices which reflect the full range of human morphology and experience? In her influential 2011 article, 'Matters of care in technoscience', Maria Puig de la Bellacasa suggests that one way to build a more equitable science would be to consider 'matters of fact as processes of entangled concerns' (Puig de la Bellacasa 2011: 89). She proposes a reformulation of 'matters of fact' to 'matters of care', stressing the ethical and affective commitments that inform the ways in which knowledge is made and represented. According to Puig de la Bellacasa, both 'concern' and 'care' derive from the Latin *cura*. Although the Oxford English Dictionary denies this common ancestor, extending etymological tendrils I find that 'accuracy' derives from the Latin *accūrāre*, 'to give attention to, to perform with care' (*OED Online* 2020). If to care suggests, as Puig de la Bellacasa proposes, 'an affective state, a material vital doing, and an ethico-political obligation,' what kinds of medical illustrations might emerge from conceiving of accuracy as a form of care and, on the part of critics, approaching visualisations as artifacts made by humans who care deeply about them (2011: 90)?

Feminist critiques of science have repeatedly called into question the false dichotomy of reason and emotion, emphasising instead the urgency of acknowledging that the 'affective entanglements of inquiry' that compel researchers to pursue their objects of study are integral to scientific ways of knowing (Myers 2015: 5). These affective and embodied investments permeate scientific endeavours, regardless of the research-er's gender; to care about what one studies is a prerequisite to all epistemic practice (Myers 2006). Acknowledging the forms that this care takes enables practitioners, users and critics of biomedical visualisations to become responsible for *how* we care.

Treating accuracy as a matter of care enables us to consider the values and hierarchies that inform which relationships and processes are deemed essential to correct knowledge. Concern for ideals like truth and humanitarianism motivates medical illustrators to express accuracy as a core value. Yet these commitments are often unrecognised, ill-defined or subsumed in instrumental mandates to 'communicate' and 'educate'. On the other hand, critiques which treat medical visuals as ready-made or machine-made reflections of biomedical knowledge misconstrue both the affective and world-making dimensions of biomedical visualisation as an epistemic practice. Conceptual decisions about what is important or necessary for 'accuracy' inform visual hierarchies throughout the process of creating medical illustrations. However, what is deemed accurate in a biomedical visualisation is contingent not only on evaluations of the current state of accepted knowledge but also on intertwined material and social relations, as well as the affective and aesthetic investments of the illustrator herself.

Understood as a form of care, accuracy does not stand in for a detached form of mechanical objectivity, at odds with emotional and subjective aesthetics. Instead, it suggests attentiveness to both the known and the unknown, negotiation of interests of both researchers and those who are affected by the research, and an acknowledgement that the illustrator's aesthetic and emotional investments are integral to her work. To perform medical illustration with care entails not merely adherence to biomedical knowledge and to the story that the commissioning researcher wants to tell about it, but also attention to and purposeful engagement with the forms of life that it renders intelligible or unthinkable. Rethinking accuracy as a form of care acknowledges not only the practical matters of material, economic and social environments in which medical illustrations are produced but also the affective mattering that anchors illustrators' deep sense of responsibility toward the ways in which their work is made to matter in medical education.

Acknowledgements

This research was made possible through a Canada Graduate Scholarship from the Social Sciences and Humanities Research Council, as well as a Dissertation Completion Award from Associated Medical Services. I wish to thank the AMI and the anonymous students, faculty and practitioners who shared their reflections and experiences with me.

References

'Accurate, adj.' (2020), *OED Online*, 3rd ed., Oxford: Oxford University Press, https://www-oed-com. ezproxy.library.yorku.ca/view/Entry/1283?redirectedFrom=accurate. Accessed 11 May 2020.

Ahmed, Sara (2012), *On Being Included: Racism and Diversity in Institutional Life*, Durham and London: Duke University Press.

Bauer, Greta R., Hammond, Rebecca, Travers, Robb, Kaay, Mathias, Hohenadel, Karin M. and Boyce, Michelle (2009), '"I don't think this is theoretical; this is our lives": How erasure impacts health care for transgender people', *Journal of the Association of Nurses in AIDS Care*, 20:5, pp. 348–61.

Brierley, Meaghan (2013), 'Dialogue and dissemination: The social practices of medical illustrators in the pharmaceutical context', Ph.D. thesis, Calgary: University of Calgary.

Daston, Lorraine and Galison, Peter (2007), *Objectivity*, New York and Cambridge: Zone Books and The MIT Press.

Mackenzie, Donald (1999), 'Nuclear missile testing and the social construction of accuracy', in M. Biagioli (ed.), *The Science Studies Reader*, New York: Routledge, pp. 342–57.

Massie, Jonathan P., Cho, Daniel Y., Kneib, Cameron J., Burns, Jacob R., Crowe, Christopher S., Lane, Megan, Shakir, Afaaf, Sobol, Danielle L., Sabin, Janice, Sousa, Janelle D., Rodriguez, Eduardo D., Satterwhite, Thomas and Morrison, Shane D. (2019), 'Patient representation in medical literature: Are we appropriately depicting diversity?', *Plastic and Reconstructive Surgery – Global Open*, 7:12, pp. 1–6.

Meynell, Letitia (2008), 'Pictures, pluralism, and feminist epistemology: Lessons from "Coming to understand"', *Hypatia*, 23:4, pp. 1–29.

Myers, Natasha (2006), 'Animating mechanism: Animations and the propagation of affect in the lively arts of protein modelling', *Science Studies*, 19:2, pp. 6–30.

Myers, Natasha (2015), *Rendering Life Molecular: Models, Modelers, and Excitable Matter, Experimental Futures: Technological Lives, Scientific Arts, Anthropological Voices*, Durham: Duke University Press.

Parker, Rhiannon B. (2016), 'The representation and production of visual gender bias in anatomy images and its effects on student attitudes', Ph.D. thesis, Wollongong: University of Wollongong.

Puig de la Bellacasa, Maria (2011), 'Matters of care in technoscience: Assembling neglected things', *Social Studies of Science*, 41:1, pp. 85–106.

Schiebinger, Londa (1990), 'The anatomy of difference: Race and sex in eighteenth-century science', *Eighteenth-Century Studies*, 23:4, pp. 387–405.

Schiebinger, Londa (1991), *The Mind Has No Sex?: Women in the Origins of Modern Science*, Cambridge: Harvard University Press.

Shapin, Steven (1984), 'Pump and circumstance: Robert Boyle's literary technology', *Social Studies of Science*, 14:4, pp. 481–520.

Shapin, Steven (1989), 'The invisible technician', *American Scientist*, 77:6, pp. 554–63.

Shapin, Steven and Schaffer, Simon (2011), *Leviathan and the Air-pump: Hobbes, Boyle, and the Experimental Life*, Princeton: Princeton University Press.

Smith, Pamela H. (2012), *The Body of the Artisan: Art and Experience in the Scientific Revolution*, Chicago: University of Chicago Press.

Suchman, Lucy A. (2007), *Human–Machine Reconfigurations: Plans and Situated Actions*, 2nd ed., Cambridge and New York: Cambridge University Press.

ILLUSTRATIONS

MATERIAL IMAGES: FLESH ON PAPER IN TWENTIETH-CENTURY SURGICAL DRAWING

Harriet Palfreyman

Images play a fundamental role in the education of surgeons. Whether as anatomy atlases or radiological scans, they teach surgeons how to distinguish health and sickness, locate pathological sites in the body, and guide their interventions into flesh. The role of images in the education of surgeons, though, goes beyond formal pedagogy and becomes a way of establishing and naturalising a specific way of seeing surgically. After conducting an ethnography of an operating theatre, sociologist Stefan Hirschauer argued that a striking feature of surgery in the late twentieth century has been the surgeon essentially making the patient body into a site resembling the anatomical illustrations through which they first learnt about the body (Hirschauer 1991). In essence, in order to render the interior of the body comprehensible and navigable, surgeons must intervene in a way that makes it resemble the drawings with which they were taught. The logical extension of this is that medical artists must therefore be able to recreate this particular view of the surgeon when producing new images. This circular relationship begs the question of just what kind of view these images require. To explore the key features of an acceptable surgical image I focus here on a drawing that depicts part of an operation to remove a cholesteatoma, a cyst affecting the bones of the ear, performed by neurosurgeon Geoffrey Jefferson in 1949 (see Figure 14.1). It was created by Dorothy Davison (1890–1984), a medical artist working in Manchester in the mid twentieth century. There is nothing particularly special about this image. There are many others like it in Davison's archive and in other collections, journals and books of the period. I have selected it because of its typicality in order to explore the ways in which it represents the surgical body. I touch on the aesthetic conventions of surgical images, but my main focus here is on the material aspects of the image-making process that allowed for the artist to produce a particularly surgical way of viewing the body. This image also allows us to access the co-operation between surgeon and artist in the creation of its final form, as Davison and Jefferson worked alongside each other at various stages of its creation. In looking at the circularity of surgical sight and surgical images, it is productive to explore the position of the surgeon in making such an image. What expectations, understandings, and aesthetics do they assume and require artists to replicate?

I suggest that the acceptable surgical image is one that not only aesthetically and compositionally renders the body intelligible but that also reflects the materiality and practices of surgery. I explore how the material processes of a particular form of drawing known as Ross Board, and of the practice of surgery, offered productive analogies between the act of drawing and performing surgery, allowing for a resolution of tensions between artist and surgeon in the production of an acceptable surgical image.

The analogy between surgery and art has been made by artists, critics, theorists and historians many times. Upon completion of her series *Hospital Drawings* in the 1940s, Barbara Hepworth noted that '[t]here is, it seems to me, a close affinity between the work and approach both of physicians and surgeons, and painters and sculptors. In both professions we have a vocation and we cannot escape the consequences of it' (Gleeson 2019: n.pag.). Hepworth's focus was on the idea of both professions as callings, but the analogy encompasses further aesthetic and material similarities. Mary Hunter has showed how art and surgery have been drawn together through a focus on the centrality of skilled handwork in both practices (Hunter 2018). Barbara Stafford has also drawn out this analogy noting the active similarities between surgical cutting and artistic etching, each of which features sharp instruments working on solid materials (Stafford 1993). Writing about medical artist Dickie Orpen (1914–2008), Sarah Casey and Gerry Davies note that Orpen's bold lines echoed the assured actions of the surgeon's scalpel adding '[s]he is not drawing what is done, but how it is done' (Casey and Davies 2020: 52).

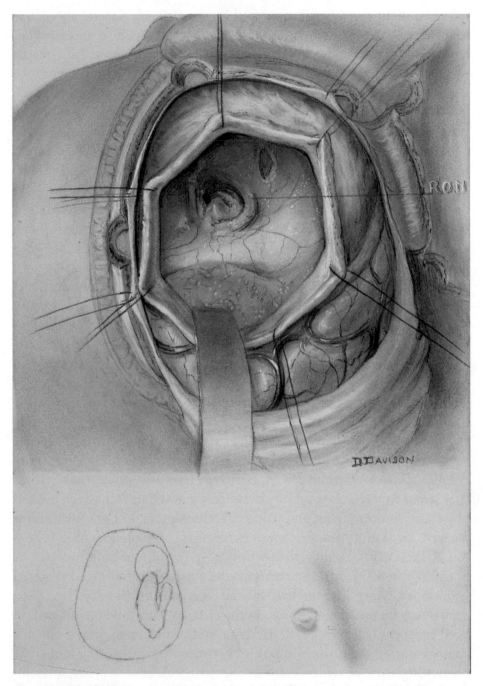

Figure 14.1: Dorothy Davison, procedure for the removal of a cholesteatomatous cyst, Ross Board drawing, (1949). With kind permission of the University of Manchester Special Collections.

Here, I build on these works and explore how Davison produced a drawing which portrayed both the materiality of the surgical subject and the material processes of the surgeon's work.

Dorothy Davison was a gifted artist with a keen interest in Egyptology. In her late twenties, she took a job at the Manchester Museum, where she often made pictures and models of Egyptian tombs and houses to illustrate talks she gave on the subject. In 1918, Professor of Anatomy at Manchester University Sir Grafton Elliot Smith (1871–1937) attended one of her talks and was particularly impressed with her copies of Egyptian wall paintings. He suggested she take up medical art and work with him at the University Medical School. Early on in her work there she encountered neurosurgeon Geoffrey Jefferson (1886–1961), who asked her if she could paint, to which she modestly replied, 'a little' (Perry 1971: 27). The two would go on to work closely together at the Manchester Royal Infirmary, with Davison producing hundreds of drawings and paintings illustrating Jefferson's neurosurgical operations and pathological specimens. At the beginning of her career at the medical school, Davison was employed on a freelance basis but, in 1939, she was officially appointed as Medical Artist at the University. In 1947, she spent time in London making links with other medical artists and went on to form the Medical Artists Association of Great Britain two years later.

This period was one of the immense professionalising efforts by medical artists. Not only was the Association started but also the *Journal of Medical and Biological Illustration* – the first journal dedicated specifically to medical illustration – was established in 1951. The mid-twentieth century also saw the establishment of special departments of medical illustration in British hospitals. The artists and photographers who worked in these departments produced images for all manner of hospital business. They made images that tracked patients' progress or decline for their hospital records; they created images and films for training medical students or for doctors to use at conferences; they visually recorded the progress of hospital research projects; and they frequently provided images for hospital publicity, annual reports, staff pictures and information literature. All this came alongside more formalised and professionalising discussion and debate over how to best represent medicine and the body.

The work of the medical artist in this period was intrinsically cooperative and they routinely worked alongside clinicians in the creation of their images. Davison herself worked closely with Jefferson and a number of others at the University Medical School and the Manchester

Royal Infirmary. Whilst most of the images she created were of pathological specimens, around 100 depict operations. These images in particular were sites of co-creation, cooperation, and frustration, as they involved a great deal of input from the surgeons themselves at various points in the process. This necessitated the negotiation of two very different, but strikingly complementary, skills. Both surgery and drawing are embodied and sensory practices often reliant on the tacit knowledge of their practitioners. Yet, the process of making such tacit knowledge explicit in order to perfect the drawing often proved difficult.

The process of creating these images began in the operating theatre, where, encumbered by a surgical gown, gloves, mask and cap, Davison would climb atop a step ladder and peer into the surgical wound to make quick preparatory sketches. Her view was often hampered by instruments, swabs, harsh lights and the pressing need to continue the surgery, she would be guided by Jefferson, hovering nearby and trying to ensure she captured the key features of the operation. Davison's frustrations with this way of working can be discerned from a series of pen and ink cartoons she made portraying Jefferson and herself at work. In one of these, Davison depicted herself in the operating theatre, balanced on her steps on her tiptoes and peering over Jefferson's shoulder. The surgeon, clearly in her way, says 'What can't see it? I can feel it' (Davison n.d.: GB 133 DDS/4/4). Following the operation, Jefferson would consult with Davison on the sketches, and she would work these up into the final image. This entailed a negotiation of the different ways of seeing of both artist and surgeon, a process which Lorraine Daston and Peter Galison have termed 'four-eyed sight' (Daston and Galison 2007: 84). The 'can't see it, I can feel it' line in Davison's cartoon suggests a fundamental tension between these ways of seeing. The elision of touch and sight the phrase suggests is revelatory of the nature of surgical sight. The surgical way of seeing is effectively a double sense, in which the haptic and the visual are inextricably entangled. The artist, meanwhile, unsterile and holding paper and pencils, had no access to this double sense and had to somehow represent visually something the surgeon could feel.

In other cartoons, Davison expressed her frustrations with trying to capture what Jefferson had seen, or perhaps felt, during the operation. In one, she showed herself and Jefferson sitting at a table and surrounded by numerous sheets of paper while she made sketches. It hints at the many stages of drafting and adjusting that were needed to produce an image which satisfied the surgeon. Jefferson is shown as saying 'you never see things the right size. The tumour was much bigger'. Then, 'that's better – perhaps a shade too large.' Finally, a third draft earns Davison a '[s]plendid, exactly as I saw it'. In another cartoon, Jefferson and Davison are again shown sitting at a table examining a drawing. Obviously unhappy with Davison's sketch, the surgeon intervened; 'Ah well, I'll go over it in red ink.' This was obviously insufficient as he then reached for his blue pen to annotate the drawings, evidently going too far with his scribblings as he then admitted that he 'can't see it myself now' and induced the artist to just read his article on the subject and work it out herself, leaving Davison with her head in her hands (Davison n.d.: GB 133 DDS/4/4).

The cartoons offer clues as to how this relationship worked. Jefferson's frustrations are evident; that Davison could not understand what he had seen in the operation, and that he himself was unable to intervene usefully enough to make the preparatory drawings clear. Davison's own frustrations, though never explicitly articulated in the cartoons, are all too obvious parallels; that Jefferson was unable to properly verbalise the way he saw the operation, and that he was incapable of helpfully marking out what he meant on her sketches. Each of their tacit skills – Jefferson's sense of touch and sight and Davison's drawing skills – were simply inaccessible to the other. In producing a final image that satisfied Jefferson, Davison had to find a way of translating the tacit, tactile knowledge of the surgeon into a finished drawing. As to how she successfully did this we must now turn to the material qualities of the drawings, for it was the material, physical and technological processes of creating the drawing that presented a productive site of mediation for the artistic and surgical views of the body.

In Figure 14.1, Davison used a particular kind of drawing, known as Ross Board. The key features of this medium are deep, almost pure black shadows and stark white highlights, with crisp lines and smooth shading that give a hyper-realistic look to the surgical subject. These features allow for the representation of the depth of the surgical incision, as well as the different textures of bodily tissues. The technique was developed in the early twentieth century by German medical artist Max Brödel (1870–1941) at Johns Hopkins University in Baltimore, Maryland and Davison herself was instrumental in adopting the technique and bringing it to the British field of medical art. This method of drawing was often favoured by the publishers of journals and books in the mid-twentieth century as it reproduced particularly well when photographed (Mohr 2017). However, I suggest that the appeal of the technique for artists working with surgeons went much deeper than this practicality. It was the material aspects of the image's production which shared productive parallels with the practice of surgery that allowed the creation of the image to act as a process of mediation between the artist's and surgeon's different ways of seeing the subject.

Ross Board drawing was a labour-intensive process requiring an extensive set of specialist tools beginning with the Ross Board itself, a thick paperboard developed in America in the late nineteenth century. The artist then needed a BB carbon pencil, a supply of carbon dust – which can be made by sandpapering the pencil lead into dust – paintbrushes, a variety of engravers' tools for scratching, a gum eraser for gently reworking shading, a chamois leather cloth for fine shading, tracing paper or parchment for protecting the drawing whilst working, and an alcohol-based fixative agent for preserving the final look of the drawing. The artist first sketched the preliminary image onto paper which was then reversed, traced and transferred to the Ross Board. Then, using a paintbrush, the artist applied layers of carbon dust to build up deep layers of shading. Blending was done with a gum eraser and chamois leather to gently work the carbon dust into the textured surface of the board. Highlights were then scratched into the drawing, the sharp engravers tools cutting away the layers of carbon and the chalk coating of the paper to reveal stark white (Clarke 1940).

We start to see, then, how the tools, materials and processes share certain comparable properties with those of surgery. Ross Board is mottled, textured and layered like skin; chamois leather literally is animal skin. The sharp tools result in light and clarity, the cuts and scratches creating stark highlights in the drawing just as the cutting edge of the surgeon's scalpel reveals the opening in the flesh. The paper is concealed and revealed strategically, with tracing paper, to avoid smudging the image. The patient's body is similarly covered and exposed by surgical drapes to keep the operative site clean and to protect the rest of the body. The artist must wield their tools carefully; a gentle touch for the smudging of shadow, and more force for the scratching of highlight. The surgeon must tread a parallel line of tension that divides the brutality of cutting into a body from the delicacy needed to intervene surgically.

To focus then on that analogy between surgery and art; for scholars such as Barbara Stafford, the acts of etching, scratching and marking carry similarities with surgical cutting and dissecting. The three-dimensionality of the Ross Board technique suggests similar analogous elements. There is the scratching away of the layers of carbon to highlight key areas, and then there is the building up of layers by brushing carbon onto paper, almost reminiscent of the final stage of the operation, in which the surgeon must bring together layers of tissue in order to repair the surgical incision. In producing an acceptable image, the artist had to grapple with how to represent the material physicality of the body, with all of its textures and depths, and the dynamic process of the operation. The Ross Board technique allowed for this by essentially recreating the materials and actions of surgery in the making of the image.

It is useful here to consider the availability of other forms of visual representation for medical artists and clinicians at this time. By the mid twentieth century, there were numerous ways to represent medical and surgical subjects visually. X-ray scan images, photography, and conceptual and technical drawings all had their places in medical teaching, research and communication. By this time, too, there were particular subfields of medicine which were thought better suited to different forms of representation. Pathology, particularly the depiction of gross specimens, lent itself better to photography. One 1960 manual of medical photography noted this centrality of photographs in the representation of pathology. Colour photographs successfully captured the varying shades and tones of gross specimens and were economical to produce. The authors even asserted that '[p]hotography is of great value in supplementing museums of pathology and color photographs have replaced many preserved museum specimens' (Smialowski and Currie 1960: 83). Photography then seemed so suited to pathological representation that, for some practitioners at least, it had the potential to not only supplant medical drawing, but also a host of other important visual and material representations.

There was, though, recognition that photography was not always a suitable medium. Often line drawings of specimens would accompany photographs to clarify certain areas. The aforementioned manual of medical photography noted that 'photomicrographs, electrocardiograms, or photographs of the appropriate region of the body may be combined with gross specimen photographs to increase their teaching value' (Smialowski and Currie 1960: 95). The addition of more visual representations accumulatively increased the value of the photographs. Thus, we see different forms of illustrative media worked more often in dialogue with each other than in resistance. Surgery was no exception to this, and surgeons employed many forms of media in their illustrations. Pertinent to our focus on Davison's 1949 image, it is interesting to note that there is an existing photograph in the archival collection that shows the same view as Figure 14.1. For Jefferson then it seems there was something not quite suitable about the photograph alone.

There are some key differences between the photograph and Davison's drawing. The photograph captures the illegible totality of the surgical incision. Drapes, clips and sutures seem almost haphazard and it is difficult to discern the minute anatomical structures of the body, or even where on the body the operation is sited. Davison's illustration is cleaner, there is less blood and fewer instruments obscuring relevant parts of the anatomy. Her close work with Jefferson and other surgeons meant they doubtless would have consulted on which parts of the photograph to highlight and which to discard. Davison's is neat, the layers of the body are defined and ordered, the shape of the wound almost as mechanically clean as the metal retractor we see parting the tissue. She has also omitted the surgical drapes and the clips keeping them in place from the drawing, allowing the viewer to see the flap of skin that has given the surgeons access. We can even see the bridge of the patient's nose in the drawing, reminding us of the location of the operation on the body.

Here the advantages of the Ross Board drawing become particularly clear. The technique far surpassed the photograph's ability to show surgical depth, textural changes in tissues and the three-dimensional materiality of the operative site. Necessity meant that photographs of surgery had to employ a depth of field that ensured everything was in focus. This could result in a rather flat-looking image, where the depth of the operation in the body and the differing textures of the body were not always evident. Davison wrote that she used Ross Board, 'because it gives texture better than any other medium, fine lines can be scratched out to show the dead white of the chalk-faced paper and gradations of tone can be obtained quickly' (Davison 1952: 234). For both artist and surgeon then, it was the technology and techniques of the Ross Board drawing which won out over photography in the creation of a superior image.

However, it was not only the artificial clarity of the Ross Board drawing that assured its acceptance in this case. Though the technique was relatively new, it allowed for the continuation of important compositional elements in surgical images that had developed since the fifteenth century and persisted into modern depictions of surgery. Indeed, the surgical view of practitioners like Jefferson was never that of a singular surgeon. After all, Jefferson and his colleagues were, as students, taught to see the surgical body from images similar to Davison's in textbooks. Thus, we also see in Figure 14.1 the presence of numerous compositional tropes from visual representations of surgery from earlier periods. These tropes celebrated surgery in its ideal form. They included the presence of sharp tools and a celebration of the penetrative qualities of surgical instrumentation; the revelatory power of the surgical touch that could open out the flesh and bone of the body with apparent ease; the active hand of the surgeon expertly wielding their instruments, locating pathology and intervening to cut and to heal; a close and intimate focus on the surgical wound, abstracted from the rest of the body, or even the idea of a patient; and finally, a paradoxical bloodlessness that illustrated anatomy but obscured the brutality and barbarism which, quite literally, represented the historic origins of surgery.

Figure 14.2 is one example of this idealised surgical view. In this image, taken from a manual of operative surgery published in 1846, we can see the hands of the surgeon expertly manipulating the cutting tools of his trade. The focus of the surgical interventions here are also hands; I hesitate to call them patient's hand as they are largely unmarked by pathological indicators, rather they are the imagined bodily object of surgery. The only difference between them and the surgeon's hand is that they are slightly paler in colour and, of course, they are the focus of the surgical work. This image speaks to a surgery based on the empirical sciences of anatomy and physiology. It recognises the manual strength and dexterity of the surgeon with the inclusion of the hands pinching and steadying the leg. It also aesthetically minimises the severity of the surgical incision. Where cuts are shown, the wounds are neat and decisive, with no blood evident. It also reclaims the use of sharp cutting tools as icons of skilful practice, rather than brutality, by showing them as clean of any blood (Palfreyman and Rabier 2018). Overall, the image seems to suggest the absence of any bodily resistance to this most extreme of operations. As Sally Frampton and Roger Kneebone (2017: 546) have shown, the large surgical incision of the second half of the nineteenth century came to be 'an iconic emblem of the power of the profession'. However, this was an icon which needed to be carefully visualised in order to avoid vivid associations with pain and brutality.

Although a hundred years separate this image from Figure 14.1, we can see the persistence of these tropes in Davison's 1949 drawing. The body in surgery's visual culture is one curiously unmarked by obvious

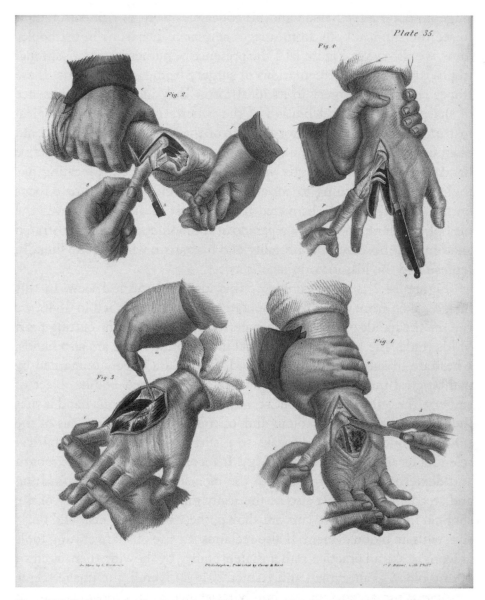

Figure 14.2: Techniques for the amputation of fingers, coloured etching, illustration for *A Treatise on Operative Surgery* (Pancost 1846: plate 36). Wellcome Collection. Attribution 4.0 International (CC BY 4.0).

pathology. It is made up of neatly delineated and recognisable anatomical structures, clean and bloodless incisions, and the presence of tools. Yet, as much as Davison's image draws from a long heritage of representation in surgery, the twentieth-century surgical body represented in these images is also a profoundly modern material. In images like

Davison's, we see the body as segmented, unnaturally neat, almost architectural in form. The images are reminiscent of the art of German doctor and artist Fritz Khan (1888–1968) that portray the body as a machine, as a factory, or an industrial structure. Michael Sappol (2017) has written about these depictions as productions of a specifically twentieth-century modernity and modernism. Indeed, the use of a very clean, almost mechanical looking cut in surgical illustrations from the same period draws not only from the wider conventions around depicting surgery but also from modernistic cultural imagery like this that understood the body as a material to be worked on, sculpted and restored to health.

Surgery posed specific challenges for medical artists. Images of surgery differ from those of gross pathology or anatomy whilst incorporating elements of both. Rather than the torpid and uncontextualised appearance of, say, a tumour removed at post-mortem, or the fixed and idealised anatomical diagram, surgical images represent particular moments of a dynamic process. Artists had to reckon with appropriately depicting the pathological focus of the image and the location of this pathology within the anatomical material as seen and experienced sensorially by the surgeon. The tensions between Davison and Jefferson's ways of seeing the same subject demonstrate that this was no easy feat. It was the artist who offered a medium that could resolve these tensions whilst still adhering to the established aesthetic traditions in which the idealised body is itself a site of tension between healthy and pathological, invaded yet bloodless. Davison's Ross Board drawing did this better than the photograph, which, in all its gory detail, threatened to upend this ideal surgical view.

Beyond the aesthetic considerations, the material analogies between surgery and Ross Board drawings allowed the creation of such images to serve as sites of unity for artists and surgeons. The medium resolved many of the tensions between the artist's visual acuity and the surgeon's senses. This allowed them to be accepted as suitable images of the surgical body to be used to elucidate and educate. Davison's drawings reify the surgical view of the body, but they also create it, as surgeons long after Jefferson viewed and learned from the drawings. Through their aesthetic and material properties, Davison's images naturalised the unnatural invasion that surgery represents, they sanitised the bloodiness and forgave the brutality of surgery. They are a reification of the surgical view of the body, a legitimation of the practice of surgery, and a key part of the identity of the mid-twentieth century surgeon.

Acknowledgements

I would like to thank my colleagues at the Centre for the History of Science, Technology and Medicine at the University of Manchester for their generous comments on an earlier version of this work. I am also grateful for the assistance of staff at the University of Manchester Special Collections, particularly Dr. James Peters, for allowing access to Davison's collection.

References

Casey, Sarah and Davies, Gerry (2020), *Drawing Investigations: Graphic Relationships with Science, Culture and Environment*, London and New York: Bloomsbury.

Clarke, Carl Dame (1940), *Illustration: Its Technique and Application to the Sciences*, Baltimore: The John D. Lucas Company.

Daston, Lorraine and Galison, Peter (2007), *Objectivity*, New York: Zone.

Davison, Dorothy (1952), 'Ross board technique', *Journal of Medical and Biological Illustration*, 2:4, pp. 233–39.

Davison, Dorothy (n.d.), *Letters and Cartoons*, Manchester: University of Manchester Special Collections, GB 133 DDS/4/4.

Frampton, Sally and Kneebone, Roger (2017), 'John Wickham's new surgery: "Minimally invasive therapy", innovation, and approaches to medical practice in twentieth-century Britain', *Social History of Medicine*, 30:3, pp. 544–66.

Gleeson, Sinéad (2019), *Constellations: Reflections from Life*, London: Picador.

Hirschauer, Stefan (1991), 'The manufacture of bodies in surgery', *Social Studies of Science*, 21:2, pp. 279–319.

Hunter, Mary (2018), 'Art and surgery: The expert hands of artists and surgeons', in T. Schlich (ed.), *The Palgrave Handbook of the History of Surgery*, Palgrave Macmillan: London, pp. 301–25.

Mohr, Peter D. (2017), 'Dorothy Davison (1890–1984): Manchester medical artist and her work for neurosurgeon Sir Geoffrey Jefferson', *Journal of Medical Biography*, 25:5, pp. 130–37.

Palfreyman, Harriet and Rabier, Christelle (2018), 'Visualizing surgery: Surgeons' use of images, 1600–Present', in T. Schlich Thomas (ed.), *The Palgrave Handbook of the History of Surgery*, London: Palgrave Macmillan, pp. 283–300.

Pancost, Joseph (1846), *A Treatise on Operative Surgery Comprising a Description of the Various Processes of the Art, Including all the New Operations; Exhibiting the State of Surgical Science in Its Present Advanced Condition; with Eighty Plates, Containing Four Hundred and Eighty-Six Separate Illustrations*, 2nd ed., revised and enlarged, Philadelphia: G.N. Loomis.

Perry, Jean (1971), 'Forty years of medical art: A biography of Dorothy Davison', *Medical and Biological Illustration*, 21:1, pp. 27–32.

Sappol, Michael (2017), *Body Modern: Fritz Kahn, Scientific Illustration and the Homuncular Subject*, Minneapolis: University of Minnesota Press.

Smialowski, Arthur and Currie, Donald J. (1960), *Photography in Medicine*, Springfield: Charles C. Thomas.

Stafford, Barbara Maria (1993), *Body Criticism: Imaging the Unseen in Enlightenment Art and Medicine*, Cambridge and London: MIT Press.

ILLUSTRATIONS

THE RADFORD COLLECTION: EXPLORING AND EXPERIENCING THE MID NINETEENTH-CENTURY MIDWIFERY LECTURE

Rebecca Whiteley

Foetuses *in utero*; maternal and infant bodies in the process of birth; pelvises with worrying distortions; developing embryos; foetal skulls; breasts; an anatomised woman with blueish skin and a mobcap; and so, so many diseased uteri. These are the things one finds in the Thomas Radford Collection of Medical Illustrations (Radford Collection) at the University of Manchester Library (UML). Belied by the neat, uniform, pearly-grey archival boxes that contain it, this collection of 276 loose images is a materially and visually diverse summation of the obstetrical and gynaecological knowledge of mid-nineteenth-century Europe. A motley bunch, the images vary in size and medium, from tiny, ragged journal pages, to large oil paintings, and encompass ink, watercolour, gouache, oil, print, pencil, paper, board and canvas. The collection also has diverse origins: some images are prints removed from books and journals; others are drawings and paintings copied from book illustrations; and others still are drawn directly from specimens or dissections.

There is almost no surviving documentation for this collection – we lack a catalogue, accompanying syllabi or any written evidence of how it was stored, displayed or understood – but the images themselves bear many traces of use. First, while they have since been cleaned and conserved, when I first began to work with them, they were fantastically dirty, indicative of a working collection regularly displayed in an industrial city in the age of coal fires and gas lighting. Second, various marks of ownership are present. Most are branded with the initials 'Dr. R'; many are stamped 'Radford Library, St. Mary's Hospital, Manchester'. Some bear round scalloped stickers with numbers, cupboard numbers and the warning 'not for circulation'. Third, the works have in various ways been prepared for display: many of those on paper have been mounted on board or edged in tape. Many are fitted with loops of pink ribbon or string, or have holes added, from which they could be hung. Finally, some bear annotations, either on the work itself, or on labels made from cut up lecture admission tickets.

What we can gather is that the images were part of the teaching collection of Dr. Thomas Radford (1793–1881), built up as a personal teaching resource, donated to St. Mary's Hospital in 1853 and subsequently employed by the hospital's lecturers. The hospital was founded in 1790 as the Manchester and Salford Lying-In Charity, with the aim of providing material necessities and midwives for poor women in childbirth. The charity also provided a team of 'man-midwives', later called surgeons, who lectured to, supervised and assisted the women midwives. Indeed, the education of these women was at the centre of the enterprise, as stated in Rule 21 of the original proposal:

> That Lectures, or Instructions be given, at the expence [sic] of this Charity, to the practicing Midwives belonging to this Institution, and to female Pupils, in order to qualify them in future, to be eligible to that Office, by one of the Men-midwives to this Charity, to be appointed by the Quarterly Board. (Anon. 1790: n.pag.)

The institution underwent many changes throughout the nineteenth century: moving multiple times to different locations; intermittently running in-patient services; changing its name, first to the Manchester and Salford Lying-In Hospital, and then in 1854 to St. Mary's Hospital; and increasingly focusing on gynaecological and paediatric as well as obstetric medicine (see Young 1964; Pickstone 1985: 31–34, 100–121). Over time, male medical students came increasingly to attend the hospital for lectures, and to train under both the surgeons and the midwives, often boarding with the latter (Young 1964: 56–57). While the suitability of the rooms provided was often debated, the hospital maintained a library, museum and space for lectures through all its moves (Young 1964).

Thomas Radford first came into contact with the hospital in 1810, when he was apprenticed to his uncle William Wood, a surgeon. He was employed as a 'man-midwife' to the hospital in 1818 and gradually rose through the ranks, becoming a consulting physician in 1841 and holding the position until his death in 1881. Alongside this work, he maintained a private practice inherited from his uncle, and he lectured to medical students at the Mount Street School and the Manchester Royal School of Medicine (Sutton and Moscucci 2004). In 1853, Radford donated his library and museum to St. Mary's, including his collection of images. The hospital had been given a museum collection by Charles White in 1808 that was 'perfectly sufficient for a complete course of lectures in Anatomy and Physiology, Pathology, Surgery and Midwifery' (Young 1964: 22–23). However, a fire in 1847 destroyed most of these original collections, making Radford's contribution likely very welcome.

Studying works in the Radford Collection that are dated, and finding the publication dates of those copied or removed from books, indicates that it was largely compiled at the beginning of Radford's career, from the 1820s to the 1850s. Core texts on obstetrics and gynaecology from the late eighteenth and early nineteenth centuries are well-represented. Radford would have used his visual collections in his lectures at various locations, where they would have been accessible to medical and midwifery students. Once deposited at St. Mary's, they would have been employed in the hospital's lectures for midwives and medical students, as well as being at least partially accessible to the public. While we do not know how long the collection remained in active use, there are indications that it was valued by the hospital's lecturers for at least a couple of decades after donation. The annual report for 1868 indicates that a catalogue was made of the collection in that year (St. Mary's Hospital 1868). And stickers on some of the images give numbers and cupboard locations, suggesting that money and effort were put into making the collection both searchable and accessible. The holes and loops of ribbon, as well as the generally dirty condition of the works indicate, moreover, that they were often removed to be studied, handled and displayed. Indeed, evidence of other contemporary teaching collections suggests that images, studied close up and hung on the walls of lecture theatres and museums, were a fundamental part of the material culture of medical education in this period (Alberti 2011; Berkowitz 2011, 2013; Hallam 2016; Slipp 2017). So we may say that the Radford Collection formed an active part of the city's midwifery lecturing scene for at least the middle part of the century, from as early as the 1820s to at least the 1870s.

The Radford Collection, therefore, is a unique and important resource for the history of medicine and its relation to visual and material culture, pedagogy and, perhaps most importantly, women's education. Yet, without accompanying textual sources, it presents some problems. While contextual evidence and a close attention to the materiality of the collection can allow us to construct part of its history, exploring exactly how it was amassed, used and experienced must inevitably be something of a speculative endeavour. This chapter aims to show what can be done by paying close attention to objects of medical pedagogy as historical resources in their own right. And it aims to demonstrate the value of more speculative thinking when addressing histories that have tended to be underexamined because of a lack of conventional sources.

Medical collections and images

As this diverse volume indicates, scholarship on medical museum collections and pedagogic objects is flourishing. In the past ten years, several excellent studies and collected volumes have focussed on such objects in the nineteenth century (Alberti 2011; Alberti and Hallam 2013; Hallam 2016; Berkowitz and Lightman 2017; Graciano 2019). These scholars have explored the ways in which different objects created knowledge, how they were used in different learning spaces and the processes of their production and display. There is also an excellent body of literature on the visual culture of medicine, largely focusing on illustrations in prestigious medical and anatomical atlases (Jordanova 1989; Kemp and Wallace 2000; McGrath 2002; Sappol 2006; Daston and Galison 2010; Berkowitz 2015). And finally, we are seeing a growing attention to collections of loose-leaf images produced by medical lecturers for teaching and research (Berkowitz 2011; Hammerschlag 2016; Hunter 2016; Slipp 2017; Wils et al. 2017; Ruiz-Gómez 2019). This last specialism has, in recent years, developed our scholarly awareness of the importance of image collections like Radford's. Indeed, such image collections were extremely common in this period, employed in almost every medical lecture and present in almost every medical museum, but they were also highly various in their content, media, sources, and proportions of original and copied images. As such, we have some way to go in fully understanding the ways in which image collections worked to form the visual, material and pedagogic culture of medicine.

As part of this endeavour, therefore, it is worth taking some time to characterise the Radford Collection. Its size and variety make this a distinct challenge, and certainly a description of every medium, source and topic covered is beyond the scope of this chapter. Instead, I propose to give a sense of the collection by emulating the way it might have been originally experienced by a student: through a selection made in order to teach on a particular topic. Pelvic distortion and obstructed labour were routinely taught in midwifery courses, and were also a particular interest of Radford's, who was an early supporter of caesarean section. The topic is also well-represented in the collection, and so while we don't know *exactly* which works might have been displayed to students, I can make a selection that showcases the variety of material on this theme, and which might plausibly have formed the visual content of a lecture on pelvic distortion:

A painting in watercolour on paper of two pelvises, the upper identified as belonging to Christie Moore. The painting was sent to Radford by a colleague and is annotated in Radford's own hand. The annotations direct the reader to linked objects in the collection, including in each case oil paintings of the entire skeletons 'suspended in the lecture theatre' and casts of the pelvises 'in the Museum […] of St. Marys Hospital'. A written account of Moore's operation also exists in the UML Archives (Radford *c*.1830s), see Figure 15.1.

Two copies of an etching by C. Pye of the distorted pelvis of Elizabeth Thompson, taken from a journal article by William Wood (Wood 1799), see Figure 15.2.

An oil painting on board of a distorted pelvis, perhaps similar to the now lost one of Moore, done by the local landscape painter John Ralston, see Figure 15.3.

A watercolour sketch of a pelvis by Radford from a specimen in the collection of his colleague Thomas Turner, annotated by Radford possibly when it was made, or later when it was donated to St. Mary's, see Figure 15.4.

A large painting on board, showing the outlets of various distorted pelvises, modelled on the illustrations in Franz Carl Nägele's *Das schräg verengte Becken* (Nägele 1839: Figures 9 and 10), see Figure 15.5.

A painting on paper, mounted on board, of a fetus passing through a distorted pelvis, copied from William Smellie's *A Sett of Anatomical Tables* (Smellie 1754: Figure 27), see Figure 15.6.

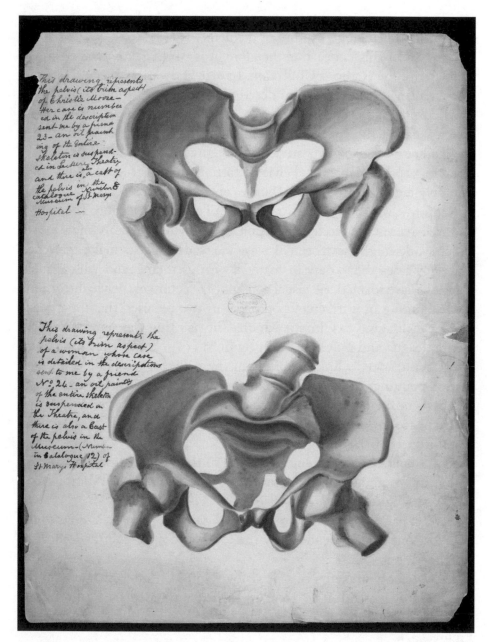

Figure 15.1: Anon., *Two Malformed Pelvises*, c.1830s, watercolour and ink on paper, 39.5 × 52 cm. The University of Manchester Library, Radford Collection, Item 9. © The University of Manchester.

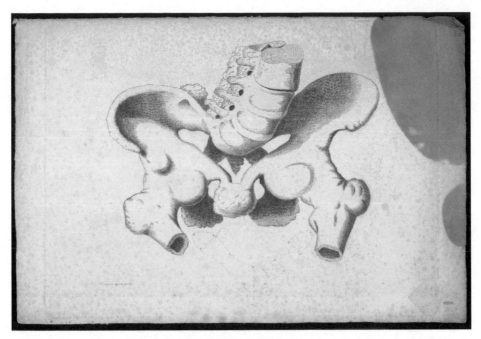

Figure 15.2: C. Pye (engraver), *Pelvis of Elizabeth Thompson*, 1799, etching on paper, 44 × 29 cm. Taken from Wood, William (1799) 'A case of Caesarean Section', *Memoirs of the Medical Society of London*, 5, pp. 463–76. The University of Manchester Library, Radford Collection, Item 13. © The University of Manchester.

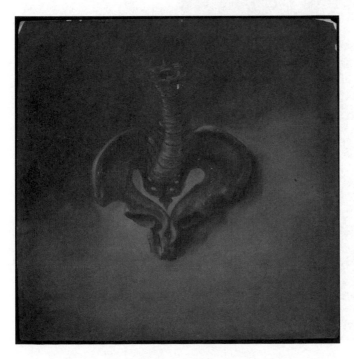

Figure 15.3: John Ralston, *Pelvis and Spine*, c.1825–33, oil on board, 46.5 × 47 cm. The University of Manchester Library, Radford Collection, Item 185. © The University of Manchester.

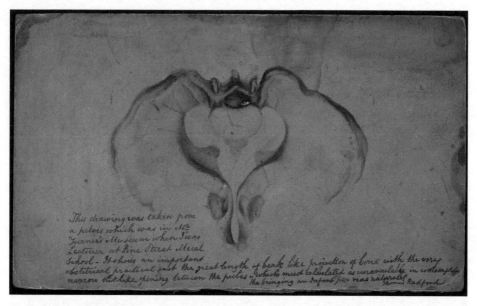

Figure 15.4: Thomas Radford, *A Pelvis in Thomas Turner's Collection*, *c.*1830s, watercolour and ink on board, 46 × 28 cm. The University of Manchester Library, Radford Collection, Item 15. © The University of Manchester.

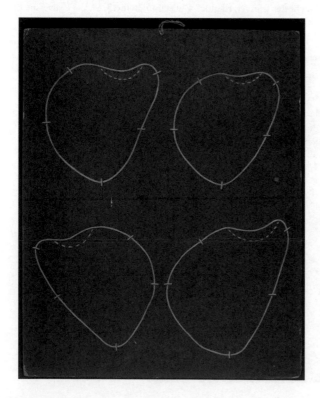

Figure 15.5: Anon., *Outlets of Four Pelvises*, *c.*1840s, gouache on board, 45.5 × 57 cm. Modelled on Figures 9 and 10 from Nägele, Franz Carl (1839), *Das Schräg Verengte Becken Nebst Einem Anhange Über Die Wichtigsten Fehler Des Weiblichen Beckens Überhaupt*, Mainz: V. von Zabern. The University of Manchester Library, Radford Collection, Item 180. © The University of Manchester.

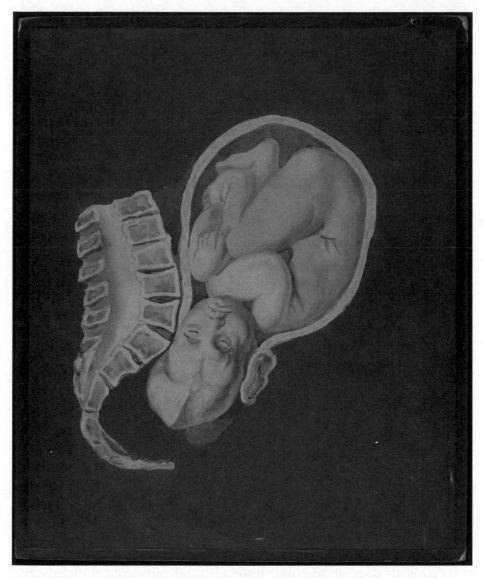

Figure 15.6: Anon., *Fetus Passing through the Pelvis*, *c.*1830–50, gouache on paper, mounted on board, 45 × 54.5 cm. Copied from Table 27, Smellie, William (1754), *A Sett of Anatomical Tables*, London: n.p. The University of Manchester Library, Radford Collection, Item 181. © The University of Manchester.

Image collections such as Radford's exemplify the great variety of learning modes that made up a nineteenth-century medical education. Some of the images refer to particular cases, and point to case notes, indicating the growing value placed on clinical observation as part of medical education (La Berge and Hannaway 1998; Foucault 2003). Other images are copies of prepared specimens and point to the importance of museum collections in training the clinical eye, and in allowing the visual and physical comparison of multiple cases. Images were an important accompaniment to wet and dry specimens in the museum because they could be made in multiples and circulated, stored more easily, and retained their colour. Finally, some images in the collection are copies of, or actual, book illustrations. This transference from book to loose-leaf image made the illustrations more mobile and comparable, allowed them to be studied collectively, and often facilitated enlargement or the addition of colour. As most medical students, particularly those below the level of the elite, would not have had access to large private libraries, exposure to book illustrations in the lecture theatre was important. Such practices, moreover, contributed to the establishment of a canon of authoritative images that taught students 'how to see', or what to look for in the complex and bewildering variety of the actual clinical body (Daston and Galison 2010: 26). Images such as those originally produced for Franz Carl Nägele and William Smellie, described previously, would have been recognisable to almost any student of midwifery in the nineteenth century, and they helped to create medical communities across the globe, standardising visual knowledge between individuals and institutions (Deblon 2017).

Image collections such as Radford's might be termed the workhorses of the medical pedagogical collection: easier and cheaper to put together than collections of specimens; more accessible through lecture courses than clinical study at teaching hospitals; and providing the authority and expertise of published works, without the necessity for private libraries or individual book study. As Carin Berkowitz has argued, image collections were central in providing 'a pedagogical programme that valued practical, formalised medical education, faced a dearth of bodies for dissection, and expanded the audience for that education to include surgeons, general practitioners, and apothecaries' and, we might add, midwives (Berkowitz 2011: 249).

Midwives and medical education

The Radford Collection was one of the resources described by Berkowitz as providing access to the intermedial and interspatial realm of nineteenth-century medical education for students lower down the medical hierarchy: midwives (who were always women); and male medical students who planned to make more modest livings as general practitioners, serving local communities and attending labours as part of a varied case load. Whether called midwifery or obstetrics, the practice of assisting women in labour remained a low-status medical practice for most of the century (Loudon 1986; Digby 1994; Nuttall 2012). As a provincial hospital, too, St. Mary's struggled for recognition, yet it situated itself as a leader in the campaign that lasted throughout the century for better and more comprehensive midwifery training and regulation for both men and women (Donnison 1977; Moscucci 1990; Nuttall 2012). Indeed, in an annual report from 1878, the governors claimed 'there is not another Hospital in Great Britain which has done more for female practitioners in midwifery, not even excepting the Rotundo Hospital in Dublin' (St. Mary's Hospital 1878: 15).

All this makes the Radford Collection a valuable resource for histories that are not particularly well covered for nineteenth-century Britain. Histories exist of the first pioneering women who qualified as doctors and surgeons in this period (Blake 1990; Furst 1997), as well as the first cohorts of women medical students at the end of the century (see Wells 2001; Dyhouse 2006). It is also widely acknowledged that women were active in nursing and midwifery throughout the century, and some part of this story, including the rise of reformed nursing (Summers 1989; Hallett 2012), and the fight for midwifery regulation, have been explored. However, with regards to midwifery, large gaps exist in the historical literature. We know, in the abstract, that while doctors worked hard to denigrate the skills of midwives, aiming to take from them all the most lucrative practice among the wealthy and as teachers and governors in hospitals and institutions, most women throughout the century were delivered by other women (see Anon. 1826; Summers 1989; Moscucci 1990). We know too that these women varied massively in their training and skill, from those with no formal training who were nonetheless respected professionals within their communities and relied upon by both local officials and doctors (Badger 2014), to medically trained professionals who held positions of authority as matrons in hospitals and lying-in charities (McIntosh 1998; Forman Cody 2004; Nuttall 2012). We know that institutions like St. Mary's in Manchester, The Rotunda in Dublin, and The British Lying-In Hospital in London also trained midwives throughout the century (Donnison 1977; Nuttall 2012), but the comprehensive and fine-grained histories of how and what such institutions taught to their women students, or the subsequent professional lives of trained midwives, remain to be written. This has all too often led to a general assumption that women were essentially excluded from medical lectures before the end of the century: that, as Susan Wells puts it, while they could work as nurses and attendants, 'they could not be authorized witnesses of the scientific rationalization of the body' (Wells 2001: 199; see also Alberti and Hallam 2013: 5). Even Jean Donnison, whose book *Midwives and Medical Men* still offers one of the most comprehensive histories of midwifery in the nineteenth century, does little more than point to the institutions that did train midwives in the period. Her analysis tends to emphasise the relatively small number of women taught in such institutions and says almost nothing about the nature of their education (Donnison 1977).

Part of the problem is that many fewer records exist for writing these histories: women, even educated professional women, have left us few of the textual sources that male medical students and doctors have in the form of notebooks, diaries, articles and other published works. Institutions, too, tended to render invisible the women who kept them running, mainly retaining records of the work undertaken by the overseeing and directing surgeons, physicians and male lecturers. The Radford Collection, as a medical museum collection amassed and employed to teach women midwives as well as medical students for at least the decades between the 1820s and the 1870s, is a unique resource for addressing these historical gaps. While we lack other resources, such as catalogues, syllabi or notes taken by the women students, the images themselves can allow us to gain a sense of the kind of medicalised midwifery education that was available to women in the mid-century, and how they might have experienced it.

It is important at this juncture to establish what we do and do not know about the attendees of the lectures at St. Mary's Hospital in the nineteenth century. Lectures for midwives was one of the original aims of the Charity, and in the annual report of 1878 it was noted that:

> Since its first foundation annual courses of lectures have been deliv-
> ered to practising midwives, and to female pupils. For several years
> they were what may be called more properly instructions, but for
> many years, at least from 1826, full courses of lectures have been giv-
> en. (St. Mary's Hospital 1878: 15)

The report suggests a shift to a more academic, medical-school style of lecture in 1826, and indeed a pamphlet published that year praised the Hospital for its training of midwives and identified Radford as the first lecturer (Anon. 1826). It was around this time that Radford also began giving midwifery lectures to medical students at Joseph Jordan's anatomy school and that he appears to have begun building up his image collection, so it is likely that the three go together, forming a corpus of visually illustrated medical lectures that were available to the city's practitioners at large. While, therefore, we have no syllabus or description that explicitly says that what was offered to the women students was academic, medical lectures illustrated with images and museum objects, we may safely assume so. A museum, as well as the lectures for women, had been features since its foundation, and indeed we know that museum objects were not forbidden to women on principle, as female members of the public were also allowed admittance to the museum, and tours were conducted for them by the matron (Alberti 2011).

From 1853, the existence of an attendance register confirms that the lectures were held yearly, over the course of twenty weeks, usually in the autumn and winter. The attendees were made up of already qualified midwives who worked for the hospital, and the women who were training under them as 'pupils' (Anon. 1853). The registers give relatively little information – just names, attendance records, reasons for absences and the outcomes of examinations. But from this, we can garner that most of the attending women were married or widowed, though unmarried women made up a significant minority, particularly among the pupils. The reasons for absences provide small snapshots of context: some women travelled from surrounding areas to study in Manchester but had to return home prematurely; others were already practicing nurses or midwives and absented themselves from the lectures in order to undertake such work. This fits with Alison Nuttall's assessment of the kind of women who attended provincial midwifery schools in the period, and while the registers give no indication, Nuttall argues that they were likely largely working class (Nuttall 2012). The pupils might attend for one or multiple years, aiming for certification, but the hospital's own midwives were expected to attend every year (Anon. 1852). What proportion of the pupils went on to have careers as professional midwives is not known, but given the diversity of practice throughout the century, it is most likely that some became highly qualified and busy midwives in their communities or at institutions, while others worked more sporadically, or combined midwifery with nursing.

Experiencing the midwifery lecture

For these women, the lectures and museum collections likely held a very different place in their working lives and their experiences of medical knowledge than they did for male medical students. In the final part of this chapter, I will explore what it might have been like as a midwife in the 1850s to experience the medical lectures at St. Mary's, and how the knowledge imparted there fitted into their wider lived experiences of practice. While such an undertaking is necessarily speculative, I argue that it is important to recognise the existence of these women's unique encounters with formalised medical education, even though they have left us without written records of that experience. Indeed, I aim to show how the Radford Collection itself can become a resource for such social and affective histories.

To begin, what would the lecture course actually cover? The Radford Collection itself suggests that embryology and gynaecology were taught, as well as the theory and practice of midwifery, with a focus on pathological complications. This would accord with the basic format of midwifery lectures that were delivered to medical students throughout the century. While the content was perpetually updated, syllabi from midwifery courses taught around Britain and throughout the century suggest that the structure tended to follow a standard pattern. Taking, for example, Edward William Murphy's *Lectures on the Principles and Practice of Midwifery*, published to accompany the lectures he gave at University College in London between 1842 and 1865 (Anon. 1877), we see a typical mixture of physiology, anatomy, pathology and medical practice, split into three sections dealing with conception and pregnancy, childbirth, and the postpartum period (Murphy 1862). A similar structure can be seen in the earlier syllabus taught to medical students at St. Mary's in 1825 by Kinder Wood (Wood 1825). While treatments changed over time, the standard difficulties including distorted pelvises, malpresentations and placenta praevia were always covered.

But did the lectures for women at St. Mary's cover all of the same material? Certainly, some women had access to the lectures I have described: Murphy's were delivered not only to men at University College but also to women at the Ladies' Medical College in the 1860s (Donnison 1977). At St. Mary's, where the pupils were of lower social status than at the London college, the content *may* have been limited or simplified to match the expected sphere of their practice. The midwives employed at St. Mary's were required to call a surgeon in 'any but Natural Presentations', but whether this was strictly adhered to is unclear (Anon. 1852: 11). Many of the midwives had a great deal of experience and were likely, as Frances Badger has argued, capable and trusted to deliver more complicated cases (Badger 2014). Indeed, the casebook of one of St. Mary's midwives – Ellen Booth – indicates that she delivered cases of breech, face presentations, twins, retained placenta and haemorrhage without assistance (Allotey 2017). This means that while the lecturer may have emphasised to his students their limits, these limits were probably not particularly narrow and the whole range of possible difficulties was likely covered, at the very least so the midwives would know when to call for assistance. Embryology might have been taught as a kind of theoretical grounding. And gynaecology might well also have been addressed, not because the women practiced in this area, but because they were likely useful in referring cases to the hospital's surgeons and physicians. Indeed, a system of 'Particular Case Cards' ensured that individual surgeons could claim particularly interesting cases (Anon. 1852: 11).

If, in terms of content, the lectures were similar to what was provided at the hospital for male medical students, they also likely had their own character, not least because the students would have been both much less and much more authoritative than their male equivalents. On the one hand, they had extensive clinical experience, already either working as a midwife or training under one. The same was not true of medical students, who were only required to attend a handful of labours in order to qualify, and who often begrudged or shirked even this small requirement (Murphy 1864). On the other hand, the women were almost certainly not accessing other forms of training or academic medical learning. Wider medical training was closed to them, and barriers of wealth, education and social expectation likely prevented them from pursuing extensive private study using books, though hospital bureaucratic requirements suggest that literacy rates were high. For them, the yearly lectures were their one entry point into the world of academic medicine, the anomaly in a career otherwise dominated by extensive practice. The lectures were a form of access and a form of gatekeeping: less like one aspect of an intermedial, interspatial and self-directed medical education, as we are used to envisioning when it comes to medical students, and more like a system for maintaining midwives who were well trained but also firmly subordinate within the medical system, as Summers has described with regard to hospital-trained nurses (Summers 1989). The lectures, I argue, likely served to combat the confidence that came with extensive practice with an awareness of the different, more socially valued medical knowledge of the male authors, lecturers and practitioners.

Given this privileged, limited, male- and institutionally controlled access to medical learning and medical collections, what might these women, pupils and midwives, have experienced in the lecture theatre at St. Mary's? Entering the lecture theatre, the women would likely have filed onto benches, facing the lecturer, an array of images and objects, and a blackboard. Their entry into the room would signal changes: some would go from respected medical professional to student, and all would feel the weight of male academic authority conferred by the architecture, the furniture and the objects in the room. For most this was not their usual place of work, but the realm of the employers and the doctors, where they came to be instructed and paid, and where they reported to the board.

Let us imagine on this day that the lecture was on pelvic distortion and that the selection of works already mentioned in this chapter was on display. How might the attendees have understood these images? Figures 15.1 and 15.2 are small works on paper that might be handed round the lecture theatre for close inspection. They show distorted pelvises, and those in Figure 15.1 each bear an annotation pointing to the specific case history, and to other objects – paintings and casts of the pelvises – in the collection. Figure 15.3, while it clearly shows a different specimen, indicates what the now lost oil painting of Moore's skeleton might have looked like, perhaps displayed on the wall as part of a series.

First, it is worth noting that for the new pupils, this very attention to the pelvis might be novel. Distorted pelvises can cause difficult labours, or even entirely obstruct the foetus from being born, but such deformities were not necessarily known about ahead of a labour. The action of examining a woman and attempting to measure the outlet of the pelvis needed to be taught, as well as the technique of mapping the haptic knowledge of a physical examination onto an abstract vision of the pelvis's shape. The images provided a look at the invisible interior of the body, and an induction into the abstract, mechanistic knowledge of the process of birth that was seen as both masculine and medicalised.

As well as presenting a new sphere of knowledge within midwifery, Figures 15.1 and 15.2 also point to the wider pedagogic collections: the large oil painting of Moore's skeleton, and casts of both pelvises which could be handled and examined and perhaps even practiced on with a foetal doll. Such objects, made up of or representing parts of the human body, are what Samuel Alberti defines as 'dividual' rather than 'individual': divorced from the identity of the living person, 'becoming metonymic for all examples of a particular malady' (Alberti 2011: 98). But it is worth considering that the women attendees may have been less inclined to divorce the specimens and images they examined from the living women from whom they originated. The midwives and their pupils, after all, spent the majority of their working lives practicing on living women, as well as caring for and knowing them both before and after their labours. Given the unscrupulous, or simply entitled ways in which specimens were often collected, the women may have been troubled by these images, by doubts over whether the women consented to their collection or production, and by speculation over how they would have felt to see parts of their bodies made so public (Alberti 2011).

Figure 15.4 is a similar kind of object, a sketch of a deformed pelvis on paper, but with the added significance that it was made by Radford himself. While Radford was no longer lecturing to the midwives by the 1850s, he would have been known to them as a consulting physician. This image may, therefore, have been presented to them as an object lesson in their more specific professional duties: not only explaining the pioneering work done by the hospital's senior physician and benefactor in the field of caesarean section, but also stressing their duty to report all relevant cases. Indeed, the hospital rules of 1852 indicate a particular interest in pelvic deformity and required that midwives summon not just the on-call surgeon, but a 'General Consultation' of all the hospital's male staff in such cases (Anon. 1852: 6).

Figures 15.5 and 15.6, both larger paintings mounted on board and clearly intended to be hung up on walls, perhaps permanently or perhaps as part of a kind of mobile and adaptable display, are both copied from illustrations from canonical published works on midwifery. Unlike the images already discussed, which derive from cases encountered by Radford and his colleagues, these images are more abstract, showing the principles of pelvic distortion and how it affects birth. Figure 15.5, more than any of the other examples discussed here, might initially have been indecipherable to the attendees. The strange amorphous shapes actually show the measurements of the outlets of four different distorted pelvises, and thus the spaces through which the foetal skull has to pass. Such an image, removed from the context of the book, would need explanation to be interpreted. Indeed, it may have been presented in combination with Figure 15.6, which shows the physical process of the fetus passing through the pelvic outlet. Here, the artist has taken care to describe the way the unfused plates of the foetal skull overlap in order to pass through the pelvis. It is unlikely that the lecturers expected the midwives to undertake private study with books, so attention to these images may have been accompanied by a kind of collective reading, with passages read aloud or summarised from Smellie's and Nägele's books.

Brought together, the different visualisations, as well as museum objects and books, build a picture of birth that incorporates technical and mechanical aspects, physical practice and pathology. This picture might have felt rather foreign to the midwives and pupils, who could not measure the women they attended as they could the images and specimens. The focus on pathological and difficult cases, too, may have felt out of step with the vast majority of standard cases that they attended. Indeed, it is also likely that the technical language used to describe childbirth in the lecture theatre was a very different one from that used in the lying-in room. But if these images represented a different realm of knowledge and one that the women had to be inducted into, it was one that likely helped them to maintain professional footing with their male colleagues, as well, perhaps, as giving them a more abstract authority with the women among whom they practiced. In being familiar with both the canonical illustrations of the discipline and the specimens within the hospital's own collection, the women gained a shared visual and technical language with which to communicate with surgeons and physicians.

Of course, responses both academic and affective must have varied greatly between different attendees, not least because while some were new to any kind of formalised medical education, others had attended the lecture course for many years. Some of the pupils may have failed to engage at all in the academic medical atmosphere and language, or have found the collections displayed disturbing or unreadable. These women may be represented in the number each year who stopped attending, or who failed to gain certification. But other pupils clearly followed the learning patterns set out for them successfully, gained certification and even won prizes.

The hospital's midwives were required to attend every year, and arguably not only in order to keep their knowledge up to date but also to keep them in their place in the medical hierarchy, perpetually reminded both of the knowledge of the lecturers and the limits of their own practice. Some may well have resented the perpetual requirement to return to the role of student, and to listen to a succession of junior surgeons (the attendance registers indicate it was usually the most junior male member of staff who lectured to the women) tell them what they already knew. On the other hand, it also likely provided them with the only access route to realms of academic medical knowledge that raised their status and earning potential. The competition for prizes and medals from the 1870s suggests that some of these midwives took pride in their engagement in the male, academic and institutional realms of medicine, and put effort into their attendance and learning. Indeed, it is possible, given the range of knowledge and experience in each cohort – from raw student to experienced professional – that some of the senior midwives acted as assistants to the lecturer, or helped their pupils to understand the lectures. The dynamics between attendees, as well as with the male lecturers and administrators, can only be guessed at. However, it is likely that the qualified midwives had vastly greater experience of normal childbirth than did any of their lecturers, and may have been able to provide a different perspective on particular conditions or practices.

Medical museum collections worked in many ways for a great diversity of students and medical practitioners in the nineteenth century. Looking at the Radford Collection and its audiences, and speculating on the ways in which it might have been used and understood, we are able to expand our stories of medical teaching and learning. Alongside the better-known story of the elite London hospital that guided its aspiring physicians in individual dissections, in walking the wards and spending long hours studying specimens in the museum and books in the library, we can place the story of the provincial lying-in hospital, which for twenty weeks each year summoned its midwives and their pupils into the edifice of learning to collectively inhabit the realm of academic medicine. For these students, the Radford Collection was deeply important. Pedagogically, it offered access to hallowed and highly masculinised realms and inducted them into identities of profession and expertise, as well as establishing their relatively humble status and the limits of their practice. In its interactions with these professional women, the Radford Collection can give us entirely new perspectives on what it meant to study medicine in the nineteenth century.

Acknowledgements

My thanks to Dr. David Shreeve for funding this research. My thanks also to the John Rylands Research Institute who have hosted my fellowship, and to the librarians, archivists, photographers and conservators at the University of Manchester Library for enabling my access to the Radford Collection under a series of adverse conditions.

References

Alberti, Samuel J. M. M. (2011), *Morbid Curiosities: Medical Museums in Nineteenth-Century Britain*, Oxford: Oxford University Press.

Alberti, Samuel J. M. M. and Hallam, Elizabeth (eds) (2013), *Medical Museums: Past, Present, Future*, London: Royal College of Surgeons of England.

Allotey, Janette (2017), 'Midwifery records of midwife Booth of Salford', *de Partu*, 27 April, https://departu.org.uk/2017/04/midwifery-records-midwife-booth-salford/. Accessed 25 August 2020.

Anon. (1790), *The Rules and Orders of the Lying-In Charity for Delivering Poor Women at their Own Habitations, and for Erecting a Lying-In Hospital in Manchester, as Soon as the Sum of £2,000 Can be Raised*, Manchester: The Author.

Anon. (1826), *An Address to the Public on the Propriety of Midwives, Instead of Surgeons, Practising Midwifery*, 2nd ed., Manchester: The Author.

Anon. (1852), *Rules of the Manchester and Salford Lying-In Hospital and Dispensary for the Diseases Peculiar to Women, and for the Diseases of Children Under Three Years of Age. Founded 1790*, Manchester: Cave & Sever.

Anon. (1853), *Register of Pupil Attendance, Lying in Hospital*, Manchester: University of Manchester Library, MMC/9/10/8/1.

Anon. (1877), 'Obituary: Edward William Murphy', *The British Medical Journal*, 1:839, p. 122.

Badger, Frances J. (2014), 'Illuminating nineteenth-century urban midwifery: The register of a coventry midwife', *Women's History Review*, 23:5, pp. 683–705.

Berkowitz, Carin (2011), 'The beauty of anatomy: Visual displays and surgical education in early-nineteenth-century London', *Bulletin of the History of Medicine*, 85:2, pp. 248–78.

Berkowitz, Carin (2013), 'Systems of display: The making of anatomical knowledge in enlightenment Britain', *The British Journal for the History of Science*, 46:3, pp. 359–87.

Berkowitz, Carin (2015), 'The illustrious anatomist: Authorship, patronage, and illustrative style in anatomy folios, 1700–1840', *Bulletin of the History of Medicine*, 89:2, pp. 171–208.

Berkowitz, Carin and Lightman, Bernard (eds) (2017), *Science Museums in Transition: Cultures of Display in Nineteenth-Century Britain and America*, Pittsburgh: University of Pittsburgh Press.

Blake, Catriona (1990), *The Charge of the Parasols: Women's Entry to the Medical Profession*, London: The Women's Press.

Daston, Lorraine and Galison, Peter (2010), *Objectivity*, New York: Zone Books.

Deblon, Veronique (2017), 'Imitating anatomy: Recycling anatomical illustrations in nineteenth-century atlases', in K. Wils, R. de Bont and S. Au (eds), *Bodies Beyond Borders: Moving Anatomies, 1750–1940*, Leuven: Leuven University Press, pp. 115–38.

Digby, Anne (1994), *Making a Medical Living: Doctors and Patients in the English Market for Medicine, 1720–1911*, Cambridge: Cambridge University Press.

Donnison, Jean (1977), *Midwives and Medical Men: A History of Inter-Professional Rivalries and Women's Rights*, London: Heinemann.

Dyhouse, Carol (2006), *Students: A Gendered History*, London: Routledge.

Forman Cody, Lisa (2004) 'Living and dying in Georgian London's lying-in hospitals', *Bulletin of the History of Medicine*, 78:2, pp. 309–48.

Foucault, Michel (2003), *The Birth of the Clinic: An Archaeology of Medical Perception* (trans. A. M. Sheridan), London: Routledge.

Furst, Lilian R. (ed.) (1997), *Women Healers and Physicians: Climbing a Long Hill*, Kentucky: University Press of Kentucky.

Graciano, Andrew (ed.) (2019), *Visualizing the Body in Art, Anatomy, and Medicine since 1800: Models and Modeling*, New York: Routledge.

Hallam, Elizabeth (2016), *Anatomy Museum: Death and the Body Displayed*, London: Reaktion Books.

Hallett, Christine E. (2012), 'Nursing, 1830–1920: Forging a profession', in A. Borsay and B. Hunter (eds), *Nursing and Midwifery in Britain Since 1700*, Basingstoke: Palgrave Macmillan, pp. 46–73.

Hammerschlag, Keren Rosa (2016), 'William Orpen (1878–1931): Looking at bodies in medicine and art', *The British Art Journal*, 17:1, pp. 78–93.

Hunter, Mary (2016), *The Face of Medicine: Visualising Medical Masculinities in Late Nineteenth-Century Paris*, Manchester: Manchester University Press.

Jordanova, Ludmilla J. (1989), *Sexual Visions: Images of Gender in Science and Medicine Between the Eighteenth and Twentieth Centuries*, New York: Harvester Wheatsheaf.

Kemp, Martin and Wallace, Marina (2000), *Spectacular Bodies: The Art and Science of the Human Body from Leonardo to Now*, Berkeley: University of California Press.

La Berge, Ann and Hannaway, Caroline (1998), 'Paris medicine: Perspectives past and present', in C. Hannaway and A. La Berge (eds), *Constructing Paris Medicine*, Amsterdam: Rodopi, pp. 1–69.

Loudon, Irvine (1986), *Medical Care and the General Practitioner 1750–1850*, Oxford: Clarendon Press.

McGrath, Roberta (2002), *Seeing Her Sex: Medical Archives and the Female Body*, Manchester: Manchester University Press.

McIntosh, Tania (1998), 'Profession, skill or domestic duty? Midwifery in Sheffield, 1881–1936', *Social History of Medicine*, 11:3, pp. 403–20.

Moscucci, Ornella (1990), *The Science of Woman: Gynaecology and Gender in England, 1800–1929*, Cambridge: Cambridge University Press.

Murphy, Edward William (1862), *Lectures on the Principles and Practice of Midwifery*, 2nd ed., London: Walton and Maberly.

Murphy, Edward William (1864), 'Introductory lecture on the history of midwifery. Delivered at University College, May 1st, 1864. By Edward W. Murphy, M.A., M.D., Professor of Midwifery', *The British Medical Journal*, 176:1, pp. 523–28.

Nägele, Franz Karl (1839), *Das schräg verengte Becken nebst einem Anhange über die wichtigsten Fehler des weiblichen Beckens überhaupt*, Mainz: V. von Zabern.

Nuttall, Alison (2012), 'Midwifery, 1800–1920: The journey to registration', in A. Borsay and B. Hunter (eds), *Nursing and Midwifery in Britain since 1700*, Basingstoke: Palgrave Macmillan, pp. 128–50.

Pickstone, John V. (1985), *Medicine and Industrial Society: A History of Hospital Development in Manchester and its Region, 1752–1946*, Manchester: Manchester University Press.

Radford, T. (c.1830s), *A Written Description of the Drawing of Three Deformed Skeletons*, M: University of Manchester Library, MMM/14/1/10.

Ruiz-Gómez, Natasha (2019), 'The model patient: Observation and illustration at the Musée Charcot', in A. Graciano (ed.), *Visualizing the Body in Art, Anatomy, and Medicine since 1800: Models and Modeling*, New York: Routledge, pp. 203–32.

Sappol, Michael (2006), *Dream Anatomy*, Washington, DC: U.S. Dept. of Health and Human Services, National Library of Medicine, National Institutes of Health.

Slipp, Naomi (2017), 'International anatomies: Teaching visual literacy in the Harvard lecture hall', in K. Wils, R. de Bont and S. Au (eds), *Bodies Beyond Borders: Moving Anatomies, 1750–1940*, Leuven: Leuven University Press, pp. 197–229.

Smellie, William (1754), *A Sett of Anatomical Tables, with Explanations, and an Abridgment, of the Practice of Midwifery, with a View to Illustrate a Treatise on that Subject, and Collection of Cases*, London: n.p.

St. Mary's Hospital (1868), *Report of St. Mary's Hospital and Dispensary for Women and Children, Quay Street, Manchester; to which is Added a Report of the Ladies' Auxiliary Society, from December 31st, 1866, to December 31st, 1867*, Manchester: Thos. Sowler and Sons.

St. Mary's Hospital (1878), *Report of St. Mary's Hospital and Dispensary for Women and Children, Quay Street, Manchester. Founded 1790. To Which is Added a Report of the Ladies' Auxiliary Society, from December 31, 1876, to December 31, 1877*. Manchester: A. Ireland & Co.

Summers, Anne (1989), 'The mysterious demise of Sarah Gamp: The domiciliary nurse and her detractors, c. 1830–1860', *Victorian Studies*, 32:3, pp. 365–86.

Sutton, C. W. and Moscucci, Ornella (2004) 'Radford, Thomas (1793–1881)', *Oxford Dictionary of National Biography*, Oxford: Oxford University Press, https://doi-org.manchester.idm.oclc.org/10.1093/ref:odnb/22999. Accessed 11 March 2020.

Wells, Susan (2001), *Out of the Dead House: Nineteenth-Century Women Physicians and the Writing of Medicine*, Madison: The University of Wisconsin Press.

Wils, Kaat, de Bont, Raf and Au, Sokhieng (eds) (2017), *Bodies Beyond Borders: Moving Anatomies, 1750–1940*, Leuven: Leuven University Press.

Wood, K. (1825), *Syllabus of a Course of Lectures on the Theory and Practice of Midwifery by Kinder Wood, Member of the Royal College of Surgeons, and of the Medico-Chirurgical Society, London, – Man-Midwife in Ordinary to the Lying-In Hospital, Manchester*, Manchester: T. Forrest [printer].

Wood, W. (1799), 'A case of caesarean section', *Memoirs of the Medical Society of London*, 5, pp. 463–76.

Young, John Harley (1964), *St. Mary's Hospitals Manchester 1790–1963*, Edinburgh and London: E. & S. Livingstone Ltd.

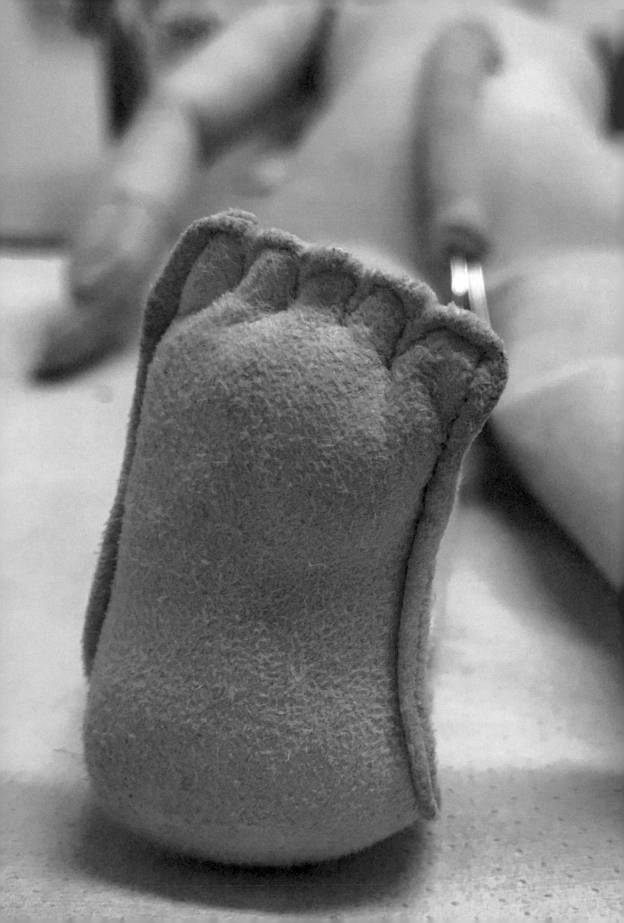

LABOUR

INVISIBLE WORK

Sally Wyatt

Medical and other education depends on huge amounts of 'invisible work', more or less well paid, more or less gendered and racialised. Cleaning is an important example, but there are other tasks, jobs and people invisible to students and their parents but nonetheless vital to everyday activities of teaching and learning. These include monitoring student numbers and progress, acquiring and cataloguing books and setting up experiments to be conducted in class or as part of research.

More than twenty years ago, Susan Leigh Star and Anselm Strauss (1999) introduced the notion of 'invisible work', that labour which is often rendered invisible in national statistics, in workplaces and in education. 'Invisible work' provides a label to something that may be familiar from our everyday lives. For example, the domestic work done by many women, especially mothers, to care for children and homes. This is unpaid and often invisible to others living in the household, a point made by feminist scholars and activists long before 1999 (Friedan 1963; Cowan 1983).

Invisible work does not only take place at home. For example, workplace cleaners are often invisible to those who start their jobs later in the day. Nor is invisible work only done by women. Many tasks essential to the functioning of everyday life are done by working class women and men, and often by migrants or racialised minorities.

In the provision of healthcare, it is not difficult to imagine the kinds of invisible work necessary for the smooth running of hospitals and clinics, again often done by low paid, racialised and gendered workers. This includes the paid work of nurses, cleaners and technicians (Mesman 2008). Healthcare

Figure TE3: A hand-stitched manikin used in obstetric simulations at Maastricht University's Skillslab. Image courtesy of Anna Harris.

systems are increasingly dependent on the invisible work of patients and their families in managing chronic conditions (Oudshoorn 2011). Not all invisible work is low paid, and certainly not all of it is low skilled, as the mention of technicians suggests.

In the opening paragraph, education is highlighted. But doing research and producing knowledge in the form of publications is also an important role for universities and is sometimes invisible (Antonijević et al. 2013). Contributions to this volume draw attention to various kinds of invisible work in the delivery of medical education and the reproduction of medical knowledge. Laboratories work has already been mentioned and, elsewhere in this volume, the reader can learn about how the craft of sewing has influenced surgery, the making of medical illustrations, the devices which facilitate the less visible work of nurses, and of the women who help medical students learn to conduct gynaecological examinations.

Paul Craddock (this volume) describes the importance of sewing skills for surgeons, telling this story through a cigarette paper. In the late nineteenth century, aspiring surgeons often learned to sew from their mothers, sisters and wives. Craddock discusses the Nobel Prize-winning vascular surgeon, Alexis Carrel, who came from a textile family, but who learned even more from the renowned embroiderer Marie Anne Leroudier. Medical knowledge is usually captured in written, published papers, thus Leroudier's contributions to Carrel's surgical innovations, namely training in delicate, craft skills, is invisible in the historical record.

The close collaboration between the artist Dorothy Davison and the surgeon Geoffrey Jefferson in early twentieth century England is analysed by Harriet Palfreyman (this volume). The importance of artists and medical illustration is discussed further elsewhere (see section on 'Objectivity, Art and Medical Images', this volume), but Palfreyman highlights how the work of the artist is decidedly invisible to the unconscious patient, but not always to the surgeons. Even if the process of creating illustrations may be visible when they are being made, the labour which went into the illustration of such medical illustrations, images and specimens may become less visible over time. Rebecca Whiteley (this volume) describes how medical images, once integral to medical education, have become separated both spatially and institutionally. In the nineteenth century, the library, museum and lecture theatre were close together, with the result that specimens, books and images circulated easily.

As already mentioned, cleaning is one of the best examples of invisible work, even though it has long been known that clean environments are essential to good medical care. David Theodore (this volume) describes how the

Nurserver was introduced into hospitals in the mid twentieth century. Designed in the 1960s by Gordon Friesen, the Nurserver is a simple, non-medical device (Faulkner 2009) that improves both hospital hygiene and workflow. Drawing on the approach widely adopted in manufacturing earlier in the twentieth century, inspired by F.W. Taylor and Henry Ford (Braverman 1974), Friesen's design circumvented the expertise and authority of doctors and architects, and paid attention to the work done by nurses and cleaners.

A final example of invisible work is provided by Kelly Underman (this volume), drawing on her own experience as a gynaecological teaching associate (GTA). Doctors-in-training learn the skills needed when examining and communicating with patients. For the latter, actors are often used. For the former, medical students often practise on themselves or on each other (Harris 2016; Wojcik forthcoming) to measure heart rates for example. Underman describes the work of GTAs, women paid to help medical students learn how to conduct pelvic exams and to communicate with the often anxious patients who have to undergo them. GTAs often provide their own gowns and gloves, set up the learning situation and undergo repeated, sometimes painful and amateurish handling.

These contributions raise interesting questions for medical education and for research about medical education, past and present. Does the invisibility of particular tasks, materials or technologies change over time or between contexts? The work and skill of Marie Anne Leroudier (Craddock, this volume) and the crafts people who produced models and other objects may suffer from a double invisibility. Their work may have been invisible during their own lifetimes, and it is also invisible in the historical record which privileges text and the written word.

The notion of 'invisible work' has provided an important reference point for scholarship in science and technology studies (STS), feminist technology studies, history of medicine and the sociology and anthropology of health. The chapters mentioned above also have implications for three recurring normative debates. First is the perennial question: for whom is this work invisible? As Star and Strauss pointed out, 'no work is inherently either visible or invisible' (1999: 9). Sometimes the people are invisible but the work is not, and sometimes it is the other way around. Certainly the work is visible to those actually doing it, and at least sometimes, also to close colleagues. Palfreyman suggests that Jefferson greatly appreciated Davison's work, and one hopes that medical students appreciate the efforts of GTAs. The bodies of the women are visible to them but the work they do in preparing for the examination may not be.

A second normative debate is about whether invisible work is necessarily undervalued and underpaid. Decisions about how much to pay cleaners in hospitals and university medical centres are largely social and political. This volume also provides examples of invisible work that is esoteric and valued, such as the work of embroiderers and illustrators.

Third, do we always want to make the invisible visible? It would be exhausting to pay constant attention to invisible work. Invisible work, rather like infrastructure, is often taken for granted until it is no longer effectively performed (Slota and Bowker 2017). Only then do the rest of us realise how much effort goes into washing and ironing clothes, putting food on supermarket shelves, cleaning the floors of office buildings, maintaining the railway network and preparing teaching for medical students. Teachers may wish to keep the mystery, and not always reveal to students the work involved in putting together a lecture or setting up a lab for students to learn about biology or anatomy.

Becoming aware of invisible work can change one's life. It can be instructive to consider the amount and types of work that need to be done to make mundane activities possible. Paying attention to the invisible work involved in medical education opens up new career possibilities (becoming a GTA or medical illustrator, e.g.), and may provide ideas for innovative medical devices (such as the Nurserver). Most importantly, awareness of invisible work fosters appreciation of the myriad people and tasks, mundane and esoteric, all of which are essential.

References

Antonijević, Smiljana, Dormans, Stefan and Wyatt, Sally (2013), 'Working in virtual knowledge: Affective labor in scholarly collaboration', in P. Wouters, A. Beaulieu, A. Scharnhorst and S. Wyatt (eds), *Virtual Knowledge. Experimenting in the Humanities and the Social Sciences*, Cambridge: The MIT Press, pp. 57–88.

Braverman, Harry (1974), *Labor and Monopoly Capital, The Degradation of Work in the Twentieth Century*, New York: Monthly Review Press.

Cowan, Ruth Schwartz (1983), *More Work for Mother: The Ironies of Household Technology from the Open Hearth to the Microwave*, New York: Basic Books.

Faulkner, Alex (2009), *Medical Technology into Healthcare and Society: A Sociology of Devices, Innovation and Governance*, Houndmills: Palgrave Macmillan.

Friedan, Betty (1963), *The Feminine Mystique*, New York: Norton.

Harris, Anna (2016). 'Listening-touch, affect and the crafting of medical bodies through percussion', *Body & Society*, 22:1, pp. 31–61.

Mesman, Jessica (2008), *Uncertainty in Medical Innovation*, Houndmills: Palgrave Macmillan.

Oudshoorn, Nelly (2011), *Telecare Technologies and the Transformation of Healthcare*, Houndmills: Palgrave Macmillan.

Slota, Stephen and Bowker, Geoffrey (2017), 'How infrastructures matter', in U. Felt, R. Fouché, C. Miller and L. Smith-Doerr (eds), *The Handbook of Science and Technology Studies*, 4th ed., Cambridge: The MIT Press, pp. 529–54.

Star, Susan Leigh and Strauss, Anselm (1999), 'Layers of silence, arenas of voice: The ecology of visible and invisible work', *Computer Supported Cooperative Work*, 8, pp. 9–30.

Wojcik, Andrea (forthcoming), 'The co-production of bodies and pedagogical technologies in medical education: An ethnographic study of skills training at a Ghanaian medical school', Ph.D. dissertation, Maastricht: Maastricht University.

MICROSCOPES

THE VIRTUAL MICROSCOPE: TRACING KNOWLEDGE OF HUMAN MICROSTRUCTURE THROUGH DIGITAL IMAGES

R. Claire Aland, Nicole Shepherd, Belinda Swyny

and Mary-Louise Roy Manchadi

Traditionally, teaching of body structure has centred around bringing material bodies together in the same physical space and time, where students learn by listening to instructors, observing role models in clinical environments, or using bodies (cadavers, biopsies, fellow students, real or simulated patients). The replacement of some learning activities with purely online delivery disrupts these traditional interactions. The absence of physical bodies and the replacement with electronic traces of the material can potentially stimulate students' imagination and facilitate deep learning. We argue that teaching histology online expands possibilities for education, and online teaching approaches should embrace these possibilities and not simply mimic the approach used in a physical classroom.

This chapter captures our reflections on a change in format to online teaching about the microstructures of the human body. We are all academics teaching into the medical programme at The University of Queensland, we teach anatomy (RCA), ethics (NS), clinical practice (BS) and pharmacology (MRM). Our institution, like many others around the world, made a rapid shift to online education in response to the COVID-19 pandemic. We explore the implications of using the virtual microscope (VM) in the online setting and have structured the chapter around the concept of trace. The *Merriam-Webster* dictionary includes in its definitions of trace: to find or discover through investigation; a minute quantity, too small to be accurately measured; the mark that indicates at some point the presence of the physical body; and to copy or trace over, to form a mental model (trace) in the mind. This common usage of trace is relevant to teaching about the microstructure of the body, as it requires students to investigate the small structures of the body, and this is done using slides created from living bodies. The aim of teaching this to students is to help them form a mental model of how the body works at a microscopic level.

At a theoretical level, we use Derrida's (1973, 1976) concept of trace as part of *différance*. *Différance* refers to distinction, deviation and spacing, and also to defer, detour, delay or relay. According to Derrida, 'the trace is not a presence but is rather the simulacrum of a presence that dislocates, displaces, and refers beyond itself' (1973: 156). When students use a VM, they perceive a static electronic trace of a material body. The image refers to more than itself, it is a representation nested in the dynamic complexity that is the human body. As suggested by Valentina Napolitano (2015), traces indicate a limit of representation, the boundary of what can be seen. Histological images are chosen to illustrate key structures, students learn to identify these features in samples yet to be seen. Students must connect the image as perceived with their memory of the microstructure of the body. A 'mental model' is a term used to refer to students' internal representation of the real world, providing an internal framework that students use to organise new learning and guide application of knowledge to problem-solving (Martindale 1993; Park and Gittelman 1995). Students using the VM can manipulate and annotate images, stimulating their imagination. In doing so, we suggest students construct a mental model of bodily processes, making connections through the in-between spaces and silences between the images, much like the gutters in-between comic strips (Liou et al. 2016).

From physical to virtual microscopy in histology teaching

Human structure is taught at both macroscopic and microscopic levels in healthcare professions education. The macroscopic is what can be seen with the eye and touched with the hand. The microscopic, in contrast, is beyond direct perception. Small parts of the body must be specially prepared and artificially coloured before interrogation. The assemblage of objects – the microscope, the hand, the eye and the prepared slides – work together to bridge the gap between perceptible and imperceptible.

Histology teaching has been traditionally located in lecture halls and laboratories, using static images (photomicrographs) and diagrams to illustrate the structure of tissues. In practical classes, students use microscopes and glass slides containing thin sections of tissues that were stained with coloured chemicals that highlighted selected structures. Such histological stains link structure with molecular and chemical composition. The physical body, in all its individual variations and imperfect forms, is thus present as a trace on the glass slides. Histology teaching uses images made of microscopic traces of the body that illustrate complex interactions of many hundreds or thousands of elements. The slides represent a moment in time, extracted from the living, functioning body. Students are expected to extrapolate from such a moment and interpret what they are seeing in terms of dynamic physiological processes, akin to extrapolating from a still shot to a movie scene.

In this approach to teaching histology, students were required to develop skills in microscope use and visual interpretation, integrating what they saw with their theoretical knowledge, to better understand structure and function (Hussein et al. 2015). To develop these skills, students worked together with tutors in a classroom or laboratory providing opportunities for the development of problem-solving and communication skills (Hightower et al. 1999). The design of most microscopes precludes more than one person working simultaneously on the same slide. A singular slide was the domain of an individual student and could not be shared between students or with teachers. Multi-head teaching microscopes permit collaboration between tutors and students, but do not scale up effectively when teaching large groups.

Approaches to teaching histology remained stable for decades, only changing with advances in chemistry or microscopy. More recently, medical educators have faced demands to reduce the time and resources used for histology teaching within crowded medical curricula (Levine et al. 1999; Drake et al. 2002; Black and Smith 2004; Bloodgood and Ogilvie 2006). Increasingly, histology has been integrated with other disciplines, such as physiology (Black and Smith 2004). Once considered essential, technical proficiency in microscope use is now required by few practitioners (Chen et al. 2011), facilitating the previously unthinkable – histology teaching without microscopes or glass slides (Paulsen et al. 2010; Jurjus et al. 2018). Instead, students can use digital tools, such as virtual microscopy. The 'virtual microscope' (VM) refers to the use of high-resolution digital images created by scanning glass slides in a digital slide scanner (Pawlina and Drake 2016). Instead of direct manipulation of the physical specimen on a microscope, students now indirectly manipulate a digital file. An advantage of the digital image is that it can be shared equally between all students and with teachers simultaneously. This expands the teaching and learning space beyond the spatial and temporal constraints of the microscope, the slide and the laboratory (Rennie and Morrison 2012).

At our university, teaching histology with VM was adopted initially by simply replacing microscopes and glass slides with computers and software within the same formal physical learning spaces. Other educators noted a similar approach in their institutions, where microscopes were simply substituted with computers, with little change in the teaching spaces or pedagogical approach (Cotter 2001; McBride and Prayson 2008). In considering the potential of new technology, the concept of affordances is useful. This term was originally introduced by Gibson (1979) and applied to technology by Norman (1988) and Hutchby (2001) to refer to the way the properties of an object emerge during the interaction between technology and the user. Conole and Dyke (2004) noted that, in general, there was little understanding of different technologies' affordances, and how those could be exploited in teaching, or supported by pedagogical theory (Conole et al. 2004). This has been true of digital histology, which often has been implemented for cost reasons without consideration of educational goals or pedagogical strategies that engage effectively with its affordances (Cotter 2001; Harris et al. 2001; Braun and Kearns 2008; McBride and Prayson 2008).

VM replicates the physically interrogative and manipulative capacities of the microscope via the mouse or touchpad (Harris et al. 2001; Braun and Kearns 2008). Knowledge construction from VM demands active engagement and manipulation of virtual samples (Mione et al. 2013, 2016). Like physical microscopy, VM fosters communication and problem solving (Plendl et al. 2009) by developing skills in manipulating the VM, using visual interpretation skills to view the tissue, combined with the interaction with other students and tutors. The advantage of multiple students working simultaneously on the same image, straightforward with VM, is difficult to achieve with traditional micro-scopes. The availability of VM outside of physical learning spaces permits extensive use in self-directed learning (Gatumu et al. 2014; Scott et al. 2017). Students are still able to discover and investigate the trace of the body, albeit now as a digital copy of the original physical specimen. One of the affordances of VM, the ease of use outside of formal physical learning spaces, makes a compelling argument for its utility in making the human body accessible online for learning in current and future education. The consideration of pedagogy alongside technological affordance is crucial here. We know that *what* students learn is directly related to *how* they learn (Marton and Säljö 1997). A risk of online teaching is that in the physical absence of teachers and fellow students, the students can fail to engage deeply with the materials, instead adopting passive and surface learning approaches (Dolan et al. 2002; Ramsden 2003). This strongly supports the requirement for human interaction in the online learning space. Using VM allows for particular collaborative and practical learning activities (Khalil et al. 2013; Ettarh 2016), which we know support deep approaches to learning (Glasersfeld 1989).

Tracing knowledge

Hirsh et al. (2007: 858) describe that one of the challenges of medical education is the lack of '[...] connection or continuity among different learning experiences'. The biomedical science curriculum, where body structure is primarily taught, is often partitioned into discrete disciplines or systems (e.g. learning about the heart separate from the lungs). This curriculum partitioning and separation of learning experiences is a reductionist approach that encourages students to learn by memorising facts as 'discrete knowable units' rather than exploring their connections (Knight and Mattick 2006). A risk of this approach is that students may not synthesise these discrete units of knowledge into an understanding of the complexity of the human body in health and disease (Marshall 2005; Bransford et al. 2000).

In addition to curricular partitioning, the models and diagrams chosen for medical texts present idealized versions of the body that students have trouble recognizing in real bodies or samples (Willan and Humpherson 1999). The vestige of the physical body is taken out of context and displayed at a magnification that rarely allows students to directly situate it back within the body or situate it within a normal range. As described in Daston and Galison (2007), scientists can select images to illustrate the perfect form, and thus be blind to variability. They argue that pursuit of scientific objectivity should instead aim to preserve 'the artifact or variation that would have been erased in the name of truth; it scruples to filter out the noise that undermines certainty' (Daston and Galison 2007: 17). In histology teaching, educators select images for the norm or typical, which rejects the variable and irregular. The ideal structure presented to the student may not exist, or may be vanishingly rare in reality. Subjective selection was less of a feature of physical microscopy and glass slides, because there are usually multiple 'copies', or sequential sections through the tissue, sometimes hundreds, which all differ slightly, and will include within them transitional regions, variations, ambiguities and artefacts introduced during processing. Subjective selection occurs with VM as the cost of digitisation, file storage and bandwidth for access initially prohibited scanning of multiple copies of the same slides. These limitations favour the selection of the most typical, representative and artefact-free slides. The omission of the variable and irregular could lead to students forming incorrect or incomplete mental models that prove a barrier to latter understanding. For example, if students only see perfectly representative sections of elastic and muscular arteries, which differ in structure and function, it is difficult for them to appreciate regions of spatial and functional continuity as the elastic artery transitions to the muscular one. Continuous temporal transitions of, for example, the uterine lining across a monthly cycle of thickening and loss are not appreciated if different phases of endometrium are only ever seen as perfectly representative snapshots, discrete in time.

Virtual microscopy is not simply a like-for-like digital replacement for physical microscopy, but rather, a new way of investigating the body. Both digital and analogue techniques visualise a trace that students use to construct their mental model of the human body. Initially, the use of ideal images was a feature of VM, but now the reduced cost and increased availability of digital storage, cheaper and faster internet access, and the advent of collaborative multi-institutional online educational resources, make it easier to present students with images that demonstrate a greater range of variability. Exposing students to this range of normality can assist them to build more robust mental models and support latter integration of complex and changing information required by life-long learning in the practice of medicine.

Separations between curricular blocks have been referred to as 'gutters' after the blank spaces between visual panels in a cartoon, where interconnectedness between panels is created by the mind of the reader, rather than explicitly by the cartoonist (Liou et al. 2016). Liou et al. (2016: 322) argued that 'playing in the gutter' is transformative – by encouraging students to work creatively within the gutters, they can more easily make those connections, and gutters become opportunities rather than barriers. Although Liou et al. (2016) were talking about larger curricular blocks, a similar idea can be applied to the distances between slides showing microscopic traces of the body, and how this relates to macroscopic structure, and the functioning or dysfunctioning of the body. Other educational researchers have examined how people make meaning from imagery. For example, Philip Yenawine (2005: 845) suggests that interpreting images calls upon 'personal association, questioning, speculating, analyzing, fact-finding, and categorizing'. Harnessing the power of technology to stimulate imagination and creativity may counter the reduction of the body by encouraging students to form connections between 'discrete knowable units' (Marshall 2005; Knight and Mattick 2006) and encourage application of knowledge into different settings (Bransford et al. 2000). Like the role of imagination in film or cartoons, to fill the gutter, students need imagination to translate that static two-dimensional snapshot of the body into the three-dimensional spatial and dynamic temporal reality of the functioning physical body. Showing a greater number of imperfect slides may help students 'fill the gutter', in the construction of more accurate mental models that bridge structure and function. Information studies researchers investigating the use of digital technologies in education have suggested that students could become 'participatory creators', rather than only consumers of pre-constructed educational materials (Meyers et al. 2013). While students could interact with textbooks by annotating them, or turning down corners of pages, VM facilitates a different kind of participatory creation, as students create their meaning of the body through digital investigation and discovery.

The rapid shift to online teaching

At The University of Queensland, histology had been taught with both online and face-to-face elements, in large repeated practical classes for the nearly 500 students in each year. Each practical class had students and teachers physically in the same space engaged in practical activities both individually and in small groups. Although VM had been introduced some years previously, the physical arrangement of the classroom was unchanged, with computers simply replacing physical microscopes. In 2020, the COVID-19 pandemic required a rapid shift to purely online delivery. The virtual body represented in digital slides was always accessible outside of class. However, the learning communities of students and tutors that had previously met in person needed to be recreated online. We did this using small group online video tutorials that permitted participants to simultaneously work with the same virtual image. In this way, the electronic trace of the body, via VM, afforded teachers and students the space in which to interact collaboratively in a way that was not possible in the physical teaching space. The small group learning space on the videoconference is now shared more equally between students and teachers. Rather than distinguishing the teacher from the students by location within the physical teaching space, online tutorials permit more equitable presence. It could be argued that with the shared body permitted by VM, and the shared online space, students now have a more substantial presence, which comes with an increased expectation of participation in learning. As a result, in 2021, our university shifted back to face-to-face teaching, but we have kept histology practical teaching online as we felt it was more effective. Virtual microscopy has been proven to be robust in the face of sudden changes in conditions, such as outbreaks which significantly impact mobility of staff and students, and continues to be a major part of a resilient teaching strategy.

Conclusion

We have traced the way that knowledge of the microstructures of the body is constructed by learners using virtual microscopy from our perspective as medical educators. When teaching histology in the physical classroom, the mental models that students form of the body are shaped by an assemblage of eye, microscope – whether physical or virtual, glass slides (material body) or their electronic trace, and textbooks. The use of 'typical' samples and textbook illustrations makes it challenging for students to apprehend the messiness and ambiguity of the real physical body. Coming back to Derrida's idea of *différance*, online teaching allows deviations and distinctions to be seen in a variety of traces of the body. Through the viewing of multiple, imperfect images, students synthesise these traces into mental models of the functioning body. We suggest that using electronic traces of the body to teach students offers new pedagogical possibilities in medicine. Using online resources means multiple views of a bodily structure can be available for viewing at a tap of a touch screen or click of a mouse. It is possible to create learning resources that integrate knowledge of the body's microstructure by bridging curricular partitions. Digital images can be viewed outside of the formal classroom or laboratory and permit collaborative learning. There is now both the pedagogical justification and the technological affordance to reintroduce errors and ambiguity to counter the reductionist tendencies of the medical curriculum. Students can discover spatial and temporal complexity, and the individuality of the physical body. They can fill the 'gutters' to form a story of the living body.

References

Black, Virginia and Smith, P. R. (2004), 'Increasing active student participation in histology', *The Anatomical Record B New Anatomist*, 278B, pp. 14–17.

Bloodgood, Robert and Ogilvie, Robert (2006), 'Trends in histology laboratory teaching in United States medical schools', *The Anatomical Record B New Anatomist*, 289:5, pp. 169–75.

Bransford, John, Brown, Ann and Cocking, Rodney (eds) (2000), *How People Learn: Brain, Mind, Experience, and School*, expanded ed., Washington, DC: National Academies Press.

Braun, Mark and Kearns, Katherine (2008), 'Improved learning efficiency and increased student collaboration through the use of virtual microscopy in the teaching of human pathology', *Anatomical Sciences Education*, 1:6, pp. 240–46.

Chen, Xiaodong, Zheng, Bin and Liu, Hong (2011), 'Optical and digital microscopic imaging techniques and applications in pathology', *Analytical Cellular Pathology*, 34:1–2, pp. 5–18.

Conole, Grainne and Dyke, Martin (2004), 'What are the affordances of information and communication technologies?', *ALT – J Research in Learning Technology*, 12:2, pp. 113–24.

Conole, Grainne, Dyke, Martin, Oliver, Martin and Seale, Jane (2004), 'Mapping pedagogy and tools for effective learning design', *Computers and Education*, 43:1–2, pp. 17–33.

Cotter, John (2001), 'Laboratory instruction in histology at the University at Buffalo: Recent replacement of microscope exercises with computer applications', *The Anatomical Record B New Anatomist*, 265:5, pp. 212–21.

Daston, Lorraine and Galison, Peter (2007), *Objectivity*, New York: Zone Books.

Derrida, Jacques (1973), *Speech and Phenomena: And Other Essays on Husserl's Theory of Signs* (trans. David B. Allison), Evanston: Northwestern University Press.

Derrida, Jacques (1976), *Of Grammatology* (trans. G. Chakravorty Spivak), Baltimore: The Johns Hopkins University Press.

Dolan, Sandra, Mallott, David and Emery, Judy (2002), 'Passive learning: A marker for the academically at risk', *Medical Teacher*, 24:6, pp. 648–49.

Drake, Richard, Lowrie, J. D. Jr. and Prewitt, Chantal (2002), 'Survey of gross anatomy, microscopic anatomy, neuroscience and embryology courses in medical school curricula in the United States', *The Anatomical Record B New Anatomist*, 269:2, pp. 118–22.

Ettarh, Rajunor (2016), 'A practical hybrid model of application, integration, and competencies at interactive table conferences in histology (ITCH)', *Anatomical Sciences Education*, 9:3, pp. 286–94.

Gatumu, Margaret, MacMillan, Frances, Langton, Philip, Headley, Max and Harris, Judy (2014), 'Evaluation of usage of virtual microscopy for the study of histology in the medical, dental, and veterinary undergraduate programs of a UK University', *Anatomical Sciences Education*, 7:5, pp. 389–98.

Gibson, James J. (1979), *The Ecological Approach to Visual Perception*, Boston: Houghton Miflin.

Glasersfeld, Ernst (1989), 'Cognition, construction of knowledge, and teaching', *Synthese*, 80:1, pp. 121–40.

Harris, Tonya, Leaven, Timothy, Heidger, Paul Jr., Kreiter, Clarence, Duncan, James and Dick, Fred (2001), 'Comparison of a virtual microscope laboratory to a regular microscope laboratory for teaching histology', *The Anatomical Record B New Anatomist*, 265:1, pp. 10–14.

Hightower, James, Boockfor, Fredric, Blake, Charles and Millette, C. F. (1999), 'The standard medical microscopic anatomy course: Histology circa 1998', *The Anatomical Record B New Anatomist*, 257:3, pp. 96–101.

Hirsh, David, Ogur, Barbara, Thibault, George and Cox, Malcom (2007), '"Continuity" as an organizing principle for clinical education reform', *New England Journal of Medicine*, 356:8, pp. 858–66.

Hussein, Inaya, Raad, Mohamad, Safa, Rawan, Jurjus, Rosalyn A. and Jurjus, Abdo (2015), 'Once upon a microscopic slide: The story of histology', *Journal of Cytology and Histology*, 6, 377, https://doi.org/10.4172/2157-7099.1000377. Accessed 18 May 2022.

Hutchby, Ian (2001), 'Technologies, texts and affordances', *Sociology*, 35:2, pp. 441–56.

Jurjus, Rosalyn, Butera, Gisela, Krum, Janette, Davis, Michelle, Mills, Alexandra and Lathan, Patricia (2018), 'Design of an online histology and pathology atlas for medical students: An instructional aid to self-directed learning', *Medical Science Educator*, 28:1, pp. 101–10.

Khalil, Mohammed, Kirkley, Debbie and Kibble, Jonathan (2013), 'Development and evaluation of an interactive electronic laboratory manual for cooperative learning of medical histology', *Anatomical Sciences Education*, 6:5, pp. 342–50.

Knight, Lynn Valerie and Mattick, Karen (2006), '"When I first came here, I thought medicine was black and white": Making sense of medical students' ways of knowing', *Social Science and Medicine*, 63:4, pp. 1084–96.

Levine, Martin, Stempak, Jerome, Conyers, Greg and Walters, Janice (1999), 'Implementing and integrating computer-based activities into a problem-based gross anatomy curriculum', *Clinical Anatomy*, 12:3, pp. 191–98.

Liou, Kevin, Jamorabo, Daniel, Dollase, Richard, Dumenco, Luba, Schiffman, Fred and Baruch, Jay (2016), '"Playing in the 'gutter': Cultivating creativity in medical education and practice', *Academic Medicine*, 91:3, pp. 322–27.

Marshall, Julia (2005), 'Connecting art, learning, and creativity: A case for curriculum integration', *Studies in Art Education*, 46, pp. 227–41.

Martindale, Michael (1993), 'Mental models and text schemas: Why computer based tutorials should be considered a communication medium', *Journal of Computer-Based Instruction*, 20, pp. 107–12.

Marton, Ference and Säljö, Roger (1997), 'Approaches to learning', in F. Marto and D. Hounsell (eds), *The Experience of Learning: Implications for Teaching and Studying in Higher Education*, Entwhistle, Edinburgh UK: Scottish Academic Press, pp. 39–58 (Chapter 3).

McBride, Jennifer M. and Prayson, Richard A. (2008), 'Development of a synergistic case-based microanatomy curriculum', *Anatomical Sciences Education*, 1:3, pp. 102–05.

'Trace, n' (n.d.), *Merriam-Webster* dictionary, https://www.merriam-webster.com/dictionary/trace. Accessed 16 August 2021.

Meyers, Eric, Erickson, Ingrid and Small, Ruth (2013), 'Digital literacy and informal learning environments: An introduction', *Learning, Media and Technology*, 38:4, pp. 355–67.

Mione, Sylvia, Valcke, Martin and Cornelissen, Maria (2013), 'Evaluation of virtual microscopy in medical histology teaching', *Anatomical Sciences Education*, 6:5, pp. 307–15.

Mione, Sylvia, Valcke, Martin and Cornelissen, Maria (2016), 'Remote histology learning from static versus dynamic microscopic images', *Anatomical Sciences Education*, 9:3, pp. 222–30.

Napolitano, Valentina (2015), 'Anthropology and traces', *Anthropological Theory*, 15:1, pp. 47–67.

Norman, Donald (1988), *The Psychology of Everyday Things*, New York: Basic Books.

Park, Ok-Choon and Gittelman, Stuart (1995), 'Dynamic characteristics of mental models and dynamic visual displays', *Instructional Science*, 23:5, pp. 303–20.

Paulsen, Friedrich, Eichhorn, Michael and Bräuer, Lars (2010), 'Virtual microscopy – The future of teaching histology in the medical curriculum?' *Annals of Anatomy*, 192:6, pp. 378–82.

Pawlina, Wojciech and Drake, Richard L. (2016), 'Authentic learning in anatomy: A primer on pragmatism', *Anatomical Sciences Education*, 9:1, pp. 5–7.

Plendl, Johanna, Bahramsoltani, Mahtab, Gemeinhardt, Ole, Hünigen, Hana, Kässmeyer, Sabine and Janczyk, Pawel (2009), 'Active participation instead of passive behaviour opens up new vistas in education of veterinary anatomy and histology', *Anatomia, Histologia, Embryologia*, 38:5, pp. 355–60.

Ramsden, Paul (2003), *Learning to Teach in Higher Education*, 2nd ed., London: Routledge Falmer.

Rennie, Frank and Morrison, Tara (2012), *e-Learning and Social Networking Handbook: Resources for Higher Education*, 2nd ed., New York: Routledge.

Scott, Ken, Morris, Anne and Marais, Ben (2017), 'Medical student use of digital learning resources', *The Clinical Teacher*, 15:1, pp. 29–33.

Willan, Peter L. T. and Humpherson, John R. (1999), '"Concepts of variation and normality in morphology": Important issues at risk of neglect in modern undergraduate medical courses', *Clinical Anatomy*, 12:3, pp. 186–90.

Yenawine, Philip (2005), 'Thoughts on visual literacy', in, Flood, James, Lapp, Diane and Heath, Shirley Brice (eds), *Handbook of Research on Teaching Literacy through the Communicative and Visual Arts*, New Jersey: Lawrence Erlbaum Associates.

MUSEUMS

THE PATHOLOGY MUSEUM AT KORLE BU[1]

Robert Kumoji and

John Nott

What follows is an edited and annotated interview between Robert Kumoji (**RK**), a Ghana Health Service pathologist based at the Korle Bu Teaching Hospital, and John Nott (**JN**), a historian of medicine. This chapter can be read simply as an interview, a tour of the museum as it stood at the start of 2019. Alternatively it can be read via the footnotes, as an analytical, material history of medical education in contemporary Ghana.

---

1. The primary health facility for what was then the Gold Coast, the hospital at Korle Bu was established in 1923, by the sea, on the edge of colonial Accra. The Korle Lagoon was intended as a buffer between the hospital complex and Jamestown, the heart of the nineteenth-century city, a role which it still serves (Addae 1996; Patterson 1981). Today, Jamestown is somewhat removed from newer centres, the neighbourhoods and commercial districts further north and east. As often seems to be the case with pathology buildings, the W. N. Laing Pathology Museum was built close to the pathology department, at the edge of the hospital complex. Named for William Neizer Laing (1929–97), Korle Bu's first Ghanaian pathologist and later medical school administrator, the museum opened in 1970 and soon grew into one of the foremost collections of pathological specimens on the continent. Although individual specimens are still used in education, by February 2019, the date of this interview, the museum has been more-or-less closed to students for the better part of a decade. To be precise, the W. N. Laing Pathology Museum is not really part of the hospital but comes under the aegis of the University of Ghana Medical School (UGMS). UGMS has shared the hospital site since it began accepting pre-clinical students in 1964 and is, today, one of foremost centres of academic medicine in Africa. The development of a medical school was an integral element of Kwame Nkrumah's vision for Ghanaian self-determination following its independence from Britain in 1957 and the President was heavily and personally involved in the foundation of the UGMS during his presidency (Easmon 1969; Patton 1996).

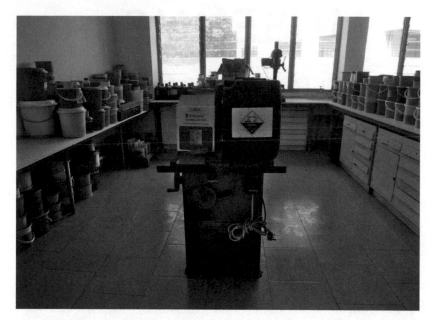

Figure 17.1: Preparation area of the W. N. Laing Pathology Museum. In the middle of the frame is the half-full container of formalin. At the rear of the frame is a drill, on which is a plaque which references the Special Commonwealth African Assistance Plan. The pots at the side are full of specimens. Courtesy of John Nott.

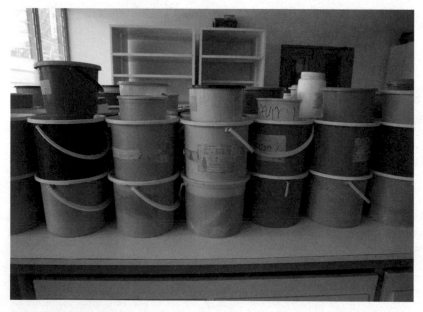

Figure 17.2: Containers full of pathology specimens, waiting to be potted up. Courtesy of John Nott.

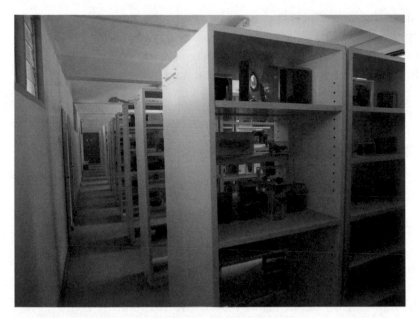

Figure 17.3: View of the main hall. Courtesy of John Nott.

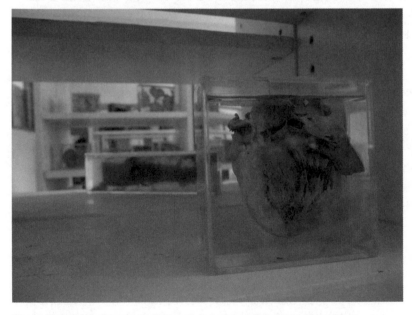

Figure 17.4: Pot in the main hall, containing a heart. Courtesy of John Nott.

RK: So this is the laboratory. It used to be an absolute mess but more recently the Head of Department insisted that the cleaning staff, who are expected to clean whatever property of the department, pay attention to this museum which had been neglected for so many years.

JN: It looks in a pretty good state.

RK: It's okay. So a few cabinets, equipment that was donated years ago by the British Government. You can still see labels. Here we go, presented by Great Britain, under the Special Commonwealth African Assistance Plan. I have no idea what that is.[2] So, these things, basically a drill to make the pots, a sander, a saw and a sealer.

Okay. These are specimens which were collected over the years and which haven't yet been potted. And I was telling you that I told our people to... Oh gosh, somebody's been... I suspected this is what would happen. Somebody has stolen the formalin (Figure 17.1). Formalin is of great value in Ghana because it's used for embalming and, as you're probably aware, there's a big fuss around dead bodies. We keep our bodies for months before we bury them. So what I had done was I had asked them to make me ten gallons of formalin to top up all these specimens, you know? This looks like something I put aside. These have my initials. The idea was to have them all topped up, so we didn't lose them forever. As I mentioned the other day, some of them are quite unique. You could spend a whole lifetime and not really see some of the samples that we will see. But the thing is that the seals are very poor. The specimens arrive in all kinds of containers. Many of them are not hermetically sealed. They don't have close fitting tops.[3] So over the years, and some of these things have been here for decades, the formalin will evaporate and you end

2. As Ghana's first medical school, and in the context of Cold War soft-power politics and Ghanaian non-alignment, UGMS received considerable assistance in terms of teaching staff and educative material from both western and Soviet states during its early years (Hecht 2011). The pathology museum, for instance, received material through the Special Commonwealth African Assistance Plan – a British-led initiative which began in 1960 in order to promote scientific training and research in former colonies across the continent. Alongside the machine tools necessary to make pots, this grant also provided materials for individual microscope study, portable tape recorders, and slide and film projection equipment for group study. This same body also provided the nucleus of the medical school library, with further donations drawn primarily from universities and charities in Western Europe and the United States (UGMS/G-52/1; UGMS/G-52/2).

up with a totally desiccated specimen because the place has been neglected. So, as I said, I asked that they top up the formalin but it now looks to me as if somebody has been stealing the formalin because these were supposed to be full.

BANGS THE CONTAINER

There's less than a fifth in each.

JN: This formalin, this would have been imported? This was imported for you?

RK: Formalin is imported, but is in common use in Ghana, largely for the embalming industry. I'm looking for a particular pot. We prepared a pot for the Fisheries Department of an octopus and it seems to have disappeared, they wanted a little collection of their own. The museum used to do work for other departments and institutions.

SOME SPECIMENS TUMBLE DOWN WITH A CRASH

Oh gosh, I'm sorry. So, you see this, the fluid is virtually... these are pots in need of rehabilitation. Look, this is completely desiccated. We've lost this. It's been dry... we can't do anything about this. Nor this. I don't know what was in this. This might be salvable, but it's unlikely. We don't have a curator, we don't have anybody to look after this. At least we're keeping the place neat and tidy.
  That would be a little office for the curator.

---

3. The period of ready access to educative materials and high state spending on science and science education was not long lived in Ghana (Osseo-Asare 2013). The growing scarcity of foreign exchange throughout the 1970s and 1980s meant that medical school budgets were quickly exhausted on imported teaching materials and laboratory consumables (PRAAD/RG/3/6/937). This was apparently a concern for medical educationists elsewhere in Africa too. Attendees at a 1987 conference in Brazzaville on *African Perspective on Medical Education* universally stressed the need for locally made textbooks and teaching tools (UG/1/3/2/2/129). Elsewhere in Ghana's scientific community, it was during this period that material improvisation became a necessary part of everyday scientific practice (Droney 2014; see also Tousignant 2013). Today, the application of advanced methods in diagnostic pathology at Korle Bu – such as the immunostaining of specific proteins or the isolation of genetic influences – continues to be hampered by the cost and availability of reagents in Ghana (Anim 2018).

JN: Where might the formalin disappear to?

RK: No place in particular. They can put it in a little polythene container and off they go. They can sell it to someone in the village. It's gold.

JN: There's that much of a market for formalin?

RK: Yes, yes, yes, yes. The thing is it's not on the open market, it's not that widely available. It's only available in select places and, it's sitting here, and somebody can make a quick fifty or a hundred Ghana Cedis out of it, so he steals it.

Looks like these are a few of my specimens. Like I said, I'm still in the habit of... you see, these are completely dry. It's gone, there's absolutely nothing in it. It's such a shame.[4]

JN: There's clearly a lot of effort that's gone into keeping these. There's a hundred, maybe more [specimens piled into various improvised temporary containers – paint buckets, jam jars, cosmetics containers and sundry other glass and plastic vessels (Figures 17.1 and 17.2)].

RK: Well, not really, it's part of a day's work. So, you're in the middle of doing a grossing, you cut up a sample and you're like 'Oh! Let's keep it!' So you just put it in the bucket and send it over here. So that's not a whole lot of work. But I'm very upset about this formalin thing.

4. The relative inaccessibility of those imported materials which are more readily available in academic hospitals in Europe – from hermetically sealed containers to laboratory chemicals – has been compounded by a pervasive, international shift away from museum collections in medical pedagogy. Elsewhere, in Britain for instance, only a handful of the more-than-80 medical museums which were open in 1950 are still operating (Hallam 2013). Those which have remained open have done so primarily because of their public appeal, rather than any pedagogic considerations or nostalgia on the part of medical educationists.

5. These same pressures have also led to a reduction in the technical and often 'invisible' labour, which is necessary to maintain delicate museum collections (Shapin 1989). Earlier, in the 1970s, UGMS had sent Dr. E. C. Christian – then a young resident pathologist and later department chair – to a specialist course held at London's Wellcome Museum, which dealt with 'the preparation, preservation and presentation of organs and tissues [...] special photographic techniques such as copying and preparation of transparencies, macro and micro photography [...] [and] maintenance of electronic equipment such as tape and cassette recorders' (UGMS/G-52 /2 1966–71: n.pag.). Similar opportunities are, today, less present and hold less value for medical schools.

This [fume cabinet] is basically, as I said, for the chemicals and stuff. This is the curators little office, in those days. The filing cabinet. I don't know...

JN: Is there anything in there?

RK: Everything's lost. We did have a young man, who was interested and the department said they'd support him. We were going to send him abroad to learn how to be a proper curator but it never happened, he hung around a while though.[5]

Is there anything in there?

JN: There's a file.

RK: I think this is... 'Vehicle'... What is this? 'Eric Manu.' Eric Manu was one of the old histo-technologists. 'Application for car loan.' What is this?[6]

I thought we might have the remnants of one of the catalogues because I know we did have the rudiments of a catalogue, something possibly Prof Laing himself had started. All that had happened was that it had been photocopied and photocopied and photocopied over the years. So there's nothing really useful. As I said, this is basically the museum laboratory. These [in piles on a counter] are teaching slides, in the days when the students would actually be given histology slides as part of their practical classes.[7]

So this is the main hall of the museum (Figures 17.3 and 17.4), it used to be twice the size. This is part of the 'renovation'. This wall, that runs all the way to the end and the doors are part of what was

---

6. By the time of this interview, the museum's laboratory was without permanent staff and had few of the materials necessary to maintain or organise the museum collection. The only piece of paper left in the curator's filing cabinet was the application for a car loan in the name of Eric Manu a technician that had previously worked in the Department.

7. Digitisation and the immediate availability of online teaching materials somewhat undermines the need for the local production of pathological specimens, as well as the preservation of extant collections. The movement towards digital histology, and the broader digitisation of audio–visual material in medical education, facilitates larger class sizes and allows for a robust medical education without the same expenditure in terms of upkeep and storage. Ready access to audio–visual materials can certainly allow for the democratisation of medical knowledge. Still, it may have been the expansion of digital histology at UGMS throughout the early twenty-first century which cost Eric Manu his job. Perhaps he even missed a few car loan repayments as a result too.

called the renovation. So, at first, the shelving extended into the other side. So, you can imagine it was so much larger. The shelving was here, so we had rows of shelves, I think there's still a few stacked down there. But this is what I meant when I said they wanted extra space for classrooms, so they split the museum down the middle and turned this into a lecture hall.

JN: So the lectures would be used in conjunction with the museum?

RK: No, it had nothing to do with the museum. The students who were being lectured here were doing courses which had a very minor pathology component. They certainly didn't need to come and examine pots.

As you can see, the museum is falling apart.[8] The metal skeleton of the concrete, when it absorbs the water, starts to rust and expands, then the concrete starts falling all over the place. So this used to be, you know, shelving all the way back. While it was being renovated, we lost a lot of the pots, many didn't come back. I estimate that we've lost at least fifty percent of the collection.

JN: And with no real idea of where they went or what's gone?

RK: No, because we didn't have the catalogue. So this is just a tiny fraction of what we had.

JN: It's a pretty expansive space, if it was twice as big...

8. Although the pathology museum at Korle Bu is deteriorating, its decline has as much to do with this recent revolution in educative technologies and pedagogic possibilities as with the specific financial and material constraints which are borne by Ghanaian universities. The question which remains, however, is what else is lost when formalin evaporates or the histology slides shatter?

9. As this book shows, the material conditions of medical education have not been fully considered by the medical humanities. Their role as drivers of medicine's globalisation and of the universalist assumptions underlie biomedical hegemony around the world are still poorly understood (see, for instance, Lock and Nguyen 2010). It might be argued that, as epistemic objects, educative materials tend to reproduce ideas and practices drawn from traditional and often imperial centres of knowledge production. Studying in conjunction with the local pathologies present in museum collections actively resists these trends.

RK: Absolutely. I forget, but it was about three quarters of the whole hall. And then the quarter had some very comfortable sofa-like chairs and a table, around which students and their tutor could sit. And they would discuss the pathology of the various pots that they were looking at. So it was a pretty comfortable place. It was air-conditioned and the classes were a lot smaller then, and they were broken into even smaller tutorial groups. So, in that quarter of the museum, maybe a little less than that, they would sit around and just discuss pathology, using the pots as teaching aids.[9] Then, over here, at the back, in here, you can't see them now, but there were little study cubicles where you could sit with your book and possibly a pot and not be disturbed. Of course, these facilitates, lavatories, male and female.

In there [a separate room at the far end of the museum space] you have seating. It's not properly cambered, you don't have a slope or anything but you have a proper blackboard or whiteboard at one end and it had heavy black curtains, so you could black the place out if you needed to project stuff. And it's also being used as a lecture hall. I suspect that's what gave them the idea to expand the lecture facilities. Because that hall was being used. Other departments were using that as a lecture facility. It was known that the Department of Pathology owned a little lecture hall that was quite comfortable. So they were already using it for lectures when they didn't have that much space.

JN: Was this the same time that pathology was moving towards audio–visual materials?

RK: This was a little before. Others were using it, you know. People were using it, they would ask for the space and use it quite often. I think they were more comfortable about turning half of it into lecture halls because they were getting a lot of good will from other departments that needed space to teach and didn't have it. So they must have thought that we could do something with the other half. So that's what happened.

JN: Are there any specimens that you think are worth mentioning, or even the way that the collection was at one point organised?

RK: As I mentioned, lots of the pots have gone missing over the years. There's far fewer than even ten years ago. I don't know where the pots went. Sometimes people take the pots for official use, you would take a pot over which you would viva a candidate. But there is no real record keeping, so you could come and take a pot and never put it back and they end up on shelves in offices or what have you and then there is a tussle over who owns those pots. Then there is the issue of people taking hearts and other human parts for traditional medical practices. I have long-suspected that this sort of thing has been going on but I have no proof of it.

JN: Has the collection changed much over the years, in terms of what pathologies are represented?

RK: There are lots of samples here which you just don't see anymore (Figure 17.5). Here are the tapeworms I was talking about the other time. That's basically providing an example. If we were keeping a catalogue – these are probably some ascaris, nematodes – but I don't think we have a proper record. So, for instance, you see in the museum that the older specimens more reflect infectious disease pathologies while more modern ones, newer specimens reflect – this is a bezoar, basically coconut, bits of coconut husk from somebody who, because of their mental condition would just keep eating coconut husks – so we don't have a record showing that transition or portraying it clearly, visually. But, from my point of view, I remember being in the autopsy suite and we would see nematodes and worms on a regular basis. The pathologists before me would keep talking about measles and older communicable diseases. And you don't see that anymore. So there is that transition, how that's being portrayed in medical education, I cannot say. Things like hydatid cyst, amoebic cysts, other infectious things aren't seen so much.[10] I just feel there's so much potential here, if each specimen were individually curated, had a little write-up, pictures, possibly histology slides.

10. As J. T. Anim, Professor of Pathology at UGMS, highlights in his recent call for the revitalisation of laboratory methods in Ghana, 'geographical pathology is essential for defining epidemiological aspects of any particular disease' (Anim 2018: 110). Binding medical education to local pathologies offers insight into endemic problems, which are poorly served by epistemic material drawn up in Europe or North America.

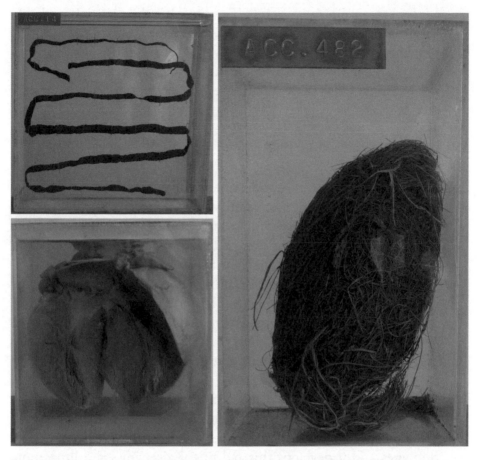

Figure 17.5: (clockwise from top left) Pot containing a tapeworm, now rarely seen in Ghana; pot containing a bezoar (more specifically, a phytobezoar) composed of coconut husk, from a patient with mental health issues; pot containing a heart showing hypertrophic cardiomyopathy, RK was the one who, as a young doctor, performed the autopsy and reserved the sample for potting, at the time, the condition was hardly (if at all) documented in Ghana. Courtesy of Robert Kumoji.

It's an extraordinary resource. Now that it's this size, it's probably about the size of the Ibadan collection. The Ibadan collection is probably better looked after so they may have more specimens. Unless they have the same problems that we do; I haven't been there, the last time I was there was in the late 1990s, so I haven't actually seen it recently.[11]

JN: How could you restore this?

RK: There would have to be commitment and a bit of money. The way I would go about it is, first of all, we would need a curator. Traditionally we have employed curators. I would say that, as an interim, we could give that job to one of the younger resident doctors in pathology, it could be part of their training.

There was a forensic section at the very end, Laing was interested in forensic pathology, I suspect we don't even know that it's the forensic section because over the years, it's dwindled to almost nothing.

JN: And how might the specimens be restored?

RK: No, these specimens are okay. You just need to change the solution. We usually use Kaiserling's solution, which is basically alcohol, glycerine and a few other things. So, over a period of time the solution ages and it develops this red tint. Kaiserling's is a little more faithful to the original colour of the sample. They will always become paler and grey and there's not a lot you can do about it. When you use pure formalin like has been used in this – I suspect this one has been restored, this is a shotgun injury to the heart, basically – this is probably not the original formalin, but it gives the samples a slightly better appearance. Just a hint. A slightly more natural ap-

---

11. It is certainly possible that the Laing collection is the largest in West Africa and, although some specimens have been lost, its new additions add material insight into the evolution of Ghana's specific disease burden. Deriving from the 1930 foundation of the Yaba College of Medicine, the Nigerian collection at the University of Ibadan has even deeper roots than the Laing Museum and faces similar pressures (Elliot 1945). Together these collections form an irreplaceable material heritage which actively promotes the localisation of biology and biomedicine, tying medical knowledge and practice to the history of health in West Africa. Their erosion in favour of audio–visual and then digital teaching materials forms part of a longer history of epistemic centralisation, standardisation and the peripheralisation of 'tropical medicine', something which is difficult to divorce from overtly imperialist applications of medical science.

pearance. The first thing is just to top up the formalin to stop them from going bad. Some of them you would change and use the Kaiserling's but once they're kept moist they're fine. The next step, some people might want to try plastination on some of these pathology specimens which is a more permanent – formalin is just as permanent, to be honest with you – but it's a little easier because you no longer have to keep the samples in a pot and worrying how the fluid is doing. So I don't think restoring them, except for the ones which are completely desiccated, like you saw on the other side, many of these can easily be restored. Those pots which are leaking need to be patched and those in which the solution has drained out need to be refilled. Then I think we should be okay.

JN: Has there been any attempt to use this with the medical students in recent years?

RK: No, not in recent years. Except with the Pathology Resident doctors, the registrars, yes, they are encouraged to spend study time with the samples here.

These [the machine tools acquired by the Special Commonwealth African Assistance Plan] all work, by the way. This doesn't, I think the element has gone [in the sealer] but it's very robustly built, I think there's a spare element in the curator's office. That works, this works, even if we don't have the sanding belts. There used to be a grinding machine here, but that was stolen about three of four years ago and nobody knows who or how it happened.

So, basically, that the Laing Museum. It's a concrete structure. Unfortunately, it doesn't seem that the construction was as robust as it could have been. Otherwise, I'd say the base of this structure would easily support a second floor. It would be easy to save, all it needs is a little commitment but the question is whether anyone wants to make that commitment. Museums are basically seen as passé.[12]

12. Addressing Ghana's specific, shifting burden of disease requires, as Ama de-Graft Aikins (2016) has suggested, a critical, interdisciplinary approach which considers both the social and biological determinants of illness. As the principle repository for the material history of disease in Ghana, the Pathology Museum at Korle Bu offers precisely this.

Acknowledgements

The authors are grateful for the insight of Dr. Afua Owusua Darkwah Abrahams, Head of Pathology at UGMS, and Prof. J. T. Anim, Professor of Pathology at UGMS. This research was conducted as part of the Making Clinical Sense project, based at Maastricht University. It has received funding from the ERC under the European Union's Horizon 2020 research and innovation programme (Grant agreement no. 678390).

References

Addae, Stephen (1996), *The Evolution of Modern Medicine in a Developing Country: Ghana 1880–1960*, Bishop Auckland: Durham Academic Press.

Aikins, Ama de-Graft (2016), *Curing Our Ills: The Psychology of Chronic Disease Risk, Experience and Care in Africa*, Accra: Sub-Saharan Publishers.

Anim, Jehoram T. (2018), 'The pathologist in Ghana and potential for research', *Ghana Medical Journal*, 52:2, pp. 103–11.

Droney, Damien (2014), 'Ironies of laboratory work during Ghana's second age of optimism', *Cultural Anthropology*, 29:2, pp. 363–84.

Easmon, Charles Odamtten (1969), 'Training of doctors in Ghana', *Ghana Medical Journal*, 8:3, pp. 208–17.

Elliot, Walter (1945), *Report of the Commission on Higher Education in West Africa*, London: HMSO.

Hallam, Elizabeth (2013), 'Disappearing museums? Medical collections at the University of Aberdeen', in E. Hallam and S. J. M. M. Alberti (eds), *Medical Museums: Past, Present, Future*, London: Royal College of Surgeons of England, pp. 44–59.

Hecht, Gabrielle (ed.) (2011), *Entangled Geographies: Empire and Technopolitics in the Global Cold War*, Cambridge: MIT Press.

Lock, Margaret and Nguyen, Vinh-Kim (2010), *An Anthropology of Biomedicine*, Oxford: Wiley-Blackwell.

Osseo-Asare, Abena Dove (2013), 'Scientific equity: Experiments in laboratory education in Ghana', *Isis*, 104:4, pp. 713–41.

Patterson, K. David (1981), *Health in Colonial Ghana: Disease, Medicine, and Socio-Economic Change, 1900–1955*, Waltham: Crossroads Press.

Patton, Adell (1996), *Physicians, Colonial Racism, and Diaspora in West Africa*, Gainesville: University Press of Florida.

Public Records and Archives Administration Department (PRAAD) (1985), Accra/RG/3/6/937, University of Ghana Medical School Foreign Exchange Budget.

Shapin, Steven (1989), 'The invisible technician', *American Scientist*, 77:6, pp. 554–63.

Tousignant, Noemi (2013), 'Broken tempos: Of means and memory in a Senegalese University laboratory', *Social Studies of Science*, 43:5, pp. 729–53.

UGMS/G-52/1 (1966), *Annual and General Reports, c. 1965–70*, Accra: Ghana Medical School Progress Report.

UGMS/G-52/2 (1966–71), *Annual and General Reports, 1971–87*, Accra: Gniversity of Ghana Medical School Library.

University of Ghana (UG), Central Archive, Legon, Accra/G/1/3/2/2/129 (1987), Medical School Agenda and Minutes of Meetings, 1988–2005, *African Perspective on Medical Education: Africa Regional Conference*, Brazzaville, 27–30 October.

NURSERVERS

THE NURSERVER

David Theodore

In modern hospital design, hospital planners devoted considerable ingenuity to creating equipment that helps nurses nurse. Up until around 1970, hospital nursing included the double sense of education and work. That is, nursing work in hospitals was carried out by nurses-in-training who were supervised by a small cadre of staff nurses (Reverby 1987). Since hospital nursing was coextensive with nursing education, any equipment designed and used for nursing work was also designed and used for nursing education. In this chapter, I explore one such piece of equipment, the Nurserver. The history of this minor piece of equipment, a material interface between the hospital supply services system and the nurse, shows how learning medicine in the modern hospital also meant becoming familiar with architecture.

Nurservers were installed in dozens of the so-called Friesen Concept hospitals across North America from roughly 1960 to 1975 (Juzwiak 1964; DeMicheal 1969). The Nurserver (see Figures 18.1 and 18.2) is little more than a metal shelving unit strategically placed on inpatient wards. The key to the Nurserver was that it could be placed *in between*:

> The Nurserver is a double-door supply cabinet between each patient's room and the corridor. The cabinet is divided vertically into clean and soiled compartments. A supply technician, standing in the corridor, can remove soiled linen and supplies from one compartment and replenish clean supplies in the other, without ever entering the patient's room or disturbing him [...] The nurse is relieved of supply-carrying duties and can use the pass-through cabinets without leaving the patient's room. (Nevitt 1968: 5)

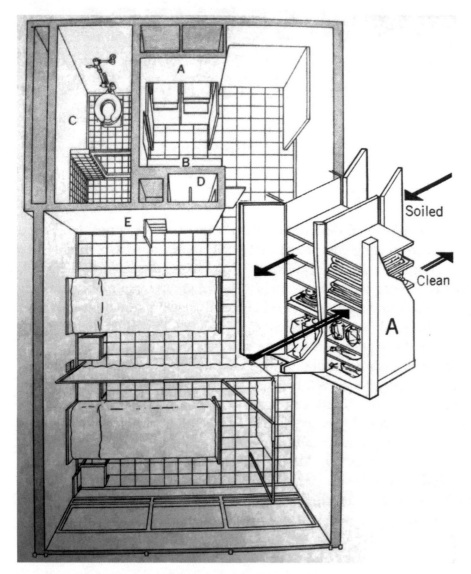

Figure 18.1: Looking into a two-bed room as you would see it with the ceiling removed. Perspective plan and axonometric drawing of a Nurserver, Marijo Juzwiak (1964), 'Glimpse of the future: The Friesen Hospital', *RN*, 27:10, p. 67.

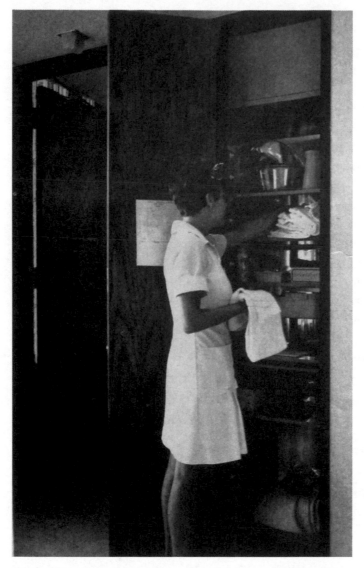

Figure 18.2: Nurse accessing a Nurserver from the corridor. 'The Interior Network', *Consulting Engineer* (October 1970): p. 108. Reprint. Library and Archives Canada, MG31 B51, Box 3.

The Nurserver is equipment used in patient care, an activity that relies not on theoretical knowledge or practical wisdom, but instead highlights 'skills that have no theoretical component at all' (Dreyfus and Dreyfus 2009: 23). Social historians of the hospital have long established a fundamental switch from care to cure at the birth of the modern institution (Jecker and Self 1991). Yet the Nurserver indicates resistance to this change from charity to science, showing that technology could serve patient care rather than medical cure, promoting nursing rather than doctoring, and showing biomedicine as a technique rather than a goal of hospital life.

Nursing education emerged in the nineteenth century as one of the key factors in the so-called invention of the modern hospital (Rosenberg 1987: 8). The professionalisation of nursing helped move medical practice out of the home and into the hospital. One new problem generated by the need for trained nurses in hospital-based modern medicine was the need to train nurses. Medicine had a tradition of theoretical and technical knowledge; nursing did not. Or to put this another way, the idea of nursing education was invented as a part of hospital history, but not necessarily as part of medical history. Instead, nursing education grew from gendered religious traditions and the contingent ways hospital life was managed and organised. Until recently, only a few staff nurses in the hospital were trained graduates. For most women – and nurses are mostly women – once trained, they left the hospital to go into private duty (Reverby 1987).

In turn, the type of hospital equipment needed for patient care was inextricable from the equipment needed to train nurses. In a 'new' type of nursing unit, advocated in 1933 by Laura Grant for the Lakeside Hospital in Cleveland, OH, planning the rooms and equipment for nursing work began with a detailed analysis of each procedure in the existing hospital (Grant 1933). This specification was then projected onto future needs, that is, present use allowed planners to estimate the quantity of nursing required in future hospital expansions. Finally, planners envisioned standardised storage modules, working areas and equipment tables, as well as places to hold bedpans, flower vases, equipment for douche and rectal procedures (private wards had their own flower rooms). It is worth citing this procedure in full:

> With the patient as the focal point of interest, the main objective in
> drawing up these specifications was to plan the location and the me-

chanical and architectural features of the space allocated for service purposes so that, first, the time and energy of the nurse might be conserved to the greatest possible degree; second, the best teaching facilities might be provided for the nurse student to the end that the patient might benefit through both the quality and quantity of service made available; and third, that the nurse and the student might find greater usefulness and satisfaction in their work through the improved facilities provided for carrying it on. (Grant 1933: 207)

Grant here gives the outline for how student nurses might become both proficient and fulfilled. Yet crucial here is the absence of a *place* for biomedical science. There is nothing in Grant's description to suggest that learning to nurse involved acquiring medical knowledge. Likewise, there is nothing to suggest that proficiently using nursing equipment requires specialised training and focused repetition. Hospital-based nurse training depended on something other than a balance between rational theory and skilled practice. It was not enough to improve nurses' ability to labour or to increase their understanding of biomedical theory: what had to be augmented through training and supported through well-placed equipment was the nurse's ability to proffer care.

Unlike most technologising tools associated with hospital medicine, then – from the stethoscope to the installation of magnetic resonance machines – the Nurserver belongs to a category that contemporaneous hospital design researchers in Britain called 'non-surgical' equipment (Lawrence 2001; Boyd Davis and Gristwood 2016). When the National Health Service began in 1948 and the government began funding hospital development, two key charitable organisations, the Nuffield Provincial Hospitals Trust and the King Edward's Hospital Fund for London recruited design researchers to create hospital equipment such as medicine trolleys and 'bed-elevators' – the mechanisms that allow the heads of the hospital beds to tilt up at an angle (Cousins 1965). In design history, the goal is to make clear the way a range of issues intersect in equipment, including safety standards, patient experience, politics, materials and manufacturing. Standardisation was a key ideology: a suitable design could be economically employed as a mass-produced object in all hospitals. But as Grant had written in 1933, design thinking also drew on the assumption that standardisation induced familiarity:

Standardization in the storage of equipment is one of the greatest factors in the success with which new nurses or students may be introduced and the ease with which they may be assimilated. Having once
learned the general plan and arrangement on one ward they know it on
all wards and, when transferred to another ward they need waste no
time in learning where things are kept. (Grant 1933: 211)

Scholars approach this kind of education – haptic, sensor-motor, embodied – through two opposed ideas (Benner et al. 2009). One is that
the nurse's body is standardised along with the equipment. The other is
that rule following, while necessary for the development of competence,
is insufficient for the development of expertise. It is, in Susan Reverby's
apt phrase, the dictum that nurses are ordered to care: for nurses to nurse,
they must care *about* their patients (rather than about the specific outcomes) and they must have institutional and material organisations that
promote their capacity to care *for* their patients. Training is focused on
learning how to position oneself in the 'general plan and arrangement',
becoming familiar with hospital material culture and architecture.

Here I give primacy to hospital architecture as a physical structure
that orders nursing activities. This is the proposition that hospital buildings are designed around nurses' work and education, rather than around
clinical encounters between patients and doctors. Most often architectural historians assess hospitals in relation to changes in architectural and medical practices, as if hospital design is primarily structured
by medical and architectural professionals (Willis et al. 2018; Adams
2007). But although the overall aim of the institution might indeed be
characterised as medical, and although transformations in professional
architectural practice undeniably influenced hospital design, nevertheless, day-to-day life in the hospital was aimed at organising nursing. In
the twentieth century, for instance, bacteriological dogma gave prominence to architectural features that visibly separated soiled materials
from clean (Kisacky 2017: 166–234). Since nurses in the patient room
are at the point of transition from clean to soiled, a concern about germs
produced a concern about where nurses are situated in the functional
diagram of all hospital activities. In addition, nurses-in-training lived
at the hospital (until around 1970). As a result, hospital architects designed important links between where nurses lived and the wards where
they worked, visible today as tunnels and bridges (Theodore 2013). The
quantification of nursing activities, often expressed as a concern for how

much 'unnecessary' walking nurses do, has also led directly to hospital planning layouts (Theodore and Vardouli 2021). Nursing work – and thus nursing training – had to be connected to the material supply systems that provided everything from bed linens and medications to food and bedside television services. Now we have in place the institutional situation in which the Nurserver arises as equipment.

The Nurserver's inventor, hospital consultant Gordon A. Friesen, was a hospital administrator who had no medical training. He is well known in medical history for his tenure as planning consultant on the United Mine Workers Welfare Fund Hospitals (Friesen 1953). Around 1960, he opened a planning consultancy in Washington, DC, and built 'Friesen concept' hospitals in Canada, the United States, Puerto Rico and Germany (Nevitt 1968). For Friesen, hospital architecture was stuck at an impasse. Existing hospitals had often first opened in the nineteenth century, and, at least, according to Friesen, new hospitals continued to be designed on the nineteenth-century principles: aseptic surgery, trained nursing, business accounting and germ theory, rather than on a clear appraisal of hospital organisation and function (DeMicheal 1969). Friesen thought hospital planning and management should not be formulated by going to staff members to find out what is needed; instead, planners should analyse the functions to be performed and design within those parameters. He used the example of the jet airplane. His claim was that it would not make sense to ask the propeller pilots how to design the jet; you needed, he argued, to design the jet and then *retrain* the pilots. The Nurserver was part of this doubled sense of training: part of the equipment necessary for a trainee to master in order to become competent, but also part of the re-training of hospital work writ large.

To explain how Friesen intended the Nurserver to perform, I turn to a series of diagrams he published in 1970. Figure 18.3 shows a diagram of how the Nurserver is located on an inpatient floor. Note that Friesen was an early advocate for having all inpatients in private rooms; the two rooms shown at the upper right in plain view are each for single patients. Note also that the specific architecture of the floor layout is not shown. It is the relations and configurations that are important, but the specific architecture would be left for the architect to design – as long as the Nurserver made it possible for the nurse to have materials to hand without leaving the inpatient room. The dotted line shows the path for clean items entering the Nurserver, and the solid line shows the path for soiled items removed from the Nurserver. The Nurserver, then, is encased within the architecture, conterminous with a wall, but connecting rather than separating corridor and room. In the centre of the floor layout is a room divided into clean and soiled areas that connects to the central supply system. This connection is shown in Figure 18.4. Here the inpatient rooms are imagined at the top of the hospital, while the bottom has receiving, laundry, stores, preparation areas and pharmacy. Figure 18.5 shows the vertical shafts that connect all of the hospital floors to this basement supply centre. The organisation of the entire hospital depends on getting materials and supplies to the nurse at the bedside.

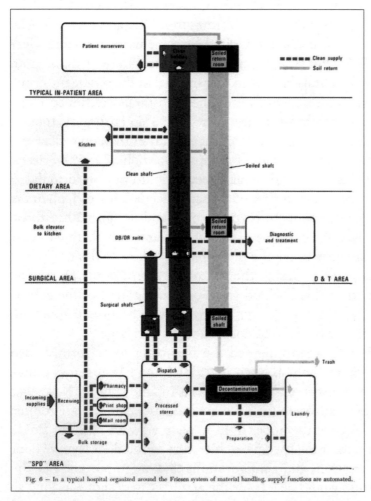

Fig. 6 — In a typical hospital organized around the Friesen system of material handling, supply functions are automated.

Figure 18.3: 'Typical Hospital organised around the Friesen system of material handling'. 'The Interior Network', *Consulting Engineer* (October 1970): p. 110. Reprint. Library and Archives Canada, MG31 B51, Box 3.

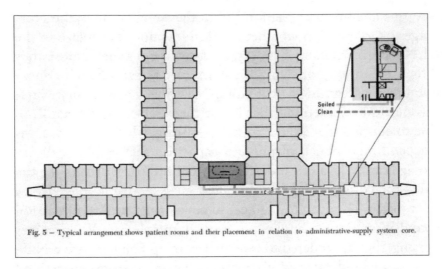

Fig. 5 – Typical arrangement shows patient rooms and their placement in relation to administrative-supply system core.

Figure 18.4: 'Typical arrangement shows patient rooms and their placement in relation to administrative-supply systems'. 'The Interior Network', *Consulting Engineer* (October 1970): p. 105. Reprint. Library and Archives Canada, MG31 B51, Box 3.

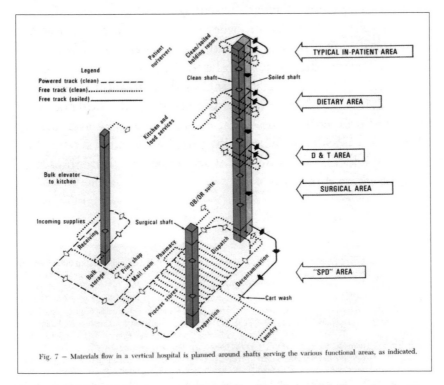

Fig. 7 – Materials flow in a vertical hospital is planned around shafts serving the various functional areas, as indicated.

Figure 18.5: 'Materials flow in a vertical hospital is planned around shafts serving the various functional areas, as indicated'. 'The Interior Network', *Consulting Engineer* (October 1970): p. 112. Reprint. Library and Archives Canada, MG31 B51, Box 3.

Given this architectural relationship to the supply system, the Nurserver urges us to question whether medical learning takes place in the hospital. Nurses-in-training clearly knew how to use a shelf before they started their education, so having the Nurserver as part of their education meant neither learning a new skill nor learning a new theory. Nursing turns out to be something that is not theorisable, and perhaps not amenable to education at all, the capacity for care, which, in turn, turns out to depend on a bunch of physical capacities that involve delivery carts, storage carts, elevators, orderlies, janitors and truck drivers. To the degree that the Nurserver educated student nurses – that it *ordered them to care* – it marks a limit to the project of conceiving medical education as the acquisition of tacit, implicit, or explicit knowledge. When nurses learn nursing, they are ordered to care by becoming familiar with a Nurserver – a specialised piece of equipment that required no specialised training to operate. For nurses-in-training, that is, medical education entailed becoming familiar with a shelf. So, while the Nurserver marks a way station on a timeline of scientific management and rationalist efficiency (Toman 2006), it is also an event on the timeline charting the material culture of care. If nursing education was meant to cultivate students' ability to separate the pathological and the normal, the Nurserver had no role. If, however, that education included the inculcation of compassion (Mol 2008), the Nurserver set the stage. In the hospital, that is, the Nurserver ordered the nurse-in-training in between and among things which were already familiar: walls, corridors, windows, beds, linens. It organised education as a matter of accumulating, through familiarity, a sense of where things are.

References

Adams, Annmarie (2007), *Medicine by Design: The Architect and the Modern Hospital, 1893–1943*, Minneapolis: University of Minnesota Press.

Benner, Patricia E., Tanner, Christine A. and Chesla, Catherine A. (eds) (2009), *Expertise in Nursing Practice: Caring, Clinical Judgment, and Ethics*, 2nd ed., New York: Springer.

Boyd Davis, Stephen and Gristwood, Simone (2016), *Early Design Research at the RCA: The Royal College of Art in the 1960s and 1970*, online exhibition commissioned by Design Research Society, http://www.drs2016.org/exhibition/. Accessed 20 September 2020.

Cousins, James (1965), 'A general purpose bedstead for hospitals', *Design*, 195, pp. 52–57.

DeMicheal, Don (1969), 'We're Practicing 20th-Century Medicine in 19th-Century Facilities', *Actual Specifying Engineer*, 21:4, pp. 88–89.

Dreyfus, Hubert L. and Dreyfus, Stuart E. (2009), 'The Relation of theory and practice in the acquisition of skill', in P. Benner, C. Tanner and C. Chesla (eds), *Expertise in Nursing Practice: Caring, Clinical Judgement and Ethics*, New York: Springer Pub, pp. 1–24.

Friesen, Gordon, (1953), 'For coal miners and their families: Chain-store hospitals', *Modern Hospital*, 83:5, pp. 54–61.

Grant, Laura M. (1933), 'A new type of nursing unit', *The American Journal of Nursing*, 33:3, pp. 207–11.

Jecker, Nancy S. and Self, Donnie J. (1991), 'Separating care and cure: An analysis of historical and contemporary images of nursing and medicine', *The Journal of Medicine and Philosophy*, 16:3, pp. 285–306.

Juzwiak, Marijo (1964), 'Glimpse of the future: The Friesen hospital', *RN*, 27:10, reprint, Ottawa: Library and Archives Archives Canada, MG31 B51 B51, Box 4.

Kisacky, Jeanne (2017), *Rise of the Modern Hospital: An Architectural History of Health and Healing, 1870–1940*, Pittsburgh: University of Pittsburgh Press.

Lawrence, Ghislaine Mary (2001), 'Hospital beds by design: A socio-historical account of the 'King's Fund Bed', 1960–1975', Ph.D. thesis, London: University of London.

Mol, Annemarie (2008), *The Logic of Care: Health and the Problem of Patient Choice*, New York: Routledge.

Nevitt, Joyce (1968), *The Gordon Friesen Concept of Hospital Design: A Symposium*, St. John's: Association of Registered Nurses of Newfoundland.

Reverby, Susan (1987), *Ordered to Care: The Dilemma of American Nursing, 1850–1945*, Cambridge: Cambridge University Press.

Rosenberg, Charles (1987), *The Care of Strangers: The Rise of America's Hospital System*, New York: Basic Books.

Theodore, David (2013), '"The fattest possible nurse": Architecture, computers, and post-war nursing', in L. Abreu and S. Sheard (eds), *Daily Life in Hospital: Theory and Practice from the Medieval to the Modern*, Oxford: Peter Lang, pp. 273–98.

Theodore, David and Vardouli, Theodora (2021), 'Walking instead of working: Space allocation, automatic architecture, and the abstraction of hospital labor', *IEEE Annals of the History of Computing*, 43:2, pp. 6–17.

Toman, Cynthia (2006), '"Body Work": Nurses and the delegation of medical technology at the Ottawa Civic Hospital, 1947–1972', *Scientia Canadensis: Canadian Journal of the History of Science, Technology and Medicine*, 29:2, pp. 155–75.

Willis, Julie, Goad, Philip and Logan, Cameron (2018), *Architecture and the Modern Hospital: Nosokomeion to Hygeia*, New York: Routledge.

PHOTOGRAPHS

TYPOLOGIES OF FATNESS: CONSTITUTIONAL PHOTOGRAPHY IN WESTERN MEDICINE, c.1930–60

Anne Katrine Kleberg Hansen

This chapter examines how, through photography, fatness has been made knowable in medicine, and how those photographs have been used as an epistemic technology which produces and reproduces knowledge. The materiality I consider are the photographs and their place within medical publications. In recent years, fat studies, scholars and fat activists have scrutinised and demonstrated the ways that terms like 'obesity' and 'overweight' medicalise and stigmatise fat bodies. Instead, they reclaim fat and fatness as neutral, descriptive terms (Wann 2009). The physicians presented in this chapter all used photography to investigate body fat, its various formations and distribution. In this way, they were heavily involved in shaping the fat body into an object of medical knowledge, termed 'obesity' or 'adipositas', and to change their terms to fatness would be a misrepresentation. I use fat and fatness as my own terms.

My analysis departs from the basic notion that visual representations contribute to, inform and form medical knowledge, rather than just reflect the state of knowledge at a given time in history. As such, differing types of medical visualisations – charts or photography, for example – are not just different ways of illustrating the same problem or phenomenon, rather they can point to the various ways in which fatness has been conceptualised historically, known and practiced within medical research. Photography was introduced to science with great expectation, due to its indexicality and promise of objectivity (Daston and Galison 1992). However, theoretical and historiographic discussions on medical photography have lately tended to focus on the failure of photography to fulfil the promise of being intrinsically scientific and objective (e.g. Mitman and Wilder 2016). In *Race and Photography*, Amos Morris-Reich (2016) insists on analysing how photographs worked as scientific evidence in their own time. The photographs in this chapter bear the mark of eugenic origins and might easily be dismissed as pseudo-science, yet I also insist that they formed part of legitimate scientific investigation in their time.

In a recent article, Lucas Engelmann (2019) argues that medical historians have failed to ask fundamental questions about medical photography and have too hastily assumed they simply served as tools of representation of disease in the clinic. Perhaps this focus on photographs as objective illustrations of disease has contributed to the conclusion that photography has failed as a medical technology. Engelmann suggests that rather 'than to ask what a medical photograph is and what disease it might show, the historian should ask when a, or rather any photograph has become a medical photograph' (Engelmann 2019: 4). In other words, it is not necessarily the clinical setting which determines the medicalness of a photograph but whether it has become utilised in medicine in some way or other – as illustration, as registration, or as exploration, for example. Engelmann analyses photographs which share the characteristic that they are not from the clinic. Still, he argues, they are medical and, drawing on Hans-Jörg Rheinberger (1999), concludes that, while some medical photography was clinical, at other times, photography formed part of experimental systems much more indebted to the investigations of more uncertain phenomenon than the illustration or showcasing of specific diseases.

In the following chapter, I discuss three different kinds of publications in order to highlight the various uses of photography in the generation and reproduction of medical knowledge. First, I will discuss the American constitutional physician William Herbert Sheldon's (1898–1977) endeavour to comprise a photographic atlas of men and the place of fatness in this attempt. Second, I will draw attention to the Danish physician Ejnar Jarløv (1888–1961), who hoped to put together a typography of fatness. This publication is a conference proceeding and, rather than displaying the finished typography, it demonstrates how Jarløv worked experimentally with clinical photography. Finally, I will consider the work of the French physician Jean Vague (1911–2003). Vague draws on the same kind of scholarship as Jarløv but the English-language publication used here is backed by years of work and previous publications of results, and Vague offers firm conclusion based on his partly photographic material.

The three physicians shared endeavour – to establish typologies of fatness – arose from a holistic strand of the early-twentieth century medicine (Lawrence and Weisz 1998). Rather than a singularly defined school, this movement was variously understood. Known as constitutional medicine and somatotyping in the US, Konstitutionslehre in Germany and biotypology in Italy, there was a shared interest in eugenics across all settings (Tracy 1992). All three physicians considered in this article shared an affinity with the Italian strand of constitutional medicine and eugenics. In contrast to German and Nordic eugenics, which favoured negative initiatives such as castration or abortion, Italian or Latin eugenics was influenced by the catholic church and a Lamarckian concept of heredity, which supported initiatives such as maternity leave to improve the quality of populations, and was less preoccupied with racial pureness (Cassata 2013; Gomes 2016). Common to this type of medicine was an emphasis on the clinic and a wish to strengthen the physician's capacity to evaluate and understand the *whole* patient. In the case of fatness, this played out in the anthropometric and photographic evaluation of the full body and its arrangement in typologies – a quest for wholeness combined with an interest in patterned variation. Rather than emphasising one basic average, when identifying what could count as *normal* from the point of view of health or medicine, constitutional physicians were convinced that humankind was clustered around several different types. Some individuals would be close to a true type, but types could also be mixed in different ways. Most often, though, it would be possible to decide upon a dominant typology present in each individual. This focus on patterned distribution, and the plurality of normal types, was a reaction to the dominant but recent trend in medicine, one which construed the normal body as singular and based on numerical averages. This approach to the normal or healthy body was developed in the last half of the nineteenth century and radically reorganised the physician's traditional focus on the individual bodies of each patient (Cryle and Stephens 2019). The popularisation of photography, however, offered constitutional physicians a material means to challenge these developments and to disperse normal bodies around a variety of typologies instead.

A typology of men and the place of fatness

In 1946, William Herbert Sheldon took over the Constitution Clinic at Columbia University (Tracy 1992). Sheldon had been trained in the tradition of Italian physical anthropology but developed his work into a much more heavily theorised, or even speculative, form of constitutional medicine (Gatlin 1998). One of Sheldon's main publications was a comprehensive *Atlas of Men* (1954), displaying an overwhelming number of photographs of young male American university students, as seen in Figure 19.1. They were all photographed in the same pose and from the same angle. Each student appeared to be almost floating in an empty space, standing on a round platform and photographed from the front, the side and the back. Their faces and genitals (if showing) were masked out with white. The key to their organisation evolved around three physical traits – endomorphy, mesomorphy and ectomorphy. Derived from the names of the three embryonic germ layers, the endomorphic trait connoted fatness and a round shape, the mesomorphic trait connoted muscularity while ectomorphic individuals were slender and long-limbed (Gatlin 1998; Vertinsky 2002). Sheldon therefore moved beyond the idea of a set of different types and instead developed a triangular spectrum in which each individual was scored according to all three traits on a scale from 1 to 7 (Vertinsky 2002: 110).

Figure 19.2 displays the most extreme varieties and offers insight into why constitutional medicine might have offered a fruitful framework to think about fatness and health. Instead of just one 'normal' man, constitutional medicine offered an understanding where individual bodies could be normal in different ways – normal according to their specific type. One reason for medical interest in identifying these different types was the assumption that they would also display different dispositions towards illnesses throughout life. As often in medical vocabulary Sheldon favoured the Greek term for body, 'soma' and coined the term 'somatotyping', thus stressing the medical implications of the different body types. However, even if humanity clustered around different types of normality, a hierarchy of normality was also apparent. This is very evident in Sheldon's description of somatotype 741, ranked 7 in endomorphy, 4 in mesomorphy and 1 in ectormorphy. 'The 741 and his permutant

471 are stupendous concentrations of human flesh. With the 651 and the 561, they embody what may be a universal animal craving for the ecstatic Dionysian binge' (Sheldon 1954: 335). Figure 19.3 displays men who all a score 7 in endomorphy, however, in the citation, it is also evident that, according to Sheldon, men could be too big from more than just fat – muscle could play a part too.

Anthropometric measures of the students were also included but except from weight, the measures were made on the carefully arranged photographs rather than taken of the individual students. These photographs were not kept in the laboratory but published in bulky, large format books brimming with photographs and measurements of bodies. *Atlas of Men* comprises pictures of around 1800 men. It can seem utterly redundant with the sheer amount of bodies looking alike in the exact same posture over and over again. But this was exactly the point: people of the same type looked alike, and the photographs served an important role of proving this. While Figure 19.3, showing the three extreme varieties of man, served as an illustration of a point, the ones systematically arranged in *Atlas of Men* served as quantification, pictorial evidence and data points. Importantly they were also a way of training the physician's eye to skilfully differentiate between somatotypes (Gatlin 1998). Constitutional medicine favoured the clinic and the importance of the sensory and visual skill to carefully evaluate and examine the patient in the consulting room. Mainstream medicine was becoming dependent on laboratory tests, which had also made it less of an art. Photographs, on the other hand, worked as a technology which supported clinical observation, instead of eroding its importance.

Experimental systems: The role of photography in the evaluation of body types

In the 1930s, the Danish physician Ejnar Jarløv conducted research in which different shapes of corporal fat, like pendulous breasts or abdomens, were the key to deciding on particular kinds of fatness (Jarløv 1932). In the early twentieth century, considerable research was conducted on how hormones affected the build and development of bod-

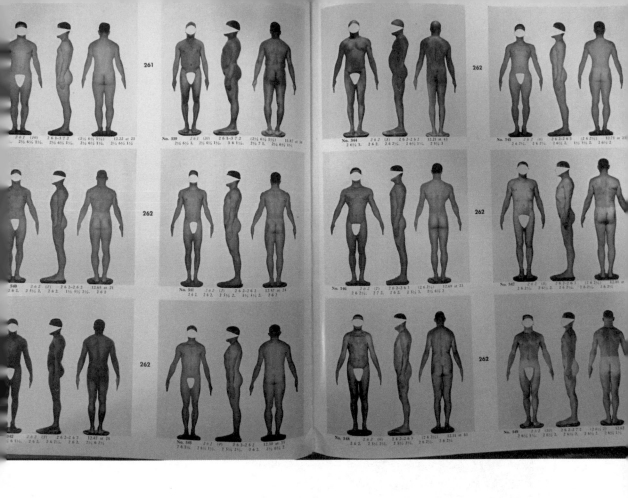

Figure 19.1: Young men of somatotype 261 or 262, meaning they scored 2 in endomorphy (fatness) 6 in mesomorphy (muscularity) and either 1 or 2 in (lankness/slenderness). The scale ranged from 1 to 7 (Sheldon 1954: 120–21).

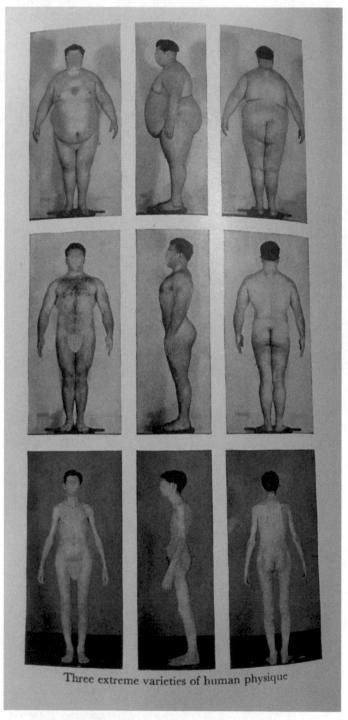

Three extreme varieties of human physique

Figure 19.2: According to Sheldon's somatotyping, these men score 711, 171 and 117, respectively (Sheldon 1940: Appendix).

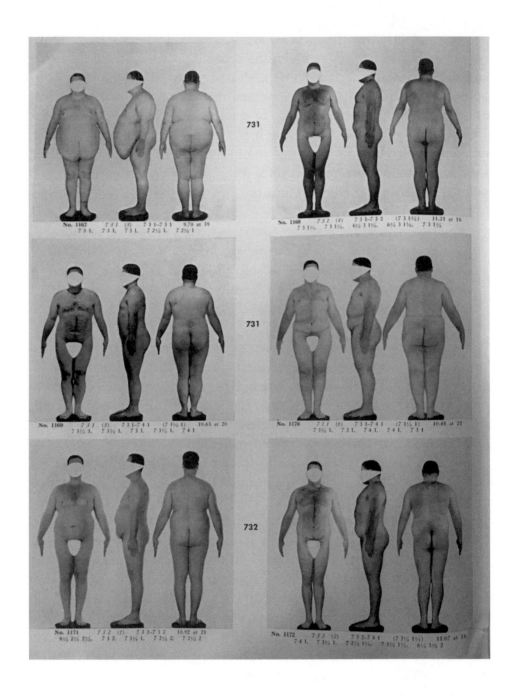

Figure 19.3: Young men all scoring 7, the highest possible rating, in endomorphy, or fatness (Sheldon 1954: 334).

ies. In connection to this, several syndromes and diseases were established, their clinical picture including specific distributions of fat tissue and often some malformation or malfunctioning of the genitals. Full-body photographs of patients appeared in medical textbooks as a way of demonstrating how the disease or syndrome looked (see e.g. Zondek 1926). Jarløv referred to this research, but he did not wish to study *special* types of obesity. He was interested in ordinary obesity. Fatness presented a difficult case for the physician since it was poorly understood but it also seemed to defy any medical definition.

> Among the many and great difficulties presenting themselves to those who desire to get a grasp of the manifold clinical features of abnormal obesity the definition itself is one of the greatest. To give concise answers to the questions: What is obesity? – and: What is abnormal obesity? – is an impossibility. (Jarløv 1932: 6)

It was important to know the difference between normal and abnormal 'ordinary' obesity because that decided whether it was a medical condition or not. But how to draw the line between normal and abnormal obesity, knowing from the clinic that humans came in so many different types, that obesity could look so different and apparently presented different health implications to different people?

Jarløv argued that while many different typologies of obesity had been suggested they offered premature hypothesises regarding aetiology and pathogeneses (Jarløv 1932: 19–29). Instead, Jarløv suggested to combine Pende's biotypology and a clinical method of nosography – the systematic classification of disease. Jarløv's ambition was to tease out the types of abnormal obesity based on the clinical picture alone: 'the nosographic statement of the clinical pictures of obesity must first and foremost be based on the pure >>clinical<< observation' (Jarløv 1932: 20). Jarløv was concerned with accuracy in the description of 'the clinical picture', a phrase that he uses repeatedly. The means to fix the clinical picture then became photography. When a typology was established, it would give clues to the underlying causes.

Jarløv based this research on outpatients. They had not necessarily consulted him due to issues related to fatness but because of other health concerns. It seems that he often took the photo himself and that he had to rely on differing degrees of consent from the patients. Some completely refused to have their pictures taken, some did not allow him to publish them, others did not fully undress or covered their parts of their bodies, and some apparently asked to have their faces anonymised. This is not done consistently, so it does not appear to be Jarløv's choice. The publications were based on a presentation and first published as a conference proceeding bearing evidence to the explorative status of Jarløv's work at this point: he is inviting his audience and readers to follow his argument unfolding, observing (some) of the same empirical evidence as himself.

Figure 19.4 is a display of faces representing a type that he was particularly satisfied with and that he named the 'uratic type'. They bore evidence of thorough morphological resemblance, even down to facial features. These men, and one woman, were not otherwise related but were so closely related in terms of typology that they even looked the same, at least to Jarløv. I suggest that these are not illustrations of a clinical type of obesity – why then focus on faces from the neck up, so little affected by fatty deposits? And why place four almost identical photographs together instead of just choosing one? I suggest Jarløv used these photographs as data, and this arrangement was his data presentation, contributing to a visual argument about similarity and suggesting a similar pattern of anamneses throughout their lives. Figure 19.5 shows the photographic representation of the whole body of the uratic type adhering to the standards of full-body anthropometric photography without much care given to include the facial features.

Not all of Jarløv's photographs followed the conventions of anthropometric or clinical photography. Figure 19.6 resembles a portrait of grandmother, mother and teenage daughter but that is not what Jarløv wanted the reader to see. These three women, related through the maternal line, displayed the same type. In Figure 19.7, the girl, aged 16, is seen full-body next to an older woman – presumably the mother or grandmother. Admittedly not fat, Jarløv conceded, the girl was

> of a marked pasty habit, which has developed during puberty and which manifests itself in her features, her mammæ, strikingly well-developed for her age, the comparatively copious fatty deposits of the nates and the femora, and in the incipient blurring of the natural contour of the small of her leg; her weight has increased very considerable in the course of a year, and she belongs to a family whose female members suffer highly from adipostias (Jarløv 1932: 49)

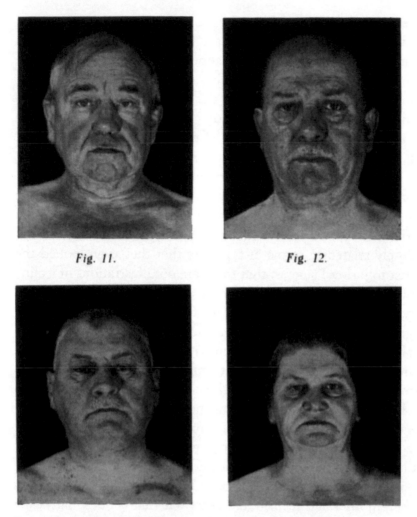

Figure 19.4: Evidence of resemblance in Jarløv's typology (Jarløv 1932: 38).

With Figures 19.6 and 19.7, Jarløv works exploratively. His arrangement of the photographs established likeness by pointing to the family line and facial resemblance and suggested a trajectory by grouping the full body photographs of the girl and the older women together. In this way, the reader was invited to observe evidence for heredity with her or his own eyes.

Jarløv published work in progress rather than a finished typology. Convinced that outer resemblance spoke of common aetiology, and insisting on the clinical nosographic method, he experimented with the arrangements of photographs and presented his most convincing results so far.

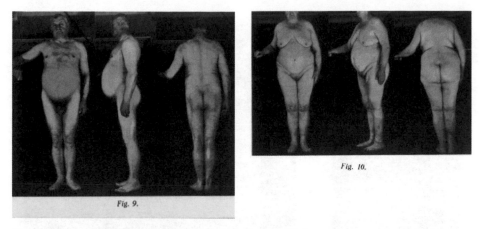

Fig. 9.

Fig. 10.

Figure 19.5: Full body display of the uratic type (Jarløv 1932: 37).

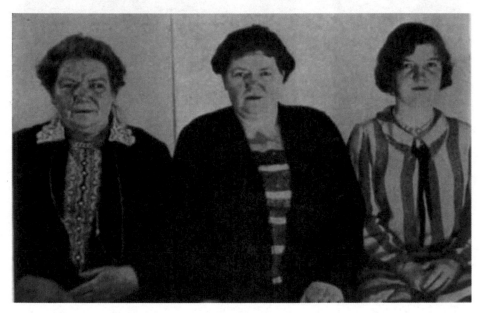

Fig. 18.

Figure 19.6: Female family members of the myxædematoid type (Jarløv 1932:48).

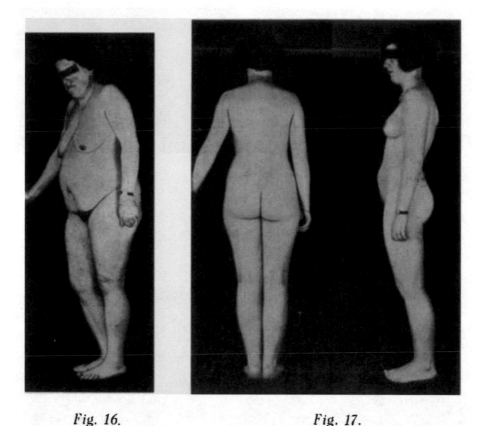

Fig. 16.   Fig. 17.

Figure 19.7: Full body and anonymised displays of the myxædematiod type (Jarløv 1932: 47).

Anthropometric measures

The French professor of medicine and endocrinologist Jean Vague was based in Marseilles, researching and teaching at the University Hospital. In the 1940s, he based his research into the bodily distribution of fat on his mostly diabetic outpatients, who consulted him for their diabetes rather than their fatness (Vague 1956). Vague was interested in patterned variation. Like Jarløv, he investigated the shapes and bodily distribution of fat based on the assumption that the different types would be susceptible to different disease. In articles published as late as the 1950s, Vague drew together work published in French in previous decades (Vague 1956, [1947] 1996). He and his students had moved beyond arranging a purely clinical typology based on outer appearance and had begun to draw confident conclusions on the relationship between body types and a predisposition to certain diseases

Vague criticised the widely accepted notion that excess body fat was just that and mainly a mechanical problem: a burden on the body, its joints and vascular system. According to Vague, the problem with body fat was not its mere accumulation:

> [I]f, instead of considering excess adiposity as an isolated always identical phenomenon, varying only in intensity, one investigates the frequency of its complications according to its chief clinical characteristics, one is immediately confronted with invaluable etiologic relationships. Experience proves, in fact, that what is important in the evolution of obesities is not so much excess adiposity per se but the activity of this excess (Vague 1956: 20)

Again, the significance of clinical experience, knowledge and reasoning is stressed. According to Vague, not all obesities were the same – they clustered around specific types according to levels of activity within the adipose tissue. To view body fat as not just a neutral deposit of energy was quite a new perspective. Hormones and other active substances in adipose tissue, however, were not easy to observe in the clinic. One of the main physiological differences effected by hormones and observable in the clinic was sex, as assigned at birth; in addition to the anthropometric characteristics, Vague's description of the patient centred on psyche, sex drive, sperm count and sex hormones. Vague and his students developed an index for masculine differentiation of the adipose tissue, in which the relation of skin folds at specific places of the body – the nape of the neck, the sacrum and the four proximal attachments of the limbs – was key to decide upon what type of fatness a patient displayed. In this case, Vague differed between android obesity, the masculine form and gynoid obesity, the feminine. Vague concluded that while it had long been known that obesity and diabetes were related, he and his research group had shown that, in adults, diabetes, atherosclerosis and uric calculous disorders were related to a masculine or android fat distribution only. Thus, obesity per se was not an issue to consider in relation to these disorders – only the specific, masculine type, characterised by a high accumulation of fat on the upper body, and which both men and women could be susceptible to, was a medical concern (Vague 1956).

Vague thus shared Sheldon and Jarløvs' focus on the importance of differentiating between different types of fatness in order to know their relationship with specific diseases. All constitutions, or types, displayed a different but type-specific pattern of disease throughout their life-course. Yet he seems to rely less on anthropometric photographs and more on anthropometric measurements. Importantly though, he still includes photographs, like those in Figure 19.8 and 19.9, but with much less mention of them in the article. Instead, they seem to serve the function of exemplars – as typical clinical expressions of gynoid and android types of obesity for the readers to consider themselves and perhaps recognise in their next clinical encounter with a patient displaying excess body fat. Another important possibility is that the many photographs utilised in constitutional medicine over the years – photographs published, arranged into typologies, presented as evidence and adhering to a strict convention of composure – had taken on a thick layer of connotations and imbedded references. Perhaps Vague did not need to present a whole catalogue of photographs because they already came with such a high number of implicit references, and because they worked within the system of all these other photographs.

Conclusion

This strand of research into fatness seems to have disappeared or become marginalised after the mid-twentieth century. Photographs also stop turning up in research on fatness. Hormones, it turned out, did not have the all-explanatory powers that was initially hoped for. Constitutional medicine, in its various forms, fell out of favour, as did eugenics, though not as instantly after the Second World War as might imagined. It has been suggested that holism in medicine in the interwar years formed part of a broader holistic revival of that period, that it survived the War but then gradually declined during the 1950s. Possible explanations include generational change, the therapeutic success of biomedicine, and less vocal criticism of modern consumer capitalism (Lawrence and Weisz 1998). Other historians have argued that fatness moved from the auspices of endocrinology – a specialisation close to the heart of constitutional medicine – to psychiatry around mid-twentieth century (Rasmussen 2012). I wonder what role these photographs themselves might have played – even if eugenics continued in some ways, could it

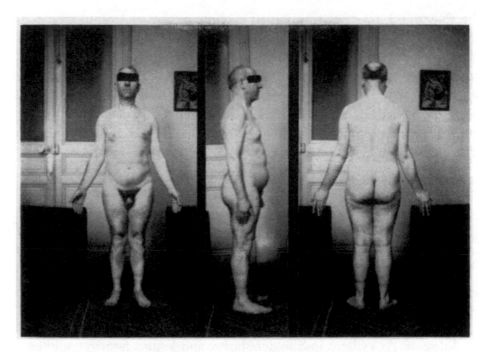

Figure 19.8: Gynoid obesity in the male (Vague 1956: 25).

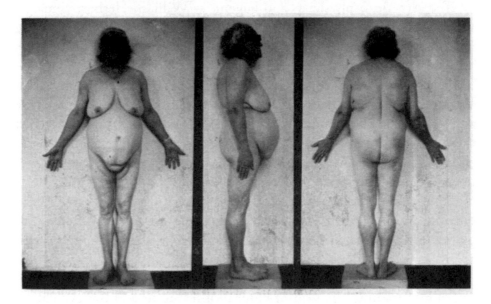

Figure 19.9: Android obesity in the female (Vague 1956: 26).

be that this kind of anthropometric photography and typology could not pass as proper medicine after the war? Morris-Reich concurs that photography lost its scientific legitimacy after the defeat of Nazism but that, before this, photography 'was conceived as a powerful, legitimate medium for the study, observation, and illustration of supraindividual differences' (Morris-Reich 2016: 32). The latter is very much the endeavour of these typologies of fatness and the role played by photography in them: they were not about portraying individuals or just representing a point or fact in the form of illustrations. The individual photographs and their arrangement into typologies were part of an investigating into generalisable patterns of adipose tissue and clusters of body types across populations. In this manner, they were invested in the exploration of what constituted physical normality and what differentiated the healthy human body from the sick one. At the same time, however, they rejected approaching the concept of normality from mere numerical averages, as was otherwise becoming the norm in biomedicine. Bodily normality existed, but in plural, and so did different ways of constituting health and disease. As evident in Sheldon, Jarløv and Vague, fatness could be a health concern, but it could also be characteristic of a natural type.

The American physician and eugenicist William Herbert Sheldon took his somatotype project to the extremes, and probably also to the margins of medicine. Yet, what is evident is his interest in the obese type. This type was part of the natural variation of man, and displayed a particular predisposition for specific illnesses, as was the case for all types. Yet a clear hierarchy between the types was also evident. Ejnar Jarløv and Jean Vague both grouped patients according to appearance based on the conviction that outward resemblances spoke of uniting underlying causes. Both found that the technology of photography gave them access to expose or demonstrate the likeness of types. I propose that these photographs worked as displays of data, sometimes in accumulated pictorial quantification, as in Sheldon, sometimes as part of an experimental explorative investigation, as in Jarløv, and sometimes as proof of argument, as in Vague. But, importantly, they all served as an invitation for other physicians to observe the phenomenon with their own eyes thus educating and training the skill of clinical observation and the evaluation of the entire body. In this, they formed part of the same project: coming to know and represent the human body through photography. The photographs both played a role in data analysis as well as in the final publications, whether they were finished typologies, experimental ones, or exemplars. In this respect, they were integral to the production of knowledge about fatness as a medical object, to the representation of fatness as a medical object and to the transmission of fatness as a medical object.

Acknowledgements

I am very thankful to professor Thorkild I. A. Sørensen for having brought the work of Jean Vague to my attention. This project has been made possible through the financial support of The Carlsberg Foundation.

References

Cassata, Fransesco (2013), *Building the New Man: Eugenics, Racial Science and Genetics in Twentieth-Century Italy*, Budapest: Central European University Press.

Cryle, Peter and Stephens, Elizabeth (2019), *Normality: A Critical Genealogy*, Chicago: University of Chicago Press.

Daston, Lorraine and Galison, Peter (1992), 'The image of objectivity', *Representations*, 40, pp. 81–128.

Edwards, Elizabeth (2001), *Raw Histories, Photographs, Anthropology and Museums*, Oxford: Berg.

Engelmann, Lukas (2019), 'Picturing the unusual: Uncertainty in the historiography of medical photography', *Social History of Medicine*, pp. 1–24.

Eraso, Yolanda (2007), 'Biotypology, endocrinology, and sterilization: The practice of eugenics in the treatment of Argentinian women during the 1930s', *Bulletin of the History of Medicine*, 81:4, pp. 793–822.

Gatlin, Stephen H. (1998), 'William H. Sheldon and the culture of the somatotype', Ph.D. thesis, Blacksburg: Virginia Polytechnic Institute and State University.

Gomes, Ana Carolina Vimiero (2016), 'Science, constitutional medicine and national bodily identity in Brazilian biotypology during the 1930s', *Social History of Medicine*, 30:1, pp. 137–57.

Jarløv, Ejnar (1932), *The Clinical Types of Abnormal Obesity*, Copenhagen: Nyt Nordisk Forlag.

Lawrence, Christopher and Weisz, George (1998), *Greater than the Parts: Holism in Biomedicine, 1920–1950*, New York: Oxford University Press.

Mitman, Gregg and Wilder, Kelly (eds) (2016), *Documenting the World: Film, Photography, and the Scientific Record*, Chicago: University of Chicago Press.

Morris-Reich, Amos (2016), *Race and Photography: Racial Photography as Scientific Evidence, 1876–1980*, Chicago and London: The University of Chicago Press.

Rasmussen, Nicolas (2012), 'Weight stigma, addiction, science, and the medication of fatness in mid-twentieth century America', *Sociology of Health & Illness*, 34:6, pp. 880–95.

Rheinberger, Hans-Jörg (1999), 'Experimental systems: Historiality, narration, and deconstruction', in M. Biagioli

(ed.), *The Science Studies Reader*, London: Taylor & Francis Books Ltd, pp. 417–29.

Sekula, Allan (1986), 'The body and the archive', *October*, 39, pp. 3–64.

Sheldon, William Herbert (1940), *The Varieties of Human Physique: An Introduction to Constitutional Psychology*, New York: Harper.

Sheldon, William Herbert (1954), *Atlas of Men: A guide for Somatotyping the Adult Male at all Ages*, New York: Harper.

Stern, Alexandra (1999), *Mestizophilia, Biotypology, and Eugenics in Post-Revolutionary Mexico: Towards a History of Science and the State, 1920–1960*, working paper series no. 4, Chicago: Center for Mexican Studies, University of Chicago.

Tracy, Sarah W. (1992), 'George Draper and American constitutional medicine, 1916–1946: Reinventing the sick man', *Bulletin of the History of Medicine*, 66:1, pp. 53–89.

Turda, Marius and Gillette, Aaron (2016), *Latin Eugenics in Comparative Perspective*, London, Oxford and New York: Bloomsbury.

Vague, Jean (1956), 'The degree of masculine differentiation of obesities: A factor determining predisposition to diabetes, atherosclerosis, gout, and uric calculous disease', *American Journal of Clinical Nutrition*, 4:1, pp. 20-34.

Vague, Jean (1996), 'Sexual differentiation: A determinant factor of the forms of obesity', *Obesity Research*, 4:2, pp. 201–03.

Vertinsky, Patricia (2002), 'Embodying normalcy: Anthropometry and the long arm of William H. Sheldon's somatotyping project', *Journal of Sport History*, 29:1, pp. 95–133.

Wann, Marilyn (2009), 'Foreword: Fat studies: An invitation to revolution', in E. D. Rothblum and S. Solovay (eds), *The Fat Studies Reader*, New York: New York University Press, pp. ix–xxv.

Zondek, Hermann (1926), *Die Krankheiten der endokrinen Drüsen; ein Lehrbuch für Studierende und Ärzte*, Berlin: Springer Berlin Heidelberg.

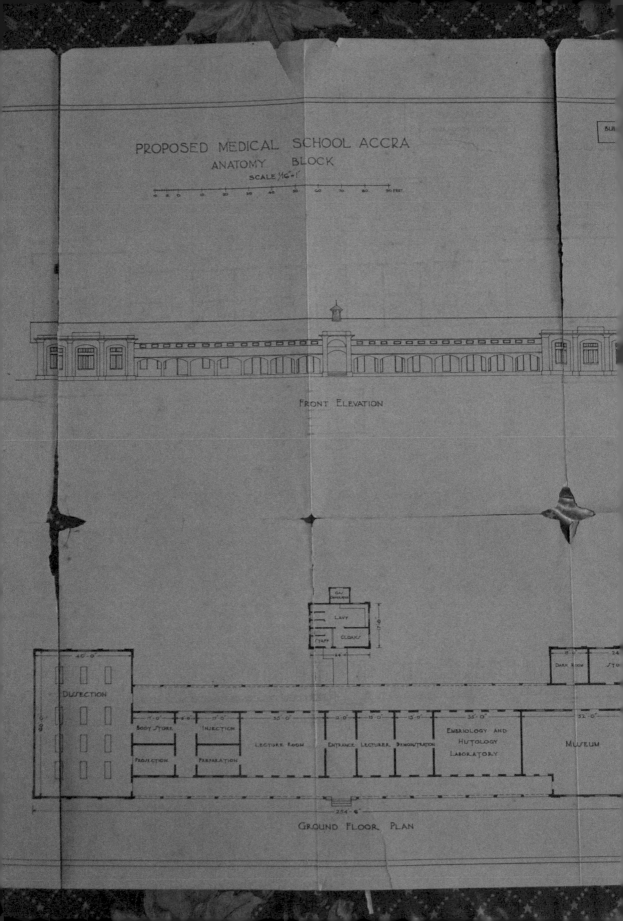

PLACE

MATTERS OF PLACE
AND AFFECT

Rachel Vaden Allison and John Nott

In a collection which considers the matter of medical reproduction, the role of place may seem an unlikely object of consideration. Yet, as many authors in this collection show, places are an important part of the socio-materiality of medical learning and knowing. The last decade of the twentieth century saw renewed interest in matters of space in the social sciences and humanities, often drawing from the insights of human geography. Anthropologists, historians, philosophers and sociologists all began to rethink and reconceptualise their fields in spatialised ways (Low and Lawrence-Zuniga 2003). Many of these accounts, however, took place as merely the backdrop, as a confluence of space and time (Ward 2003). Yet, as Edward Casey has forcefully explained, we do not live in space, we live in places; while human experience may begin in space and time, it naturally proceeds to place (Casey 1996). Place is, as such, the most essential characteristic for human being and knowing. Such a phenomenological approach requires a radical departure from the description of place as a geography or ecology external to the human subject. Instead, 'place is constituted, experienced and relational' (Ward 2003: 83). According to Kathleen Stewart, the experiential nature of place derives from 'its sensory materiality [...] [thrown] together in moments, things, in aesthetic sensibilities and affective charges' (Stewart 2012: 519).

Figure TE4: Blueprint for an unbuilt Anatomy Block, part of a larger medical school complex proposed for construction in colonial-era Accra, in what is now Ghana, c.1928. Image courtesy of Public Records and Archives Administration Department (PRAAD), Accra, ADM/5/3/26.

As many of the chapters in this collection show, medicine is learned, taught and reproduced in place, and in relation to the materials which proffer knowledge of the body and which make these spaces so affecting. As spaces which are firmly associated with death and debility, recovery and rehabilitation, hospitals and medical schools are laden with sensations and emotions that exist often beyond conscious consideration. These are places which Casey would describe as 'thick spaces' which resist the globalising effects that have seen 'places become thinned out' (Casey 2001: 684). Yet these places can also be considered as spatialisations of political authority and epistemic tradition, contributing to what Nigel Thrift has described as the 'engineering of affect' through design (Thrift 2007: 235). In this respect, these spaces form part of an 'affective infrastructure' (Street 2012: 44) of biomedical practice.

These dual pressures of place are apparent, for instance, in Annmarie Adams's (this volume) architectural history of McGill's pathology institute. The construction, in 1920s Montreal, of a distinct space for pathology spoke to the nascent development of academic pathology as a distinct discipline; its appendage onto McGill's older clinical buildings suggested the necessity of pathology for curative medicine. Yet this space has long outlived the moment of its construction, today presenting an enduring, affective link with a historical conception of disciplinary distinction at a time when extensive, practical pathology is being routinely removed from basic medical education. These are the sort of developments which might be said to promote cultural-homogeneity and the thinning out of place, especially in the ever-expanding digital spaces of the internet. The digitalisation of teaching materials, as Claire Aland et al. (this volume) detail with regard to the virtual microscope, disrupts modes of teaching which had, for decades, brought the material bodies of patient and practitioner together in the same physical space. In their discussion of the pathology museum at the University of Ghana, Robert Kumoji and John Nott (this volume) question whether the displacement of medical education threatens the localisation of pathology in favour of an abstracted universal conceptualisation of disease.

Yet this digital dis-placement is also the most valuable affordance of virtual microscopy – knowledge of the human body freed from spatial and material constraints. As other chapters in this collection also show, technology allows affective insight into spaces which had previously been inaccessible. Looking again at pathology, Christian Bonah and Joël Danet (this volume) show, for instance, how the development and distribution of autopsy films also provided affective access to the autopsy room. Rebecca

Whiteley (this volume) details a collection of obstetric illustrations from a Manchester lying-in hospital which offered a similar utility for British midwives in the mid nineteenth century. Of course, the affective weight of place also had a disciplinary function. Midwives' yearly invitation into the lecture theatre served to combat 'the confidence that came with extensive practice with an awareness of the different, more socially valued medical knowledge of the male authors, lecturers and practitioners' (Whiteley, this volume: 260). Yet access to illustrations offered women working in provincial cities free insight into the elite, exclusionary and exclusively male spaces in which medical knowledge was traditionally transmitted.

Jessica M. Dandona (this volume) presents a collection of photographs which detail the more comprehensive transgression of these gendered spaces later in the nineteenth century. Scrapbooks from Pennsylvania's Woman's Medical College – the first American institution to grant women medical degrees – emphasise that this was a place of industry, compositions are crowded with diligent students, anatomical prints and the tools necessary for the dissection of cadavers. While the development of photography proffered objective, scientific insight, the 'indeterminacy, ambiguities and lack of clarity [in these photographs] do not reaffirm the power relations established by the clinical gaze but instead reveal its instability' (Dandona, this volume: 122). The affective influence of place means that spatial change still has the potential to unsettle biomedical tradition. Stacey Langwick and Mary Mosha (this volume) detail how the Uzima Collective began experimenting with the construction of a garden at the heart of a Tanzanian medical school. Filled with therapeutic foods and herbal remedies, the garden forms a site of resistance against the pervasive pharmceuticalisation of health. As an epistemic space, the garden invites students to consider Tanzania's therapeutic sovereignty with a mind to its history and emplacement within an East African ecology.

In the thick, affective spaces which make up the Euro-American heart of biomedicine, medical tradition is not so readily questioned. David Theodore's (this volume) focus on the Nurserver, a relatively simple piece of hospital furniture, emphasises that medicine continues to be made in experiential relation to place and the material history of biomedicine. Designed in pursuit of efficiency in the postwar hospital, the development of the Nurserver highlights the ways in which medical knowledge – in a practical sense – is arbitrated by the emplaced materiality of medical care. Existing in between the nurse and the hospital's supply of clean and sterilised materials, this everyday piece of hospital equipment illustrates how learning medicine in the modern hospital also requires learning to submit to the places in which medicine is practiced. Place, as all these chapters show, is integral to the development of known and knowing bodies in biomedicine – as Edward Casey again explains, 'we are placelings, and our very perceptual apparatus, or our sensing body, reflects the kind of places we inhabit' (Casey 1996: 19).

References

Casey, Edward S. (1996), 'How to get from space to place in a fairly short stretch of time: Phenomenological prolegomena', in S. Feld and K. H. Basso (eds), *Senses of Place*, Santa Fe: School of American Research Press, pp. 13–52.

Casey, Edward S. (2001), 'Between geography and philosophy: What does it mean to be in the place-world?', *Annals of the Association of American Geographers*, 91:4, pp. 683–93.

Low, Setha M. and Lawrence-Zuniga, Denise (2003), 'Locating culture', in S. M. Low and D. Lawrence-Zuniga (eds), *Anthropology of Space and Place: Locating Culture*, Oxford: Wiley-Blackwell, pp. 1–46.

Stewart, Kathleen (2012), 'Precarity's forms', *Cultural Anthropology*, 27:3, pp. 518–25.

Street, Alice (2012), 'Affective infrastructure: Hospital landscapes of hope and failure', *Space and Culture*, 15:1, pp. 44–56.

Thrift, Nigel (2007), *Non-representational Theory: Space, Politics, Affect*, London: Routledge.

Ward, Sally (2003), 'On shifting ground: Changing formulations of place in anthropology', *The Australian Journal of Anthropology*, 14:1, pp. 80–96.

PROPS

PROPS IN BREAKING BAD NEWS SIMULATION

Kaisu Koski and Kirsten Ostherr

This chapter discusses the utilisation of various props in 'breaking bad news' simulations with standardised patients. Standardised patients (SP) are individuals who have been trained to portray characteristics of a real patient to provide medical students the opportunity to practice their clinical and interpersonal skills before taking their licensing exams. While SPs perform a large variety of clinical scenarios, the context of breaking bad news is considered among the most challenging, requiring a portrayal of a realistic emotional tone, and including an appropriate level of student confrontation. SP work has been previously considered in terms of dramatic arts (Smith et al. 2014). However, the specific material aspects of utilising props in simulation encounters have been left unexplored. Instead, if mentioned at all, props are typically overlooked as unspecified objects to 'produce [the] illusion of authenticity' (Sanko et al. 2013: 217). This is not surprising, as the SPs themselves are often considered as objects (assessment instruments, physical models) within a larger medical education enterprise (MacNaughton 2012: 7), instead of being seen as co-creators of simulation encounters or as medical educators. This chapter argues that intentional utilisation of everyday objects and furniture in simulation education can provide valuable lessons that contribute not only to patient satisfaction and outcome but assist the medical student in transitioning between different stages of a consultation as well. In contrast to the props that are utilised in scenarios involving physical examination and interventions, the props in the breaking bad news scenario are less spectacular. As a result, the bareness of the scenario allows the student to practice subtleties in their non-verbal communication, and 'being' with a patient instead of 'doing' medicine, thus laying a necessary foundation for other types of consultations as well. We begin by introducing our framework and study procedure, moving subsequently to examine the props as they appear in a breaking bad news simulation, to conclude with a discussion on the props' educational functions.

In this chapter, we look at props through theories developed to analyse performer–object interaction in a theatrical performance, acknowledging a fundamental complementarity between an object and a performer (Paavolainen 2012). Such consideration includes not only the three-dimensionality of objects as material participants in the stage action but also the spatial dimension (how props move in concrete stage space) and the temporal dimension (how props move through linear stage time) (Sofer 2003). We are thus using a scenographic-performative lens to discuss the materiality and spatiality that are related to the props, such as their various locations and moments of utilisation, their being present but purposefully unused, or the objects being mistakenly absent altogether.

The props in the breaking bad news simulation discussed here are seemingly everyday objects and do not include clinical instruments. Some of the scenario's props are used by the SP, some by the student and some by both of them. The main props in this simulation consist of a consultation room door, two chairs, a tissue box, a CT scan result sheet and miscellaneous props from the SPs lifeworld. These props have different purposes and moments of importance, such as announcing entrance, anchoring the bodies within the space, materialising clinical evidence and comforting the patient. While a door or a chair could also be considered as part of a set design or scenography, we here consider them as props. In this view, a prop is an object that is physically moved or altered in some way as a result of the actor's physical intervention (Sofer 2003). Thus, since the door in this scenario has an important function in indicating the spatial and temporal borders of the interaction, and the students are required to knock on, open, and close it, we here consider the door as one of the key props of the simulation. Similarly, the physician's chair and its movement (on wheels) has a crucial role in alignment with the patient's emotions. This definition of a prop, however, frames one iconic accessory of clinical practice, the white coat, beyond the scope of analysis. It is nonetheless worth noting that while most students wear a white coat in the class, this is not instructed in the script. Accordingly, none of the SP characters responds to the absence or presence of the coat. Besides actual utilisation of the props though, we will identify absences of particular actions that the props would call for. In doing so, we will differentiate *showing* from *telling* (Rabinowitz 2005), by distinguishing an actual usage of an object, as opposed to merely saying one would use it.

The aim of the exploratory reading is to identify currently overlooked mechanisms and meanings of prop utilisation in breaking bad news simulations, and their role in teaching about doctor–patient relationships. We also contribute to exploration of cultural codes embedded in prop utilisation in breaking bad news encounters, emphasising the encounters' constructed nature. We identify ways authenticity of clinical practice is imagined and performed through props. We raise questions about both the controversy and the power imbalances that are related to the props, including reasons for refusing to use them, and the challenges faced in the unintended absence of certain props. Finally, and more broadly, we contribute to understanding of the ways in which material objects help construct particular feelings and meanings in clinical settings.

Study description

As part of this film-based inquiry, we observed, recorded and transcribed three 90-minute sessions of a breaking bad news class for third-year students in the United States medical school where this study was conducted. We subsequently conducted open-ended interviews with three SPs specialising in the case. In each class, three students volunteer, one at a time, to perform a resident doctor's role in a breaking bad news scenario in front of a large classroom with peers and faculty. The breaking bad news scenario utilised by the medical school where we conducted this study was developed based on standards established by the Southern California Macy Consortium (Morrison and Barrows 1994) and adapted by the clinical faculty. There are two (confidential) scripts for this simulation; one for the SPs and one for the students. None of the props were mentioned in the students' one-page script as a preparation for the simulation. The students also do not receive other specific training in how to break bad news prior to the class. The SP script is nine pages long, including suggestions for possible reactions to the student behaviour. It briefly mentions a purse, tissues, and chair, but does not specify their spatial or temporal utilisation or meaning.

In all of the sessions, an SP portrays the role of a character called 'Ms. Kelly', each time using a different personality type: sad, angry or unfocused. Ms. Kelly arrives at the doctor's office expecting simply to pick up a pre-employment health form, but instead receives the news that a CT scan of her lungs, taken as part of her complete physical exam, shows a large mass. The same two female SPs have portrayed this scenario for over a decade now, and they have co-developed aspects of the prop utilisation (or purposeful non-utilisation) by observing and reviewing each others' performances. However, they have also developed their individual styles and have their own sets of props, and excel in performing different personality types. To prepare the set, they stack their props and accessories next to their chair and behind the table, to be able to change these quickly in-between the student encounters. As part of this study, Kaisu Koski directed the documentary film *Scenes of Disclosure* (2017), from which the images in this chapter originate.

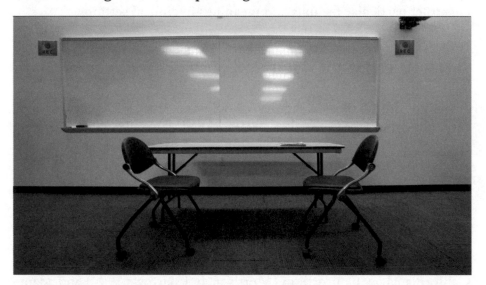

Figure 20.1: The initial set design for a breaking bad news simulation. Kaisu Koski (dir.), *Scenes of Disclosure*, 2017. USA. Copyright Kaisu Koski.

The breaking bad news scenario as prop utilisation

In this section, we describe the progression of the breaking bad news scenario through the props that are being utilised. The props have a typical dramaturgical order of appearance, although some of them are used in several steps of the encounter. Even though we look at the scenario's props in the order of their appearance, certain props which appear as the emotion mounts in the scene (i.e. towards the end) take on added importance. We introduce excerpts of the dialogue between the SPs, medical students and faculty, to illustrate how the props are mentioned both in the actual simulation and the class feedback.

Door (Entrance)

The simulation scenario is considered to begin from behind the classroom door; the door is thus a boundary between an onstage and offstage area. The student typically announces that they are entering by knocking on the door, and subsequently opening the door and entering the room. This is an unscripted rule, but it is normative training within American medicine and in the breaking bad news scenario, this rule is monitored by the 'social control' of the SPs, faculty and peers. In a case when one student did not pass through the classroom door before beginning the encounter, and instead went to sit directly in his chair in front of the SP, he was asked to begin again from behind the door before the session could proceed. The door itself is situated behind the SP, so they cannot comfortably see who is entering the room (Figure 20.2).

While door-knocking is an everyday skill that is typically not paid attention, not all styles of interacting with the door are suitable in a clinical context. An example of this is a situation in which knocking was actually absent, and the student said 'knock knock' instead. The SP chose to ignore this, with a dismissive expression in her face. She waited in silence until the student actually knocked on the door and only then responded with 'come in'. There is thus a difference between saying and doing; the simulation is not an airy imagination exercise and the SP here seems to guard its realness being rooted in its materiality. The SPs thus monitor the student's required suspension of disbelief, refusing to allow the exercise to turn into mimicking.

Chair/s

According to the SP script, they 'are seated in a chair at the front of a small lecture hall. Across from you is an empty chair'. It is not specified who sits on which side, but in this medical school the performers always sit on the same sides; student on the left, SP on the right. Interestingly, one of the SP personas ignores the scripted advice and does not sit down to wait for the doctor to enter the room; the 'unfocused' Ms. Kelly (as interpreted by one SP) walks back and forth in the front of the stage talking on her cell phone when the student doctor enters. She continues her phone call and walks around for two more minutes as the student attempts to herd her to a seat (Figure 20.3). Here, the empty chair becomes a focal point of this wandering choreography, as the student tries to steer the SP closer and closer to it. This is not a 'felt absence' of an object (Sofer 2003: 27) but is, in fact, a felt absence of an appropriate utilisation of it: we know the chair needs to be occupied before the encounter can continue. In this scene, the chair has been transformed from a mundane stage object to a centrifugal site directing movement onstage without any manipulation of it.

Another moment when a chair becomes a prop is if the student decides to pull their chair closer to the SP as a gesture of consolation. The chairs in this classroom are light weight and have wheels; moving them does not require a lot of physical effort. A chair may also become a prop when (unconsciously) utilised in an unusual way. That is, normally we do not hold the chair when we sit on it. This will thus look odd and communicates the seated person's uneven emotional state. The dialogue excerpt below is from the tutor feedback afterwards.

> **Tutor:** I think that's when you started getting nervous.
> **Student:** Right.
> **Tutor:** You were fiddling with your fingers and you were talking about that and you were holding the chair.

Miscellaneous SP props

The three personality types portrayed by the SPs have their own dedicated props. Some of these are mentioned in the SP script (tissues, purse), and some are devised by the SPs. The dedicated props not only make it easier for the SP to quickly shift between the personality types but these props have an important pedagogical function. Specifically, the props are barriers to a smooth scenario progression, as the SP script instructs them 'not to be too easy on the student'. Props used for such a purpose particularly include a purse, magazine (they have been flipping through it while they wait), sunglasses, phone and a hand mirror. The SP script mentions the purse in the context of looking for tissues and the patient attempting to leave, instructing the SP, 'you can pick up your purse'. However, the angry Ms. Kelly is clutching the purse in her lap throughout the entire exchange (Figure 20.4). The purse becomes thus not only a physical barrier between their body and the physician, but as the SP explains in an interview, it is a sign of preparedness to leave at any moment; the student should feel a sense of time pressure as a result of this. Some of the props, however, are used as clues of Ms. Kelly's lifeworld, which could be beneficial for the student to understand. For instance, the unfocused character sometimes shows the doctor a photo of a grandchild in the beginning of the simulation. While this may seem like an insignificant distraction in the process of getting into the test results, it offers a valuable entrance for the student later in the conversation. The SP tells about this in an interview:

> SP: I showed this photo of my grandbaby to the student and said, 'I know everybody thinks their grandbaby is the most beautiful grandbaby in world,' and then we went on. As it turns out this person has had a horrible experience with cancer and is really doubting whether she even wants to know if she has cancer. The student just reaches over and he picks that picture [of the grandbaby] and he says, 'This is why you should have that biopsy.'

CT scan result sheet

The student typically enters the simulation holding the CT scan results in their hand. During the dialogue, the paper usually rests on the table, but occasionally the SP may request to have a look at it. The test result paper is the key prop in this simulation, representing the voice of medicine (Mishler 1984) in the form of clinical evidence. It is a so-called 'speaking' prop that relays information to the patient that would otherwise require the presence of a messenger (Sofer 2003: 22), in this case the radiologist. In a temporal sense, the test result sheet is a snapshot of a past moment, likely to be followed by more results (in a linear order in a patient folder), always having a delay, unlike real-time imaging. This prop signals a larger offstage world beyond the simulation, and channels the radiologist's voice, as well as the CT scan's machine vision.

The absence or presence of the results sheet is central to the scenario from the very beginning: the patient is coming to the office thinking to pick up a piece of paper that actually proves that she is healthy. Instead, she is presented a paper that suggests an abnormality. The student script does not specifically instruct them to have the test result sheet at hand, but when one student does not have the papers with them, the angry

Ms. Kelly reacts to it strongly. When evidence of the results was missing, the student had nothing to hold on to, no details to double check and read out loud.

> **SP:** So, that's what this report, I mean you don't even have everything with you or you are just...
> **Student:** It was on a computer.
> **SP:** Oh! It was on the computer?
> **Student:** Yeah, I was reading on the computer.
> **SP:** Oh! All right so I was just supposed to trust your memory like there was nothing concerning about what you saw besides that it might be cancer?

Tissue box

Utilisation of particular props asks for specific verbal and nonverbal gestures. For instance, offering the patient a box of tissues is only appropriate as a gesture of consolation, in response to the patient's emotions. Utilisation of a tissue box has an impact on the chair and body position of the doctor: by offering tissues it may be more natural to move closer to the patient. The SP script advices them to 'look for tissues in your purse' if needed, instead of waiting for the doctor to offer it. Typically a tissue box is, however, prepared on the table, half way between the doctor and the patient. In one breaking bad news session, no one had prepared the tissue box, but a student nevertheless decided to pretend it was there and offered an imaginary tissue box to the SP. Though a mere arm gesture, the SP in this occasion accepted it much as a performative improviser would do (always accept what your co-improviser offers), meaning that the absence of a prop, such as the test result paper, does not always cause an interruption of the scene, but rather, is context dependent. The class feedback after the offer of imaginary tissues addresses this, with humour:

> **SP:** That felt very, I felt nurtured when she did it, even with the fake tissues.
> **Tutor 1:** All right, that was our fault, we usually have tissues.
> **Tutor 2:** We thought we would use the, your shawl.
> **SP:** I was getting ready to.

Door (Exit)

The function of the door at the end of the simulation has other connotations than it has in the beginning. While it still represents a border between the onstage and offstage areas, there are now specific references made to the offstage areas as a result of planning the next steps for the patient. Here, similar to saying 'knock knock' in the beginning, the student should be aware of whether they are saying or imagining that they will do something, or actually doing something. Typically, the encounter ends with discussion of next steps and the need for the SP to make a new appointment at the front desk, while the performers remain seated until the very end. However, a spontaneous performative variation one student created of this, and the subsequent SP feedback, demonstrate the educational potential hidden in this scenario; seemingly ordinary interactions with the stage props may have long lasting impacts on the patient's experience.

> **SP:** At the very end when I said, 'I think I need to go because I need to think about this.' I mean this person is just overwhelmed. I loved that you stood up and you said, 'Okay, I'll go with you.' I think you are the first student I've ever seen in ten years actually get up and walk to the door with me when I walk out of the room. You wanted to make sure I was okay. You were kind of following me out to make sure I've got what I needed and then I could talk to somebody.

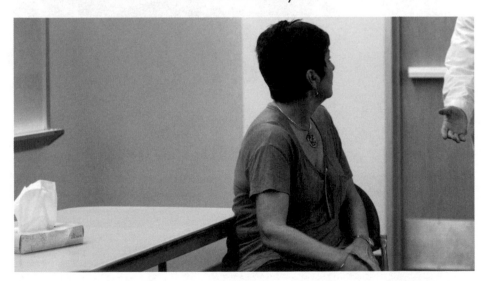

Figure 20.2: The student is required to enter the stage from outside the classroom (standardised patient: Katie Gruner). Kaisu Koski (dir.), *Scenes of Disclosure*, 2017. USA. Copyright Kaisu Koski.

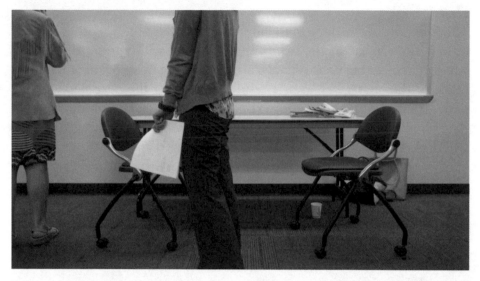

Figure 20.3: The unfocused personality type of Ms. Kelly is talking to her phone when the student enters. Kaisu Koski (dir.), *Scenes of Disclosure*, 2017. USA. Copyright Kaisu Koski.

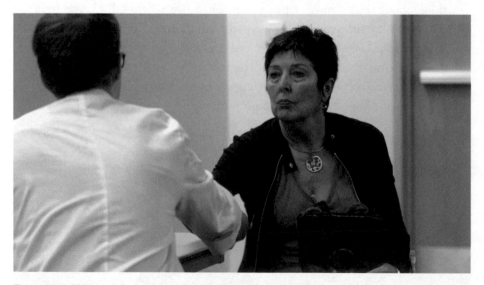

Figure 20.4: When performing an angry Ms. Kelly the standardised patient (Katie Gruner) holds a purse during the entire encounter. Kaisu Koski (dir.), *Scenes of Disclosure*, 2017. USA. Copyright Kaisu Koski.

The props' educational functions

Simulations utilising material objects such as anatomical models are central in training clinical or surgical skills. However, this chapter suggests that everyday objects have important roles in medical training as well. We have discussed the props used in the breaking bad news simulation in light of their dramaturgical functions and meanings at different stages of the encounter. All of these props are, with some variations, present in actual clinical practice and thus have existing conventions of utilisation and user behaviour. Sometimes, however, their utilisation or appearance is purposefully different in the simulation than in actual clinical practice. In this discussion, we consider the (present or absent) props' educational functions. We have identified several previously obscured ways their utilisation advances learning about doctor–patient communication, and how they materialise and refine simulation-based learning.

First, the props contribute to *setting boundaries of appropriate professional performance*, and the SPs assess and define these boundaries in real time through their performance. They let the student know when, in their assessment, the student has crossed a boundary, such as insensitive behaviour and lack of listening, vagueness or giving false hope. For instance, saying 'knock knock' may be used in everyday life when a door is already open, but here, when entering the consultation room from behind a closed door, it is not considered appropriate. The SP's refusal of the student's verbal knock thus sets boundaries to what is seen as professional clinical behaviour. Furthermore, while the simulation could be considered to start with the student doctor sitting in front of the patient, it is here considered significant that it begins from behind the consultation room door. The SP emphasises this in their feedback: 'I mean not just now, but ten years from now, fifteen years from now, you always have to be prepared every time you walk in the door'. Needing to physically enter through the door stimulates the student to acknowledge the importance of transitioning from one space to another in a medical realm, when, for instance, encountering one patient after another in their future practice. While the skill of transitioning between the patients and between the different steps of a consultation is always important, in different cultural and clinical settings, the doctor may be inside the room, welcoming the patient to enter from a waiting room, instead of entering while patient is waiting. This would invite developing a variation on the choreography of the door.

The props' second educational function *accentuates the relationship between clinical evidence and the student's translation thereof.* In fact, in this simulation, the CT scan result sheet appears as an emblematic of clinical evidence and the voice of medicine (Mishler 1984), which includes pictures of medical imaging as well. In the breaking bad news simulation as portrayed in this study, it is not possible to conduct the encounter in a satisfactory manner in the absence of the test result sheet. Most students are aware of this and enter the simulation holding their script (simulating the simulated test results). However, having evidence with them may be the easiest part of the student's responsibility; at the core of this scenario lies the task of translating the voice of medicine into appropriate patient dialogue without sounding robotic. In particular, the problems often arise from a polyphony amongst the results and their interpretation: depending on the character demeanour, the SPs reacted either positively or negatively if the student's narrative deviated from the test result narrative. Furthermore, even when the student's story and the test result sheet were in unison, the angry SP character disbelieved the doctor's voice alone and required to see proof, pinpointing the power of image or 'black on white' over spoken word. The student is thus not only carrying the piece of paper with them, but they may be asked to read the results word-by-word by the SP. Therefore, they should know about the result sheet layout and to quickly find answers to the SPs questions. The CT scan results sheet also demonstrates a case for learning from the absence of an object, as one student was missing the result sheet altogether. The absence of the sheet may, in some sense, be a more realistic situation; physicians may not walk around carrying patients' tests results in their hands for confidentiality reasons. Instead, most consultation rooms include a computer. Yet, the lesson that the test result sheet introduces relates to the presence of evidence in supporting the physician's narrative, whether a digital or paper file.

The third educational role the props have is to *provide vehicles for adjusting appropriate proximity and orientation*, manifesting in the chairs on wheels in this simulation. In general, the layout of the consultation room has an impact on interpersonal communication. For instance, equal access to the laptop computer screen has been proven to improve information exchange (Ajiboye et al. 2015). Furthermore, the physician's non-verbal behaviour, such as leaning forward and adjusting proximity to the patient, has been shown to improve patient satisfaction (Larsen and Smith 1981; Griffith et al. 2003). The impact of positioning chairs next to each other, instead of opposing each other, thus extends beyond information exchange, especially when viewing unfavourable test result images. As one physician adviser to this study noted, in those situations he purposefully sits next to the patient and they face the image (and its consequences) together. This would be possible in the breaking bad news simulation setting as well, if the student would choose to lay the test result sheet on the table and invite the SP to look at it together.

The fourth educational value of the everyday props emerges from their capacity to *highlight the distinction between an embodied action and imagined behavior*. Regarding the door in particular, the students often *say* that they will walk the patient to the front desk, but they remain seated instead. The meaning of actual walking with the patient should not be underestimated. In fact, it could be seen as a small performative manifestation of the model of medicine in which the patient is accompanied (Vegni et al 2001). Instead of sending the patient away alone, the physical accompaniment, at least during the very first steps after receiving bad news, may support a sense of emotional accompaniment as well. Breaking bad news simulation in this study thus expands, albeit intuitively, the repertoire of the student's non-verbal communication both spatially and temporally by including the entrance and exit to the encounter, as well as the student's awareness of the proximity between what they say and what they do.

The relationship between the everyday props and non-verbal communication is often left without much attention in medical education, and the advice on non-verbal communication may appear abstract to the student. However, observing the student's utilisation of everyday props may help formulate detailed feedback on non-verbal behaviour. Accordingly, the breaking bad news class tutors commented on the chair utilisation in particular, including how to get the patient to sit down, the impact of the doctor gripping the chair, and the usage of the chair in varying proximity to the patient. The learning stimulated by the props has further relevance for clinical practice; while non-verbal behavior has wide-ranging effects on patients' social, psychological and physiological outcomes (Robinson 2006), a mismatch between the doctor's verbal and nonverbal behavior may, in fact, have negative consequences for the patients' health outcomes. Specifically, a large gap between what a healthcare provider says and does has been found to be a barrier for optimal pain relief (Dihle et al. 2006). Yet, the timing of the action is a skill to be developed as well; a doctor can be too 'proactive' and focused on the prop only. While some patients may experience tissue-offering as patronising, nudging the tissue box towards the patient is especially insulting in the absence of actual tears (Gardner 2015); the cue for tissues should be tears and not the other way around.

In the absence of clinical instruments and interventions, the breaking bad news simulation lays the bare essence of a clinical consultation visible. In fact, it allows space and close examination of the everyday objects: if there was a blood pressure cuff involved, for instance, the feedback would likely concern its usage instead of door-knocking and other everyday elements of medical interaction. This bareness has a capacity to increase the students' awareness and sensitivity to subtleties of everyday objects and associated choreography and gestures that make the patient feel accompanied. By absence or dysfunction of props, or excess of patient props, the simulation increases their skills in problem-solving. It trains the student in decision-making about the appropriate timing of moving forward and pausing, highlighting the value of observation and listening in order to identify valuable cues from the patient's lifeworld. We suggest that awareness of the subtleties in behaviours and meanings associated with everyday props advances a future medical education in which *being* with and accompanying the patient will be considered essential skills.

Acknowledgements

The authors wish to thank the faculty, staff and students involved in the Breaking Bad News teaching at the medical school where this study was conducted. Warm thanks to the director and team in the Standardized Patients programme in the Surgical & Clinical Skills Center. This project has been financially supported by the Academy of Finland, Tampere University and the Rice University Humanities Research Center. The Committee for the Protection of Human Subjects at the medical school where this study was conducted has provided ethical approval for this this study (IRB number: HSC-MS-18-0083).

References

Ajiboye, Folaranmi, Dong, Fanglong, Moore, Justin, Kallail, James K. and Baughman, Allison (2015), 'Effects of revised consultation room design on patient–physician communication', *HERD: Health Environments Research & Design Journal*, 8:2, pp. 8–17.

Dihle, Alfhild, Bjølseth, Gunnar and Helseth, Sølvi (2006), 'The gap between saying and doing in postoperative pain management', *Journal of Clinical Nursing*, 15:4, pp. 469–79.

Gardner, Caleb (2015), 'Medicine's uncanny valley: The problem of standardising empathy', *The Lancet*, 386:9998, pp. 1032–33.

Griffith, Charles H. III, Wilson, John F., Langer, Shelby and Haist, Steven A. (2003), 'House staff nonverbal communication skills and standardized patient satisfaction', *Journal of General Internal Medicine*, 18:3, pp. 170–74.

Koski, Kaisu (2017), *Scenes of Disclosure*, US and Finland: Rice University and Tampere University [Trailer available at: https://vimeo.com/227863178. Accessed 11 January 2022.].

Larsen, Kathryn M. and Smith, Charles K. (1981), 'Assessment of nonverbal communication in the patient–physician interview', *Journal of Family Practice*, 12, pp. 481–88.

MacNaughton, Nancy (2012), 'A theoretical analysis of the field of human simulation and the role of emotion and affect in the work of standardized patients', Ph.D. thesis, Toronto: University of Toronto.

Mishler, Elliot G. (1984), *The Discourse of Medicine : Dialectics of Medical Interviews*, Norwood: Ablex.

Morrison, Linda J. and Barrows, Howard S. (1994), 'Developing consortia for clinical practice exams: The Macy project', *Teaching and Learning in Medicine*, 6:1, pp. 23–27.

Paavolainen, Teemu (2012), *Theatre/Ecology/Cognition. Theorizing Performer-Object Interaction in Grotowski, Kantor, and Meyerhold*, Basingstoke: Palgrave Macmillan.

Rabinowitz, Peter J. (2005), 'Showing vs. telling', in D. Herman, J. Manfred and M. L. Ryan (eds), *The Routledge Encyclopedia of Narrative Theory*, London: Routledge, pp. 530–31.

Robinson, Jeffrey D. (2006), 'Nonverbal communication and physician–patient interaction: Review and new directions', in V. Manusov and M. L. Patterson (eds), *The SAGE Handbook of Nonverbal Communication*, Thousand Oaks: SAGE Publications Inc., pp. 437–60.

Sanko, Jill S., Shekhter, Ilya, Kyle, Richard R., Di Benedetto, Stephen and Birnbach, David J. (2013), 'Establishing a convention for acting in healthcare simulation: Merging art and science', *Simulation in Healthcare*, 8:4, pp. 215–20.

Smith, Cathy M., Edlington, Tanya L., Lawton, Richard and Nestel, Debra (2014), 'The dramatic arts and simulated patient methodology', in D. Nestel and M. Bearman (eds), *Simulated Patient Methodology: Theory, Evidence and Practice*, West Sussex: John Wiley & Sons, pp. 39–45.

Sofer, Andrew (2003), *The Stage Life of Props*, Ann Arbor: University of Michigan Press.

Vegni, Elena, Zannini, Lucia, Visioli, Sonia and Moja, Egidio (2001), 'Giving bad news: A GP's narrative perspective', *Supportive Care in Cancer*, 9:5, pp. 390–96.

RADIOGRAPHS

LASERS, SCREENS AND MODELS: THE MATERIAL ASSEMBLAGES OF LEARNING PATTERN RECOGNITION IN RADIOGRAPHY EDUCATION

Peter D. Winter

This chapter focuses on how materials are used to help radiography students learn to see patterns in X-ray images. The discussion is grounded in three vignettes from training interactions where diagnostic radiography students learn pattern recognition as a part of first-year training and workplace preparation. It explores how radiography professionals engage students with materials to make sense of patterns in X-ray anatomy. I present the rationale for the use of pattern recognition as a way of looking at medical images and show how pattern recognition can be understood as a sensory understanding of visual–material sources. I then describe three ways in which pattern recognition is delivered to students via three material means in the radiography degree, which builds up this sensory knowledge: the laser pointer, the computer screen and the 3D anatomical model all contribute to the building of sensory knowledge. Video footage is included to show how an assemblage of laser pointers, computer screens and 3D anatomical models makes this type of seeing possible. Such specification immediately opens up the question: how do students learn to see patterns in X-ray images? The question is significant, since sharing this 'assemblage' are other materials, other technologies, other people and their materials too, bringing into question the constitution of seeing, showing and perceiving. I argue that each material context offers a means of learning X-ray anatomy through concrete sensory detail. These, in turn, affect their knowing in order to build towards an 'observational-embodied look' (Fountain 2010: 49).

Pattern recognition

The identification of patterns in medical image interpretation is called pattern recognition. It is a general term for the instantaneous comprehension of different forms, shapes, configurations or 'patterns' whereby an individual can identify whether or not a medical image is 'normal' or 'abnormal' for diagnostic purposes (Swinburne 1971; Corr 2011). There are many examples of pattern recognition in medical image interpretation. Instant pattern recognition, for example, grew out of the cognitive psychology discourse and offers the opportunity to compare medical imaging information with similar previous examples from memory (van der Gijp et al. 2017). Other prominent examples of the application of pattern recognition include the ability to recognise abnormalities rather than to interpret findings based on a formal set of rules (Chen et al. 2017), the 'description' of, for example, imaging appearances for professionals who require anatomic closure (Williams et al. 2019), and how it is a form of 'non-systematic' reasoning so as to allow professionals to quickly look at whatever attracts their attention (Kok et al. 2015). In addition, patterned recognition capabilities are used to generate diagnostic decisions, a mental representational form of problem solving that is often framed as the connection between individual perception and cognition (Bloomer 1990; Custers et al. 1996).

Often this research focuses on a comparison of visual competence between experts (e.g. Williams et al. 2019) or, to a lesser extent, between experts and undergraduate students (e.g. Eisen et al. 2006). These accounts, however, neglect the learning process and how knowledge of these patterns are learnt or built in the first place. To begin to understand how professionals learn to see patterns in medical images we must turn our attention to the speciality of pathology – the ability to diagnose illness via macroscopic or microscopic means – in order to get a better picture of the learning process. For example, in their study on the development of visual expertise in pathology, Crowley et al. (2003) compare the visual diagnostic process of novices, intermediates and expert pathologists in order to highlight the basic cognitive processes underlying their expertise. In doing so, Crowley et al. (2003) identify five processes of learning to see – as types of 'cognitive' categories – during a microscopic investigation: (1) data examination, (2) data exploration and explanation, (3) data interpretation, (4) control processes and (5) operational processes. They state that these five parts entail the *novice's perception of parts* to the *expert's recognition of patterns*. Such a study is important for several reasons. First, it shows how pattern recognition consists of having learned a perception of parts of the pathology which over time and practice builds to a holistic mode of recognising the pattern of pathology. Second, it demonstrates how prolonged exposure to a diverse range of pathologies and their microdetails can generate an understanding of patterns. Third, any specific amount of time spent on each category can show whether the pathologist is a novice or expert. Fourth, it serves as a springboard for showing how the learning process can be unpacked and broken up for analysis.

However, overly attributing the learning process to cognition that is rooted in mental processes has taken for granted the unique sphere of the social and material aspects involved in the social process of learning to see. This really comes as no surprise: the 'cognitive' approach to research has helped constitute a learning model based on description and taxonomic representation of anatomic appearances (Lesgold et al. 1988; Crowley et al. 2003; van der Gijp et al. 2017); a focus that has narrowed the development of visual expertise to a form of information-processing and measurement of competence, with social process and material arrangements stripped away. In the nature of sociological analysis, however, we are able to analyse the learning process as part of an ongoing action constellated by the distinctive conditions, strategies, and practices engaged in by humans and their material 'things' (Clarke 2003). Prentice (2013: 88) in her study of surgical training discusses how this focus on a material approach to learning actually involves nesting students in an assemblage of educational hardware and expert knowledge and proceduralisms 'in order to be able to reason anatomically as a physician'. Fenwick (2014) also discussed the role of materials in assemblages of medical training as a way of learning through material engagement; a process of learning that allows humans to 'attune very closely' to the micro-details of concern. A combination of all these factors – the value placed on seeking structure within the material and manipulating the information to make sense of it – may highlight how students come to successfully memorise, understand and visualise anatomy. This process of learning to see is an example of 'deep learning' as opposed to 'surface learning', where students are able to develop a personal framework of understanding spatial relationships between structures (Pandey and Zimitat 2006: 8; Turney 2007).

These discussions of material engagement also highlight the embodied and sensory knowledge as parts of the assemblage that enable different ways of seeing. Goodwin (1994), for instance, has also long advocated the use of bodies, visual texts and material objects to teach visual expertise (or professional vision in the terms of Goodwin). In medical education, the growing interest in the tacit dimension of visual expertise (Polanyi 1958; Engel 2008; Saunders 2008; Friedrich 2010; Fountain 2014; Friis 2017; Gegenfurtner et al. 2019) exhibits the view that material and visual evidence are useful tools for developing an embodied relationship to underlying features of parts or patterns in medical images. Prominent here has been the work of Kenny Fountain (2014), for whom an important part of the value of visualisation and material practices in medical education is its capacity to embody anatomical information. What these various uses of material and visual resources recognise is the power of people to embody features or patterns as both haptic experience and anatomical knowledge of the human body. This insight is not new. As Fountain (2010) has noted, the nineteenth century conception of western medicine emphasised its social, haptic character: 'by the eye, by the touch, by the measurement from some fixed point, by line, or by percussion' (Fountain 2010: 50). The capacity that pattern recognition can be generated by different forms of tacit knowledge is, however, distinctive. As the next section points out, pattern recognition is generated in part by three key materials and their role in delivering a special kind of sensory training.

Important for this book, materials and material practice is a central part of this process of ensuring anatomical understanding and building medical knowledge of the human body. I will argue that these three processes materials (lasers, screens and 3D models) not only build language and structure of anatomical knowledge but it also works towards sensory knowledge and embodiment among learners. That is, before students can competently make decisions about normal patterns in an image, then students must learn to accomplish an 'observational-embodied look' (Fountain 2010). This learning of pattern recognition is accomplished largely through the use of an elaborately constructed material assemblage and demonstrated *from* the hand *to* the head. Learning pattern recognition involves placing students in an affective space of materials, visual practices and discourse that can be used for learning recognition of the normal. Drawing on Goodwin's highlighting and coding practices as two socially organised modes of seeing within transcriptions of video footage helps reveal this. Goodwin (1994: 606) identifies highlighting and coding practices as central to the development of professional vision where it becomes necessary, upon occasion, to code and highlight phenomena; coding 'transforms phenomena observed in a specific setting into the objects of knowledge that animate the discourse of a profession', whereas highlighting 'makes specific phenomena in a complex perceptual field salient by marking them in some fashion'. I also include the use of gesture through which seeing is enabled and sustained to represent content. Brackets are used in an analytical way to link the visual practice to the talk in order to show how talk, highlighting, coding and gesture mutually elaborate each other within a framework of action (Goodwin 1994).

In the examples that follow, I aim to use video ethnographic vignettes to describe three ways in which pattern recognition, comprised of seeing patterns in medical images on display, is learned. These vignettes draw attention to how pattern recognition is learned by placing students in an affective space of lasers, screens and 3D models. I first focus on a professional radiographer teaching a large class of around 50 radiography students in the first week of their degree just starting to learn about pattern recognition in radiographs. The teaching takes places in the 'Introduction to X-ray Image Interpretation' class, which focuses on a presentation of a basic selection of bones and a light-hearted introduction to image interpretation: my concern here is the material use of a laser pointer, with its illustrative ways of seeing and analysability, particularly how it highlights the visual experience to that aspect. The process of learning in this instance begins with the laser pointer.

The second focus of this chapter takes place in the 'Application of Imaging 1' class in which the aim of the module is to provide a foundation in X-ray anatomy, and introduces students to taxonomical terminologies of anatomy in the context of X-ray images. My concern here is the material use of computer screens – how pattern recognition, particularly through touching, labelling and spelling out the subtle parts of radiographic anatomy displayed on screen, is gained piecemeal as a material–practical activity. The process of learning in this instance continues with a focus on the detailed practices with computer screens, cross-referenced images and PowerPoint tools that allow students to 'see for themselves' and learn from each other in which they can share their personal experience (Polanyi 1958).

The third focus of this chapter also takes places in the 'Application of Imaging 1' class – this time, however, the practices with computer screens enlists a 3D anatomical model to help the students label the image. With the addition of the model into the mix, they create a means of understanding and deepening their appreciation of anatomical parts, such as cavities and surface markings. These parts accumulate to trigger a perception of a certain pattern in the image (Friis 2017) in order to understand the parts as a whole or 'overall picture' (Pandey and Zimitat 2006; Prentice 2013).

Lasering the trabecular pattern

The first type of pattern that the radiography students were introduced to – in the class 'Introduction to X-Ray Image Interpretation' – was a bone pattern, the trabecular pattern. Here a professional radiographer (Mrs. Campbell) presents the pattern as a significant feature of bone-based or musculoskeletal (MSK) radiographs. As we join the scene, Mrs. Campbell stands in front of a large projector screen and next to a computer in a room dimmed by windows with blinds; the large class of students sit down around a room full of tables listening to her talk and see the images on screen. She describes how the trabecular pattern must be *'smooth'*, a figurative description that transpires in the student's perception of the image in terms of its material and haptic evidence of touch and texture. In doing so, the exact moment of the word is coordinated with the use of a material technological object – the laser pointer – to 'highlight' (Goodwin 1994) the location of the pattern:

> **Mrs. Campbell:** So, trabecular pattern. Has anybody heard of the word 'trabecular pattern'?
> **Marco:** I heard it the other day
> **Mrs. Campbell:** That's the word for today then, trabecular pattern [Gesture: both hands rub the air in a smooth manual action like a windscreen wiper]. Sometimes you can't see a fracture, but you can see disruption in the trabecular pattern [Highlighting: lasers the disrupted pattern on the radius bone]. So, you can see how *smooth* this is

[Highlighting: lasers the bone in a straight line as if to mimic the patterns smoothness]. But then you can see that it's *not* [Highlighting: lasers the bone in a straight line until it gets to the disrupted pattern]. It's disrupted here [Highlighting: lasers the bone in a jagged way as if to mimic the disruption in the pattern], the trabecular pattern.

In order to explain the smoothness of the trabecular pattern, Mrs. Campbell uses a laser pointer to highlight the smoothness of the trabecular pattern, which in part is due to the textural distinction between the smooth and the not so smooth. In doing so, she not only directs attention to the features on the two bones (disruption, smooth) but also how the smoothness is associated with a straight laser movement and disruption is associated with a jagged laser movement. This finding reflects how the use of laser pointers compliments speech and how its movements are always involved in the process of understanding the meaning of others (Knoblauch and Tuma 2011). In this sense, Mrs. Campbell helps to identify how smoothness is associated with what may be defined as normal and disruption as abnormal.

In addition to highlighting the normal and abnormal patterns of the arm, Mrs. Campbell also does a lot to lay the ground for sensory description and sensory means of learning X-ray anatomy. For instance, the word *'smooth'* is captured by the connotations of learning the pattern through the hands and the tactile experience, highlighting the sensory attunement of the professional's body. Mrs. Campbell's understanding of smoothness comes from translating knowledge of the bone's texture, which remains tacit, to her own body. The interaction clarifies that the normal texture of the anatomy on the surface of the bone has somehow become familiar to Mrs. Campbell, allowing her to describe anatomical information in common-sense terms familiar to students from their everyday lives.

Computer screens and the labelling of radiographs

The computer room is a small L-shaped room containing nine desktop computers, a large LCD screen and a large green 'bone box'. The bone box contained 3D anatomical models of different body parts: the upper and lower limbs, thorax, abdomen, shoulder, spine and pelvis. These models were indicative of developing an understanding of which X-ray anatomies the radiography students needed to learn and the types of radiographs they needed to produce/interpret. Four classes of between twelve and fifteen radiography students were split into groups of two or three in front of two computer screens. One computer screen displayed a PowerPoint presentation with radiographs that represented each body part and provided a variety of digital tools for the students to label the image and/or change its contrast. The second computer screen displayed internet searches of visual information about the radiographs displayed in the PowerPoint presentation. Both screens were used for comparative purposes – a cross-referential approach which draws relation between the anatomies in the PowerPoint radiograph and schematic diagrams/radiographs of the normal anatomy available online. This observation connects with the findings of other research studies on the radiological interpretive process and learning to see (Pasveer 1989; Prasad 2005; Dussauge 2008; Winter 2019). To begin, radiographer Mr. Jim Richards, gives a 10-minute presentation on the five basic densities in a radiograph. He states:

> bone is generally white [...] normally fat would be not quite as white so that will be light grey [...] so soft tissues would be a mid-grey and then fluids, blood and things, are a dark grey and air is nearly almost black.

After the presentation, Mr. Richards presents the final PowerPoint slide that reads: 'Look at the images and compare them with the bones. Can you work out which part of the bones makes which patterns on the image?' and asks the students to label the PowerPoint radiographs using relevant online sources and anatomical models of the bones in question.

As across all the four classes, the looking and touching of computer screens was central to their vision of learning pattern recognition, particularly what appeared to be significant locations, cavities and surface features of bones. The accounts that I offer in the two labelling activities below shows the process of the student's perception of parts and the beginning of a holistic vision of patterns; accounts that stress the interdependencies between different kinds of subtle and micro anatomical forms. This might be thought of as a cumulative mode of pattern recognition, and this is the underlying attunement and adjustment which results in the fitting together of parts into a perceived pattern (Crowley et al. 2003; Friis 2017). In Pandey and Zimitat's (2006: 13) words, it is: 'the overall picture' and part of the deep learning approach. We will see this understanding in the final vignette but, before we do, let us see how this understanding begins by way of two radiography students (Carrie and Joanne) and their tactile use of two computer screens. The left computer screen offers a schematic diagram of the anatomy of the lower leg, while the right computer screen exhibits an actual radiograph of the lower leg. We join Carrie and Joanne having correctly labelled the two main bones of the lower leg ('tibia' and 'fibula') and who now look to label its more subtle features, beginning with the 'tibial tuberosity':

> **Joanne:** Are you going to label these bits up here? [Highlighting: left hand points at the 'tibial tuberosity' on the radiograph (screen 2)] *Looking at the leg illustration on screen 1*
> That's the tibial–
> **Carrie:** What is it?
> **Joanne:** *Reads the schematic illustration on screen 1*
> Tibial, tibial tuberosity
> **Carrie:** [Coding 1: creates 'text box' and types 'tibial tuberosity']
> **Joanne:** The bit that kind of sticks out [Highlighting: left hand rubs tibial tuberosity on screen 2]
> **Carrie:** Oh yeah! Which bit, here? [Highlighting: cursor hovers around the region of the tibial tuberosity on screen 2]
> **Joanne:** Yeah, you know where it kind of bridges out? [Highlighting: left hand rubs a prominent area of the proximal tibia]
> **Carrie:** [Coding: repositions label to where Joanne pointed] this bit here?
> **Joanne:** It's down, I think? It's this point right here [Highlighting: right hand rubs the proximal tibia on screen 2]
> **Carrie:** [Highlighting: places cursor over the location of Joanne's finger]
> **Joanne:** Yeah
> **Carrie:** [Coding: final adjustment of the 'tibial tuberosity' label]

This exchange exhibits the many steps in learning the position and feature of the 'tibial tuberosity'. First, leg anatomy must be recognised from the radiograph (screen two) and its schematic equivalent searched for online (screen one). Digital tools are then used on screen two to inscribe and label the tibial tuberosity. The label being produced on the radiograph in screen two is cross-referenced with the position of the tuberosity within the diagram on screen one. Because Joanne is in close proximity to the schematic diagram, she is able to direct the 'labelling the anatomy' activity through cross-referencing the radiograph. Carrie labels the tuberosity, its anatomical form, as well as its location through directed learning and in collaboration with Joanne. This venture continues the acculturation of radiography students to anatomical language and initiates them into the culture of pattern recognition in which 'anatomical terms are the lingua franca' (Prentice 2013: 42). In her tacit application of 'highlighting', there is a *salient* logic to Joanne's finger rubbing which shows both the anatomic location of the tibial tuberosity and its form or texture on the radiograph. Each label (comprising of 'text box' and 'arrow') on the radiograph, itself a 'coding' practice (Goodwin 1994), has a classificatory logic that builds up the 'idea' of the tibial tuberosity through cross-referencing with the diagram.

3D model anatomies and the labelling of radiographs

In this vignette, the previous experiences of learning subtle or small amounts of visual information is built upon. It is built upon through the use of a 3D model anatomy of the radiograph that is under focus and present in the PowerPoint slides. In order to help describe the locations of the anatomy in the flat 2D radiograph, the anatomical model can help students gain spatial detail of locations and subtle textures of the anatomy that the simple act of looking at images does not provide (Prentice 2013). It seeks to bring closer their descriptive detachment of the anatomy in the previous examples by a 'deep' approach to learning. This deep approach is said to build up a personal interrelationship between facts and the ability to develop a relational view of structure and function; spatial understanding is learned in this process by 'seeking a structure within the material and manipulating the information to make sense of it in relation to what is known of the subject matter' (Pandey and Zimitat 2006: 8). To consider this spatial skill, we join a group in which three radiography students (Amar, Vakul and Niha) label a radiograph of the elbow. Having labelled the two main bones of the elbow (ulna and radius), albeit incorrectly, the group now turn their attention to the more subtler features of each bone, beginning with the ulnar's 'epicondyle'.

The subtlety of the form or pattern of the epicondyle is commonly dealt with in a way that echoes Joanne and Carrie's labelling practice above. Niha's (left) task is to manually label the PowerPoint images via the keyboard whilst Amar and Vakul are at hand consulting schematic images or diagrams via a second screen. However, this time Vakul consults the 3D model of the left human arm and shoulder in order to answer his question about the location of the epicondyle:

> Vakul: The epicondyle is going to be this thing here [Highlighting: right hand points at epicondyle on screen 1, see Figure 21.1] that bone sticking out there
>
> Niha: [Coding: creates text box and labels it 'epicondyle']
>
> Vakul: So, if you look at it this way [Gesture: right hand grips the model arm so that it is held in place for the others to see]
>
> Niha: Mhm [Coding: creates arrow and positions it near the epicondyle]
>
> Vakul: And you can see there [Highlighting: left hand rubs the 'medial epicondyle' on the model elbow] that groove there [Highlighting: left hand index finger rubs the cavity of the 'medial epicondyle' on screen 1] is about here [Highlighting: left hand rubs the 'medial epicondyle' on the model arm, see Figure 21.2]
>
> Amar: Yeah, yeah [Coding: adjusts arrow to the text 'epicondyle' on screen two]
>
> Vakul: Obviously we don't really know much yet so when we look at this [Highlighting: left hand traces the uneven outline or bump of the lateral epicondyle on screen two] and think 'hang on a sec, he's got a few bumps on that bit here' [Highlighting: rubs the lateral epicondyle on the model]. Have a feel of it
>
> Amar: [Highlighting: Amar rubs the lateral epicondyle on the model arm, see Figure 21.3]
>
> Niha: It looks actually like that
>
> Vakul: And you'll just see that this is normal. This is just how it is
>
> Amar: Yeah
>
> Niha: Yeah
>
> Amar: It's just the positioning of the bone
>
> Vakul: Exactly, yeah, so that should be basically normal in almost everyone

First, Vakul delivers information about the epicondyle that highlights its location and explains the location of the epicondyle. When referring to

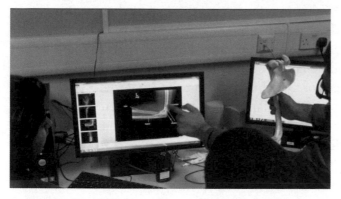

Figure 21.1: Vakul 'points' to the location of the lateral epicondyle on the radiograph (screen one).

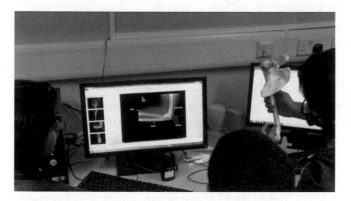

Figure 21.2: Vakul 'rubs' the 'lateral epicondyle' on the model.

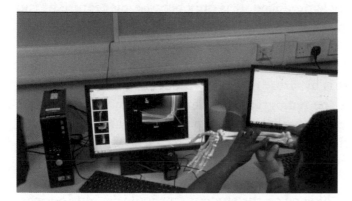

Figure 21.3: Amar (left) and Vakul (right) 'rubbing' the bumps of the lateral epicondyle on the ulna shaft of the model.

the *'bone sticking out'* Vakul is referring to the round elevation or bump on the outside (lateral) of the ulna bone which is said to characterise the lateral epicondyle. Second, Vakul becomes attuned to directing another feature of the epicondyle and describes it as *'that groove there'* as his fingers rub both the locations of the cavity on the image and then inside the cavity belonging to the medial (middle) epicondyle on the 3D model. In an iterative sense, Vakul then returns to the bump of the lateral epicondyle but this time invites Amar to *'have a feel of it'* to seek in what he means. In both instances, there is a very simple processing of visual information and how students go about building recognition of patterns. Both examples have consequences for seeing the epicondyle as a *'bone sticking out'* or *'bumps on that bit there'* (lateral epicondyle) and *'that groove there'* (medial epicondyle). This language and haptic experience (the act of rubbing) has consequences for seeing the epicondyle in a way that is familiar to Amar and Niha (assuming that both know the meaning of 'bumps' and 'groove'). Here, the anatomical model is used by Vakul to help him ascribe both the appearance and the texture of the bumps and groove, allowing him to both feel and sense the subtle differences in the epicondyle. In doing so, he creates a path to perception of the epicondyle pattern for Niha and Amar to recognise by shifting between model and radiograph, a performance that coordinates their sense of the epicondyle on the model with the epicondyle on the computer screen.

Although Vakul does not verbally state the epicondyle as having medial and lateral aspects, his figurative language and tacit engagement allows us to explicate this distinction in reference to the canon of anatomical literature. Importantly, and like in the examples above, a descriptive sense of normality is produced. It is only because the feature of the lateral epicondyle (on the model) is 'bumpy' that they are able to decipher that the ulna on the radiograph is not anatomically different, or abnormal. Indeed, Vakul encapsulates this point eloquently when he says: *'this is just how it is'*. It is by virtue of the 3D model and the gathering of this information that the radiography students come to recognise that the bone is *'basically normal'*. Through this process of handling-and-describing, Vakul uses the model to mediate the tacit knowledge of participants in a community of practice (Lave and Wenger 1991). Within this dialogue, Vakul's role in constructing Amar and Niha's knowledge about 'what's normal' can be likened to the student archaeologist in Goodwin (1994) and her ability to perceive differences in colour, consistency and texture in the dirt with the use of a representational resource. Not unlike the archaeologist's colour chart, the anatomical model is an essential instrument for seeing, interpreting and *feeling* the bone as normal and is itself a practice of coding (Goodwin 1994). In this way, the students are said to be embodying the properties of the anatomy in the radiograph as part of 'classification work' (Hirschauer 1991: 279).

Conclusion

This analysis of the sociomaterial assemblages of radiography education has explored how materials, visual practices, gesture and everyday discourse are concurrently asserted in the seeing, showing and perceiving of patterns in X-ray images. Through this process, students 'attune to what matters' (Fenwick 2014), where the insights afforded by a material approach to learning are portrayed as a route to sensory knowledge. Each vignette shows how a vision of pattern recognition is built; most notably by the three main material elements of the assemblage: the laser pointer, the computer screen and the 3D anatomical model. I show how the process of learning forms, shapes, configurations or 'patterns' in X-ray anatomy involves not simply a cognitive approach of mental memorisation but an assemblage of materials, gesture, visual practices and everyday discourse. Doing so acknowledges how learning pattern recognition cannot be solely understood in terms of the brain without taking into account the body and the sociocultural world that it experiences (Goodwin 1994).

An 'observational-embodied look' (Fountain 2019: 53) is expressed in the enduring emphasis on 3D anatomical models as full of potentially significant textures – cavities and surface markings – that only a material approach can reveal. Radiography students can follow how a flat 2D anatomical structure *'should be basically normal'*; visual and haptic evidence, garnered through hands-on action, allows the student to make sense of X-ray anatomy. This type of sensory knowledge is recognised as being a significant step in making sense of problems within anatomy and/or problems which may arise in the production of X-ray images, such as optical illusion, superimposition and size distortion/ magnification (Winter 2019). Nonetheless, the observational-embodied look occupies a sensory way of learning to see that makes observations and interrogations possible, a process that involves both 'looking at and feeling objects and then figuring out what one is actually seeing and touching' (Fountain 2010: 53). In this way, visual and material resources not only have the power to deliver anatomical knowledge regarding pattern recognition, but to manifest a shared perception of the image with a kinaesthetic and tactile experience. This observation contributes to our understanding of the sensorality and materiality of learning, particularly with regards to medical images.

Acknowledgements

The research conducted for this chapter was supported by a Ph.D. studentship in Sociology (STS pathway), funded by the Economic and Research Council (ESRC) (award: 149372004/1 awarded to Peter Winter) and sponsored by the University of Sheffield, UK. Special gratitude to the radiography professionals and students who kindly granted me access to video record their x-ray image interpretation classes.

References

Bloomer, Carolyn (1990), *Principles of Visual Perception*, 2nd ed., New York: Design Press.

Chen, W., HolcDorf, D., McCusker, Mark, Gaillard, F. and Howe, P. (2017), 'Perceptual training to improve hip fracture identification in conventional radiographs', *PLoS ONE*, 12:12, p. e0189192, https://doi.org/10.1371/journal.pone.0189192. Accessed 11 January 2022.

Clarke, Adele (2003), 'Situational analyses: Grounded theory mapping after the postmodern turn', *Symbolic Interaction*, 26: 4, pp. 553–76.

Corr, Peter (2011), *Pattern Recognition in Diagnostic Imaging*, Geneva: World Health Organization.

Crowley, Rebecca, Naus, Gregory, Stewart, Jimmie and Friedman, Charles (2003), 'Development of visual diagnostic visual expertise in pathology: An information processing-study', *Journal of the American Medical Informatics Association*, 10:1, pp. 39–51.

Custers, Eugene, Regehr, Glenn and Norman, Geoffrey (1996), 'Mental representations of medical diagnostic knowledge: A review', *Academic Medicine*, 71:10, pp. S55–S61.

Dussauge, Isabelle (2008), *Technomedical Visions: Magnetic Resonance Imaging in 1980s Sweden*, Stockholm: Division of History of Science and Technology Royal Institute of Technology, KTH, Stockholm papers in the History and Philosophy of Technology.

Engel, Peter (2008), 'Tacit knowledge and visual expertise in medical diagnostic reasoning: Implications for medical education', *Medical Teacher*, 30:7, pp. 184–88.

Eisen, Lewis, Berger, J., Hegde, Abhijith and Schneider, R. (2006), 'Competency in chest radiography. A comparison of medical students, residents, and fellows', *Journal of General Internal Medicine*, 21:5, pp. 460–65.

Fenwick, Tara (2014), Sociomateriality in medical practice and learning: Attuning to what matters, *Medical Education*, 48:1, pp. 44–52.

Fountain, Kenny, T. (2010), Anatomy education and the observational-embodied look, *Medicine Studies*, 2, pp. 49–69.

Fountain, Kenny, T. (2014), *Rhetoric in the Flesh: Trained Vision, Technical Expertise, and the Gross Anatomy Lab*, New York and London: Routledge.

Friedrich, Kathrin (2010), '"Sehkollectiv": Sight styles in diagnostic computed tomography', *Medicine Studies*, 2:3, pp. 185–95.

Friis, Jan Kyrre Berge (2017), 'Gestalt descriptions embodiments and medical image interpretation', *AI & Society*, 32, pp. 209–18.

Gegenfurtner, Andreas, Lehtinen, Erno, Helle, Laura, Nivala, Markus, Svedström, Erkki and Säljö, Roger (2019), 'Learning to see like an expert: On professional vision and visual practices', *International Journal of Educational Research*, 98, pp. 280–91.

Goodwin, Charles (1994), 'Professional vision', *American Anthropologist*, 96:3, pp. 606–33.

Hirschauer, Stefan (1991), 'The manufacture of bodies in surgery', *Social Studies of Science*, 21: 2, pp. 279–319.

Knoblauch, Hubert and Tuma, René (2011), 'Videography: An interpretive approach to video-recorded micro-social interaction', in E. Margolis and L. Pauwels (eds), *The SAGE Handbook of Visual Research Methods*. Los Angeles: SAGE, pp. 414–30.

Lave, Jean and Wenger, Etienne (1991), *Situated Learning: Legitimate Peripheral Participation*, Cambridge: Cambridge University Press.

Lesgold, Alan, Glaser, R., Rubinson, H., Klopfer, D., Feltovich, P. and Wang, Y. (1988), 'Expertise in a complex skill: Diagnosing x-ray pictures', in M. T. H. Chi, R. Glaser and M. Farr (eds), *The Nature of Expertise*, Hillsdale: Erlbaum, pp. 311–42.

Pandey, Priti and Zimitat, Craig (2006), 'Medical students' learning of anatomy: Memorisation, understanding, and visualisation', *Medical Education*, 41:1, pp. 7–14.

Pasveer, Bernike (1989), 'Knowledge of shadows: The introduction of X-ray images in medicine', *Sociology of Health and Illness*, 11:4, pp. 360–81.

Polanyi, Michael (1958), *Personal Knowledge: Toward a Post-critical Philosophy*, Chicago: University of Chicago Press.

Prasad, Amit (2005), 'Making images/making bodies: Visibilizing and disciplining through magnetic resonance imaging (MRI)', *Science, Technology, & Human Values*, 30:2, pp. 291–316.

Prentice, Rachel (2013), *Bodies in Formation: An Ethnography of Anatomy and Surgery Education*, Durham: Duke University Press.

Saunders, Barry (2008), *CT Suite: The Work of Diagnosis in the Age of Noninvasive Cutting*, London: Duke University Press.

Swinburne, K. (1971), 'Pattern recognition for radiographers', *The Lancet*, i, pp. 589–90.

Turney, Ben (2007), 'Anatomy in a modern medical curriculum', *Annals of the Royal College of Surgeons of England*, 89:2, pp. 104–07.

Van der Gijp, Anouk., Vincken, Koen, Boscardin, Christy, Webb, Emily, ten Cate, Olle and Naeger, David (2017), 'The effect of teaching search strategies on perceptual performance', *Academic Radiology*, 24:6, pp. 762–67.

Williams, Imelda, Baird, M. and Schneider, M. (2019), 'Improvement of radiographer commenting accuracy of the appendicular skeleton following a short course in plain radiography image interpretation: A pilot study', *Journal of Medical Imaging and Radiation Sciences*, 66, pp. 14–19.

Winter, Peter (2019), '"Bodies of Seeing": A video ethnography of academic X-ray image interpretation in undergraduate radiology and radiography education', Ph.D. thesis, Sheffield: University of Sheffield.

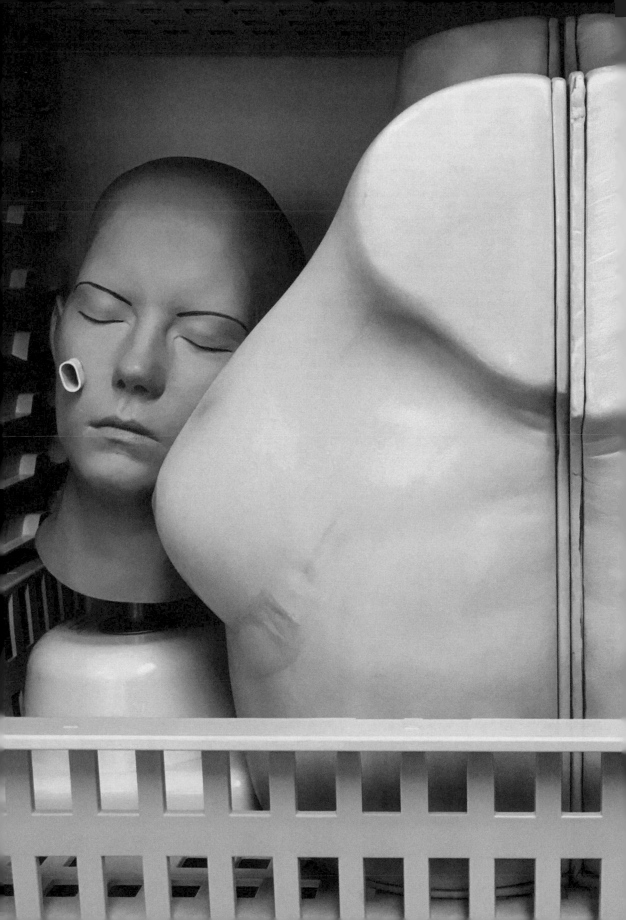

SIMULATION

SIMULATIONS IN HEALTH PROFESSIONS EDUCATION

Andrea Wojcik

As I write this essay, the word 'simulation' in combination with 'health professions education' may prompt associations with virtual reality – something like video games for surgeons (Johnson 2007; Prentice 2013). But if '*simulation imitates one process by another process*,' where 'the term "process" refers solely to some object or system whose state changes over time' (Hartmann 1996: 83, original emphasis), then even a cursory glance at medical education, past and present, reveals more than digital simulations. Historically, obstetric manikins have been made from leather, basketwork and human remains (Owen 2016); more contemporary uteri might be knitted or made from porcelain (Nott and Harris 2020); and healthy volunteers are often employed to act as patients (Guarrasi 2015; Taylor 2011; Underman 2015). Even the centuries-old practice of dissecting the dead may be understood as a simulation of the living body. Many of the authors in this collection are intrigued by similarly non-digital, often improvised, simulations in health professions education, and readers who follow the thread of simulation through this collection will gain insight into the persistence of non-digital simulations in twenty-first century classrooms.

The authors writing about simulations in this collection are acutely aware of a point Sherry Turkle (2009) emphasised in *Simulations and its Discontents* – simulations inevitably simplify reality. In other words, a simulation's fidelity, or its faithfulness to real-world happenings, is always partial. Turkle

Figure TE5: Manikins used to practice physical examination skills, in storage at Maastricht University's Skillslab. Image courtesy of Anna Harris.

reminded readers that partial fidelity can be dangerous, particularly when it is forgotten, but she also showed that partial fidelity can be simulation's strength. Some authors in this collection expand on the value of partial fidelity by demonstrating its pedagogical value. Christine Den Harder and Anna Harris (this volume), for instance, suggest that a semi-transparent balloon partially filled with water creates a 'sensory analogy' that helps students visualise, feel and hear fluid collecting in a patient's abdomen. Paul Craddock (this volume) similarly describes how a modest cigarette paper mimics the sensory experience of stitching vascular arteries. In both pieces, the objects used to simulate healthcare practices could not be mistaken for actual patients, and yet they help to facilitate changes in practitioners' perception, a shifting bodily awareness that some have argued is central to learning (see e.g. Ingold 2017). These subtle differences in perception are also notoriously difficult to verbalise. Taken together, Den Harder, Harris and Craddock (this volume) suggest that, in a time when health professions students most often spend their first years of study away from patients, in classrooms, lecture halls, laboratories and dissection theatres, the goal of simulation is not always to create a virtual reality of the clinic. Instead, medical educators can and do lean into simulations' inevitable simplification in order to tease clinical practices apart – to slow them down, enable repetition and make them tangible as well as visible.

The value of simplification does not necessarily explain the persistence of the non-digital. In fact, when Turkle (2009) wrote about the promises and dangers of simulations, she referred explicitly to the digital. The persistence of the non-digital, then, requires some additional consideration. To this end, some chapters in this collection both implicitly and explicitly speak to the concept of 'affordances', often credited to James Gibson (1986) but further developed by authors in various disciplines. One such author writing about medical education, Anneke van der Niet (2018), defined affordances as 'possibilities for *action*, which derive from our individual relationship to objects and other persons' (363). For instance, Rachel Vaden Allison (this volume) explains that the various sounds produced by an anatomy teacher drawing with chalk recalls different bodily textures encountered during dissection. In a way, drawing on a chalkboard offers a synaesthetic simulation of dissection precluded by more contemporary whiteboards and smartboards.

Where van der Niet (2018) suggested that medical education teachers play an important role in guiding students to notice differences, and thereby perceive new possibilities for action in the environment, Allison (this volume) and other contributors to this collection emphasise that it is not only teachers that guide students but also the materials used in simulations, for materials have possibilities as well as limitations (Rietveld and Kiverstein 2014). Kaisu Koski and Kristen Ostherr (this volume), for instance, demonstrate the indispensability of everyday objects when re-enacting patient interactions. Without doors, purses and tissues, the simulation, in which students learn to break bad news, fails. Peter Winter (this volume) writes about learning to interpret digital X-rays, reminding readers that even when the digital is present, human bodies and models often help translate a three-dimensional body into a two-dimensional image. In Denielle Elliott with Dominic Halls's chapter (this volume), the authors also show how patient histories, the famous neurological case of Phineas Gage in this instance, can also be materialised, such as a three-dimensional printed skull. In other words, the digital is informed by the material, tangible world (see also Myers 2015). When read alongside each other, these contributions can be interpreted as a (re)discovery of the complexity of the non-digital and as a plea for medical educators and curriculum designers to carefully consider material affordances.

If some of the pieces touching on simulation in this collection can be read as a reminder for health professions education programmes to value the non-digital, others provide reminders that the non-digital is also sometimes problematic. Andrea Wojcik et al. (this volume) question which skills a rather gruesome looking silicone wound allows medical students to demonstrate in formal assessments and conclude that a shammy cloth stapled over sponge might sometimes provide a more suitable simulation. In her account of the material assemblages required in the performance of a simulated patient, Ivana Guarrasi's chapter (this volume) shows the complexity involved in simulating a pathological 'heart' in the body of a healthy actor. Rachel Prentice's contribution (this volume) is a reminder that the non-digital can also be complicit in confusing the simulated for the real. Like John Nott and Anna Harris (2020), Prentice raises questions about the undesirable legacies of simulations that continue to 'stick' to contemporary education programmes. In considering dissection as an exercise in understanding the living body, she argues that the (historical) prominence of the cadaver in medicine and medical education has shaped biomedical knowledge, including approaches to healthcare provision and treatment. In other words, approximating the living body via the cadaver has shaped the reality of contemporary medical practice, possibly for the worse.

Taken as a whole, authors writing about or around simulation in this collection offer a cautiously enthusiastic endorsement of non-digital simulations in health professions education. They point to the unacknowledged potential of commonplace materials, which has important implications for health professions education programmes. For one, it shows that simple, affordable materials can legitimately facilitate learning, potentially allowing programmes to opt out of acquiring the newest and most expensive simulation technology. It also invites teachers and curriculum designers to imagine other possible simulations that might address the shortcomings of inherited simulation practices as well as prompting a return to older collaborations between medicine and art. As Erik Rietveld and Julian Kiverstein (2014) suggested, and as Roger Kneebone and Fleur Oakes (this volume) demonstrate, with the introduction of embroidery in surgical education, finding new potentials in materials may require turning to people with different skills and expertise. This potential, however, does not mean that creating effective simulations with everyday objects is an easy task, or without cost. While some options may not demand much capital, they might instead rely on invisible forms of labour (Wyatt, this volume). Someone would have to take the time to carefully assess a classroom's material environment and experiment with making analogies to the human body. For all the enthusiasm for the possibilities of non-digital simulation in this volume, contributors also remind us that a critical eye always remains necessary.

References

Gibson, James J. (1986), *The Ecological Approach to Visual Perception*, Hillsdale: Lawrence Erlbaum Associates.

Guarrasi, Ivana (2015), 'Residual categories in medical simulation: The role of affect in the performance of disease', *Mind, Culture, and Activity*, 22:2, pp. 112–28.

Hartmann, Stephan (1996), 'The world as a process: Simulations in the natural and social sciences', in R. Hegselmann, U. Müller and K. G. Troitzsch (eds.), *Modelling and Simulation in the Social Sciences from the Philosophy of Science Point of View*, Dordrecht: Kluwer, pp. 77–100.

Ingold, Tim (2017), *Anthropology and/as Education*, Abingdon: Routledge.

Johnson, Ericka (2007), 'Surgical simulators and simulated surgeons: Reconstituting medical practice and practitioners in simulations', *Social Studies of Science*, 37:4, pp. 585–608.

Myers, Natasha (2015), *Rendering Life Molecular: Models, Modelers, and Excitable Matter*, Durham: Duke University Press.

Nott, John and Harris, Anna (2020), 'Sticky models: History as friction in obstetric education', *Medicine Anthropology Theory*, 7:1, pp. 44–65.

Owen, Harry (2016), *Simulation in Healthcare Education: An Extensive History*, Cham: Springer.

Prentice, Rachel (2013), *Bodies in Formation: An Ethnography of Anatomy and Surgery Education*, Durham: Duke University Press.

Rietveld, Erik and Kiverstein, Julian (2014), 'A rich landscape of affordances', *Ecological Psychology*, 26:4, pp. 325–52.

Taylor, Janelle S. (2011), 'The moral aesthetics of simulated suffering in standardized patient performances', *Culture, Medicine, Psychiatry*, 35:2, pp. 134–62.

Turkle, Sherry (2009), *Simulation and Its Discontents*, Cambridge: MIT press.

Underman, Kelly (2015), 'Playing doctor: Simulation in medical school as affective practice', *Social Science Medicine*, 136–37, pp. 180–88.

Van der Niet, Anneke G. (2018), 'When I say… affordance perception', *Medical Education*, 52:4, pp. 362–63.

SKULLS

MEDICAL MUSEUMS, MATERIALITY AND THE TRAUMATIC BRAIN INJURY OF PHINEAS GAGE

Denielle Elliott with Dominic Hall

On 13 September 1848, a young man, Phineas Gage, was working on the railroad in Cavendish, Vermont (USA) tamping an explosive charge for blasting when the charge prematurely detonated, sending his tamping iron (3 cm in diameter and 1 m long) through his neurocranium, before landing about 20–25 m away. Gage was assisted by other workers who carried him to the road where he was placed on an ox cart and then taken to town. There, he stood up on his own and walked into the Inn, where he waited to see the doctor (MacMillan 2002; Bigelow 1850). This accident, and his rather astonishing recovery (Gage survived, though died twelve years later from epileptic seizures that were most likely related to the injury), shaped understandings of the brain and influenced theories of brain function and structure in neurology. Gage remains one of the most important clinical cases shaping the history of medical education in neurology and psychology. His wound and recovery shaped how neurologists and psychologists understand the impact of brain injury in terms of personality, memory, inhibition, frontal lobe behavior and sense of self. His injury, but especially his survival from the brain trauma, became an exemplar that also shaped the history and development of brain surgery in the late 1800s (MacMillan 2002). His case is still discussed in contemporary neurological education textbooks and taught in anatomy and psychology classes (for instance, see Stuss and Knight 2013; Zauld and Rauch 2006, among many others).

Gage's skull and the tamping iron that passed through it are on display at the Warren Anatomical Museum in Boston, MA, as part of the Center for the History of Medicine at Harvard Medical School, and under the protection of curator Dominic Hall (see Figure 22.1). This chapter reflects on the use and meaning of Gage's medical case, his skull and the tamping iron in medicine broadly. I am particularly interested in the material power of Gage in his death, a power that comes alive through a curated collection of objects held at the museum including his skull, a life cast, photographs, scans and a 3D model. Here I consider a few questions. What scientific and medical work is being done by Gage's remains? Who visits the exhibit? How is his skull and new models taken up in contemporary medical education? This chapter draws on archival medical journal papers, a conversation with the Warren Anatomical Museum curator Dominic Hall and a virtual visit to the museum's holdings in order to consider these questions. This chapter was proposed, researched and written by its first author (Elliott), but acknowledges the contribution of Dominic Hall, using 'with' (rather than 'and') to signal the collaborative nature of its production.

Though only his skull and the iron have been preserved, the intense interest that they have drawn over the years emerges from what they (might) tell us about the brain. The desire to preserve the skull, in other words, is not as part of archaeological or osteological collections that help us understand the biological differences in evolution, nor a study in physiognomy, nor the historical study of anthropometry, but arises from the recovery of Gage and reported long term effects that he experienced as a result of the brain injury. And thus, I situate my understanding of this particular collection as a question about the curation of brains and brain specimens particularly in medical museums (see Kwint and Wingate 2013; Coleborne and MacKinnon 2017; Gere 2013; Alberti 2011), in addition to the larger questions being explored in this volume about the material objects of medical education.

Gage's story is often told as an exceptional example of what the brain can sustain and recover from. In other words, its plasticity, the way in which neuronal pathways are rerouted and regenerated, with minimal impact on cognition, executive function and working memory. But it is also the story of discovery within medicine: a mid to late nineteenth century example of how medical professionals came to understand cellular recovery, the consequences of traumatic brain injury on cognition, personality and mobility, and theories of localised function within the brain.

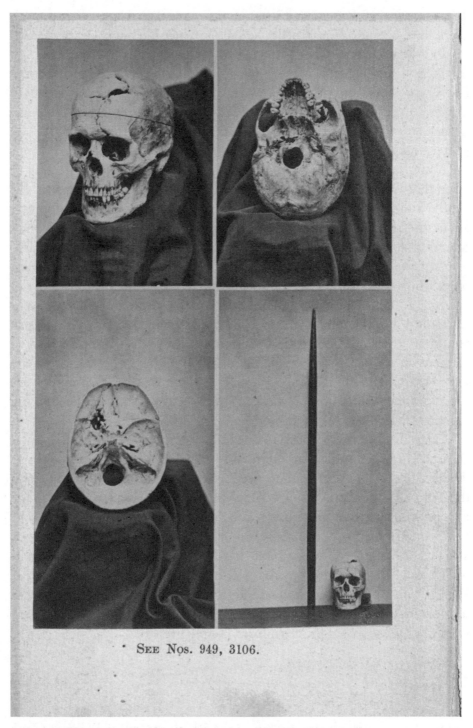

SEE NOS. 949, 3106.

Figure 22.1: Gage's skull and tamping iron. Courtesy of Warren Anatomical Museum, Center for the History of Medicine in the Francis A. Countway Library of Medicine.

There are few, if any, cases written about more than Gage, even though there have been dozens of other equally remarkable brain injury cases.

In an edited book about the 'matter' of medical education, what are the ethical implications of focusing on human remains? Can we redefine Gage's skull and his case, away from its role as material artefact (in death) to think about its liveliness as matter, as an extension of Gage, with a force to still shape biomedical knowledge? Shaped in part by post-humanist and feminist materialist approaches to objects and things including Jane Bennett (2010) and Karen Barad (2003), I write this in hope that we might exercise a more caring encounter with Gage in his death. Such recent feminist materialisms force us to think differently about the relationality of these objects, that is the way in which such matter shapes relations, knowledge and affect. This approach demands we think about his skull *relationally* rather than as a curious anatomical object. In Barad's view, matter is 'not a thing, but a doing, a congealing of agency' (2003: 822). She expands, 'matter refers to the materiality/materialization of phenomena' (Barad 2003: 822). Such an approach helps us reanimate the skull from a fixed museum exhibit or scientific artefact to Gage as an important actor who has shaped the history of neuro-scientific research and clinical encounters. In a sense then, this gives him life again as we consider how his skull is entangled with knowledge-making practices in neurology and related fields.

Gage has become almost a caricature within medicine and popular culture. There are endless accounts of him, video re-enactments, animations, high school videos online, even a Lego animation of his injury on the railroad. Even in Malcolm MacMillan's exhaustive accounts, Gage is portrayed as a case or a puzzle to be solved, rather than the life story of a worker and his occupational injury. There is a sense that Gage as a man has been forgotten, a man that clearly struggled after the event with a long-term brain injury that left him changed, for better or worse. While it may be an occupational tactic within medicine to focus on the immediate injury and interventions, rather than the whole patient, here I consider what we might learn from Gage's life story.

Phineas Gage

Many readers may already be familiar with the story of Phineas Gage but as a reminder, I will quickly summarise what has been established about Gage. Little is known with any certainty, but a number of scholars have attempted to piece together information so we might have a more complete understanding of Gage before and after his accident. Most notable is the work of Malcolm MacMillan who continues to solicit information via a website, asking people to contact him if they might have any additional information on Gage or his family members (MacMillan 2000, 2002). I rely largely on MacMillan here who has constructed the most accurate image of Gage's life even as he writes, 'Next to nothing is known about his birth, his education, his personality characteristics, and his working life before and after the accident that thrust him into fame' (2002: 369). Unfortunately, we never hear from Gage himself; there are no diaries, or letters written by him, except for a note written to the museum when he requested that they return the iron bar he had donated. All information about the medical case is read through descriptions and accounts about him and the accident or conjecture based on other sources. A sense of what Gage was like is drawn solely from the records of the doctors who saw Gage after the accident – Edward Williams, the first doctor to see Gage, John Harlow, who arrived an hour after, and Henry Bigelow, a surgeon who became interested in the case after reading about it. Combined, their papers, testimonies and records provide the basis for most inferences made about Gage as a person (who he was before the injury), the brain injury, and the effects of the injury on Gage as he healed, in particular papers written by Harlow (1848 and 1868) and Bigelow in 1850 (these have been reprinted by MacMillan in his monograph), both of which are held at the Warren Anatomical Museum.

According to MacMillan (2002), Gage was an eighth-generation American, a descendant of kin from County Suffolk who immigrated to Salem in 1630. The Gage family lived in Massachusetts for the first three generations, and then moved to New Hampshire in 1772. Phineas was the oldest of five children, probably born 9 July 1823, may be in Lebanon, New Hampshire. There is little information on his schooling, family life or even where he actually lived, but MacMillan suggests he attended high school and worked the farm of his grandfather in Grafton, a town nearby. How he came to be working on the railroad is also a mystery. As MacMillan reminds his readers, Gage was not employed by the Rutland and Burlington Railroad company but by a local outfit contracted to prepare the ground for the laying of the steel tracks, near Cavendish in Vermont.

Harlow and Williams, the first attending doctor, seem to have known Gage a little, but any reflections on his character and personality would have been based on relatively infrequent or brief encounters in Cavendish prior to the accident. Williams recounts that as he first arrived at the Cavendish Inn, Gage said, 'Doctor, here is business enough for you' (Bigelow 1950: 16). And Harlow reported, 'he recognized me at once, and said he hoped he was not much hurt' (1848: 390), which suggests that they were at least acquainted. According to Harlow's first paper published about Gage on 13 December 1848, Gage was 'a foreman, engaged in building the road, 25 years of age, of middle stature, vigorous physical organization, temperate habits, and possessed of considerable character' (1848: 20). Harlow's knowledge of Gage prior to the accident is important to this story because it has implications for how the brain injury comes to be understood by neurologists (as a baseline that is used for comparison postinjury).

As mentioned, Gage was preparing a hole for blasting when he tamped the powder, it exploded suddenly and forcefully shot the 13.5 lb tamping iron through the zygomatic and maxilla bones, exiting out of his frontal bone. Harlow explained,

> I am informed that the patient was thrown upon his back, and gave a few convulsive motions of the extremities, but spoke in a few minutes. His men (with whom he was a great favorite) took him in their arms and carried him to the road, only a few rods distant, and sat him into an ox cart, in the road, sitting erect, full three quarters of a mile, to the hotel of Mr. Joseph Adams, in this village. He got out of the cart himself, and with a little assistance walked up a long flight of stairs, into the hall, where he was dressed. (1848: 389–90)

Harlow admits how gruesome he found the sight was, how unprepared he was for such a case and apologises for omitting a lot of detail from his notes. What I am interested in here for the purpose of this chapter is how the attending doctors perceived and characterised Gage. During the examination of Gage, Williams reported that Gage 'was relating the manner in which he was injured to the bystanders; he talked so rationally and was so willing to answer questions, that I directed my questions to him' (Bigelow 1850: 16). And Harlow stated, 'the patient bore his sufferings with the most heroic firmness' (1868: 390). Later in the evening, Harlow notes that Gage 'does not wish to see his friends, as he shall be at work in a day or two. Tells me where they live, their names, etc.' (1868: 391). Gage comes across as gracious, kind, and stoic. It is not until the 22nd of September that we see Gage is scared and feeling unwell (when it seems he has developed an infection). Harlow reports that Gage says that 'he shall not live long so' (Harlow 1868: 391). Henry Bigelow was the surgeon who became involved in the case a few days after, hearing an account of it from another colleague. Bigelow's (1850) paper offers more description of the event and Gage himself, referring to him as 'shrewd and intelligent' (1850: 14). He repeats this sentiment in a letter sent to Dr Jewett written the 12 May 1868 (one of the holdings at the Warren Anatomical Museum). We also hear from the three doctors that Gage was liked by his colleagues and considered a reliable worker.

He stays in the Inn and recovers eventually, something which seems miraculous in part because of the injury but more so because of the crude medical interventions that were used to help heal him – castor oil, 'a cathartic of calomel and rhubarb,' and nitrate of silver. Gage's ability to recover is a testament to his strength and perseverance, and the ability of the brain to recover even with extreme trauma. But most of the descriptions around Gage are about how horrific his injury is, how unbelievable the story of recovery is, and about the miracles of medicine. Perhaps understandably for the time the injury becomes sensationalised. His medical case becomes a matter of interest for its shock value and thus as time passes, Gage the patient becomes less important to the story. Bigelow writes, 'this is the sort of accident that happens in the pantomime at the theatre, but not elsewhere' (Bigelow 1850: 19).

After Gage departs from the Inn on 25 November 1848, little is known about what he does, where he goes, or how he is feeling. Mac-Millan (2002) surmises that he spent 1849 at his parents' home recovering, then traveling to Boston in November to be examined by Bigelow, who presented Gage to 'the Boston Society for Medical Improvement, and also to the medical class at the hospital' at Harvard, at which time he states that Gage is 'now perfectly healed' (2002: 20). During this visit, Bigelow creates the cast of Gage's head that remains today in the museum collection. In April 1849, he returns to see Harlow who reports that 'his physical health is good, and I am inclined to say that he has recovered. He has no pain in head, but says it has *a queer feeling which he is not able to describe*' (1868: 339, emphasis added). He writes that Gage has reapplied to this position of Foreman with the contract company 'but is undecided whether to work or travel' (Bigelow 1868: 339).

Though MacMillan is clearly intent on trying to correct the errors in our understanding of Gage and his injury, much of what has been fictionalised, distorted, and simply made up, he too relies on conjecture to some degree. MacMillan writes, 'Phineas recovered physically, surviving for eleven and a half years, but was so changed psychologically that he never worked at the level of a foreman again' (2000: 47). Yet, we do not actually know why Gage did not return to work as a foreman. Perhaps it was the physical scarring, perhaps it was a near death experience, perhaps it was a fear of another explosion. We really do not know how 'changed psychologically' he was (2000: 47). In 1849, when Harlow sees Gage again, he writes about what he perceives as a dramatic shift in Gage's personality.

> Previous to his injury, though untrained in the schools, he possessed a well-balanced mind, and was looked upon by those who knew him as a shrewd, smart business man, very energetic and persistent in executing all his plans of operation. In this regard his mind was radically changed, so decidedly that his friends and acquaintances said he was 'no longer Gage.' (Harlow 1868: 415)

Harlow or Bigelow does not mention if Gage reported feeling changed or if he was aware of changes in his personality, and, if so, if he understood them as a result of tissue damage in his brain, a life-changing event, or the physical scarring – aside from his report of a 'queer feeling' that he cannot explain. Yet, one of the key reasons that Gage's skull and the tamping iron are held in a medical anatomy museum and the reason his case is mentioned in countless psychology, anatomy and neurology textbooks is because it is believed his personality changes as a result of the brain injury. This has led credit to the theory of functional localisation in neurology which ascribes particular areas of the brain to particular functions (for instance, the frontal lobe is associated with personality, speech and language with Broca's area, and so on). But given the lack of account from Gage, missing medical records and limited reportage, a significant degree of uncertainty exists.

Harlow reports that Gage started to travel regionally (Boston and New York) and there is evidence to suggest that he then travelled to South America. One source reported that 'after his recovery he travelled about with his bar, and exhibited himself in several of the large cities in this country' (Jackson 1870: 147), and another suggests he joined

Barnum's American Museum in New York for a while. In 1851, he took work in a livery stable and then, in 1852, he left the east coast of the USA and went to Chile, 'to establish a line of coaches in Valparaiso' (1868: 340), where he stayed for approximately eight years driving horse-drawn coaches. He apparently was not well in Chile and thus returned to San Francisco where his mother, Hannah Trussell Swetland Gage, and sister were living. Harlow corresponded with Gage's mother who reported he returned from Chile ill, suffering from epileptic seizures (MacMillan 2002). Seizures are a common condition for those who have suffered traumatic brain injuries and it is not atypical that the onset of seizures occurs many years after the initial injury. According to Harlow (as he learned from a letter from Gage's mother), Gage had a serious seizure (probably a grand mal) on 20 May and died the next day on 21 May 1860. He was buried in San Francisco.

There was no autopsy when Gage died. His body was exhumed, probably late in 1867, with consent from his family and his skull given to Harlow in early 1868. The bar was donated first in 1850 by Gage who then later requested the iron be returned to him (the handwritten note by Gage is in the museum's collection). Harlow retrieved it the same time he retrieved the skull and donated it to the museum for a second time. The Warren Anatomical Museum reimbursed Harlow some of the expenses of exhuming Gage, suggesting a somewhat more complex relationship between the university, Harlow and the family. Of course, by the time it has been exhumed the brain tissue had completely decomposed and so all conclusions about any brain damage caused from the injury rely on the publications, letters, the skull and, more recently, new digital reproductions. The medical records are dated, medical knowledge was relatively limited at that time, and technological limitations of existing technology for creating and recording images or preserving biological samples mean that the historical evidence is partial at best.

Though there have been many similar dramatic, accidental brain injuries since the mid 1800s, Gage remains one of the most well-known and publicised cases, if only as a curiosity for many. It is beyond the scope of this brief chapter, but MacMillan and many others have highlighted how Gage shaped understandings of frontal lobe damage, emotions, semantic memory, disinhibited behavior and impulsivity, along with shaped how neuroscientists thought about the theory of functional localisation (Shelley 2016; MacMillan 2002, 2004; Damasio 2000). Gage and his injury have been central to medical education since shortly after his injury. MacMillan (2008) recounts that in 1849, a year after the injury, Gage travelled to Boston where he met with medical students at Harvard University with surgeon Henry Bigelow. Gage's standing in the collection of the Warren Anatomical Museum has ensured that his pedagogic role continued long after his death.

Warren Anatomical Museum

He who attempts to teach anatomy without a museum strictly deserves the name of imposter. (Frederick J. Knox cited in Alberti 2011: 56)

Museums have been critical in the historical teaching of medicine and anatomy. The Warren Anatomical Museum was just one of thousands operating in the late nineteenth century, often attached to medical schools. Human organs, pathology specimens, other anatomical remains, and medical and surgical instruments and artefacts, memorabilia, alongside of images and texts were essential to the way in which medicine was taught and practiced beginning in the sixteenth century until the mid to late 1900s. As many have noted, there has since been a decline in medical museums due to a move towards new technological pedagogical practices, issues of space allocation on campuses and expenses associated with maintaining the collections and keeping them relevant to contemporary medicine (Marreez et al. 2010; Wakefield 2007). Medical and anatomical museums have faced funding shortages, declining visitor numbers and challenges acquiring new materials. Museums have also struggled to embrace new pedagogical practices in medical education (Wakefield 2007; Marreez et al. 2010). Many museums have been closed, but others, like the Warren Anatomical Museum, are being redesigned and their role in medical education revisited (Marreez et al. 2010).

The Warren Anatomical Museum is the home of the Gage exhibit, which includes a collection of materials: the skull, the tamping iron, the life cast, photographs of Gage, written materials and reproductions of the scans (see Figures 22.2–22.4). At the Warren Anatomical Museum, Dominic Hall reported that Gage remains the main attraction, drawing medical students, student groups (from middle school until postgraduate), graduate students in anatomy, psychology and the neurosciences, as well as the scientifically curious public. The museum is part of the admissions tour offered by the medical school at Harvard University.

The gallery that exhibited Gage was in the Library, and the tours would stop in the gallery specifically to see Gage. In 2020, the Museum's collections are closed as it undergoes a major renovation, opening again in the fall 2022. I had the chance to talk with Hall about the Gage exhibit and what he knew about Gage. One of the things that most struck me during our conversation was that Hall referred to him by his first name – as *Phinaes* – like a friend. I sensed that Hall had a sort of affective attachment for Gage and that he feels a deep ethical responsibility in caring for the Gage collection, but also in how Gage's story is shared with the world and used in medical education today. He spoke to me about concerns regarding consent, the reproduction of Gage's skull through new 3D printing machines, and how Gage's case is taken up in medical and anatomy education at Harvard.

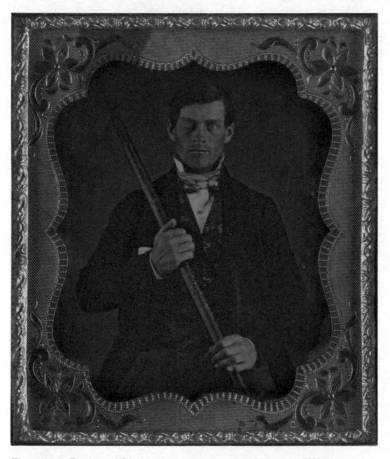

Figure 22.2: Portrait of Gage with his tamping iron. Courtsey of Warren Anatomical Museum, Center for the History of Medicine in the Francis A. Countway Library of Medicine; Gift of Jack and Beverly Wilgus.

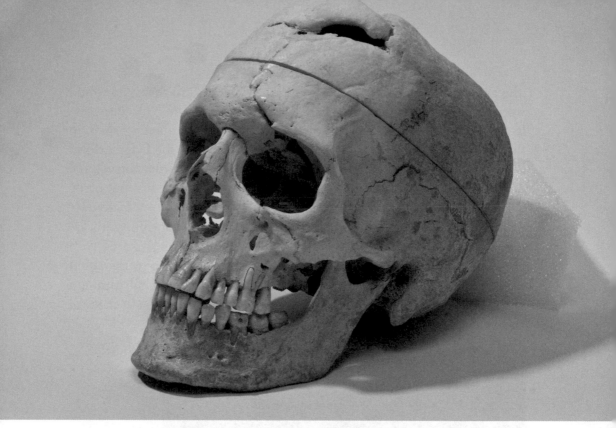

Figure 22.3: Gage's skull. Courtesy of Warren Anatomical Museum, Center for the History of Medicine in the Francis A. Countway Library of Medicine.

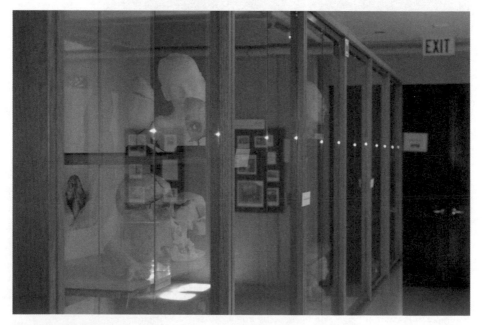

Figure 22.4: Warren Museum exhibit. Courtesy of Warren Anatomical Museum, Center for the History of Medicine in the Francis A. Countway Library of Medicine.

As Hall explained, one of the areas of concern with displaying the skull of Gage is the ethics of displaying human remains in contemporary museums, even for medical or educational purposes (Lohman and Goodnow 2006). Such issues have been particularly dominant among archaeologists and medical museums with holdings collected under colonial initiatives (Daehnke and Lonetree 2016; DeBlock 2019; Jenkins 2008), where human remains were stolen or removed without consent. There have now been a number of high-profile cases where human remains have been restituted to homelands. Saartjie Baartman's remains, for instance, which had been held in Paris at the National Museum of Natural History, were returned to South Africa (Daley 2002). In 1990, the Native American Graves Protection and Repatriation Act (NAGPRA) outlined policies and directions for human remains to be returned to Native American and Alaskan Native communities when requested (Ousley et al. 2005; Kakaliouras 2012). The holding of Gage's skull in some ways resembles osteo-archaeological collections of skeletal remains that are held in museums around the world. The use of human remains in medical education is a contested field and not everyone agrees that human remains still have a place in medical education (Champney et al. 2019; Coman et al. 2019). In Gage's case, his mother agreed to donate his skull and iron to the Warren Anatomical Museum. We have no evidence that Gage agreed to this donation in advance of his death but, as Hall noted, Gage did seem to participate in the performative display of himself while alive so perhaps he would have been pleased to know there was a large influential exhibit about him.

The 2000–20 exhibit – with Gage's skull, the cast and the iron – was rather uninspiring. Like many older anatomy museums, the iron, skull and cast were set on shelves behind a glass casing. Some of these curatorial decisions are limited by concerns about preservation (for instance, breakage, temperature and humidity control). Plans for the new exhibit are still underway but Hall suggests something more interactive and dynamic, including audio-recordings and other multimedia. New digital technologies have resulted in exhibits that are more interactive, using digitally remastered videos (Ratiu and Talos 2004), CT scans (Van Horn et al. 2012), virtual models (Thiebaut de Schotten et al. 2015) and rapid prototyping technology (Kelley et al. 2007), and even offer medical students a chance to handle a near identical replicate of Gage's skull (see Figures 22.5 and 22.6). Gage has had a rather nominal role in the formal medical or anatomical curricula at Harvard University (and other regional medical education centres), which makes sense given the limits around student interaction with the skull. New technologies are changing the possibilities for student engagement with the material remains of Gage and more broadly with him as patient.

Three-dimensional visual models of the brain

The story of Phineas Gage continues to stir interest across fields of medicine and researchers are now using new digital technologies to offer new interpretations of the injury. In 2004, Peter Ratiu and Ion-Florin Talos, borrowing the skull from the museum, created a visual using computed tomographic imaging of the skull and generated a three-dimensional visual model of a brain in order to ascertain with more certainty the angle of the iron rod, the damage to the skull and the possible extent of the brain injury (see Figure 22.5). They concluded, 'the brain injury must have been limited to the left frontal lobe and spared the superior sagittal sinus' (Ratiu and Talos 2004: 21). These computer imaging techniques have developed a model brain to sit within the reconstruction of the skull so that they can imagine what actual brain injury *may* have resulted from the iron bar (Thiebaut de Schotten et al. 2015). Such digital reconstructions based on the CT images of the skull allow us to see the entry and exit point of the tamping iron and neurologists can *surmise* the damage it might have caused to his brain but the one thing neuroscientists always agree on is how little we know or understand about the brain. Gage's case became a model for understanding localisation theory and the orthodox sensory-motor frameworks in medicine and these new computer-mediated technologies help undo some of the misunderstandings.

A limitation of visual models, and with a skull preserved behind glass, is that the possibility for multisensorial learning is impeded, they can't touch or feel the bone. As others have well documented, students of anatomy have relied on sensory education since medicine began (Fountain 2010; Richardson 2000; Harris 2020). Such embodied learning, through cadavers, 'living models' (Fountain 2010), or knitted uteruses (Nott and Harris 2020) has been critical to pedagogical practice for how students learn to use their own bodies as part of their practice (through their hands, sense of touch and sight). Concerns about preserving Gage's skull has meant that students have been unable to hold the skull, to run their fingers across the healed fractures, to feel the weight of his injury in their hands. But innovations in rapid prototyping has changed that.

In 2019, Dominic Hall collaborated with colleagues at Harvard Medical School's anatomy programme to create a three-dimensionally printed model for first-year medical students studying general head and neck anatomy, so that students could hold a replica of Gage in their hands as they studied facial musculature, optics nerves and bone structure (see Figure 22.6). This has meant that Gage has been formally re-introduced to the anatomy curricula at Harvard, a shift made possible by new computer technologies. Feeling, touching, tracing Gage's skull allows for a more haptic interface with bone anatomy and for learning that is important for how students learn to use their own bodies in medicine (Prentice 2005; Fountain 2010). These new 3D models could be considered a variation of what Rachel Prentice has called 'body objects', which act as 'teaching tools, diagrams, and models' (2005: 847). Though Prentice's body objects 'inhabit computers', these 3D print products are only born of computers. They are similarly 'hybrid objects' as both 'medical and computational or engineered objects' (Prentice 2005: 847).

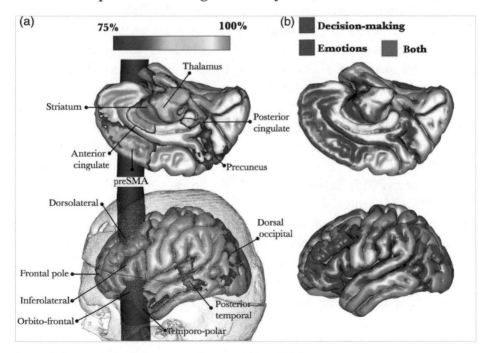

Figure 22.5: Gage's affected brain areas (Ratiu and Talos 2004).

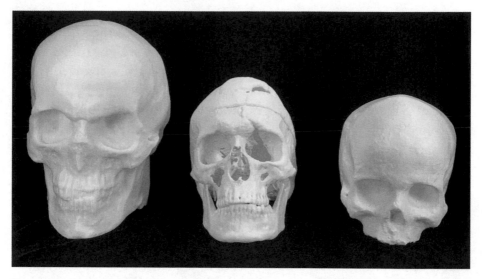

Figure 22.6: Gage's skull (middle), created with a 3D printer, alongside other 3D-printed skulls from the Warren Anatomical Museum Collection.

Rapid prototyping refers to a range of new technologies, including 3D printing, which use CT and MRI scans (DICOM data, or digital imaging and communications in medicine), computer-aided design and printing machines that generate 3D models. The 3D models are produced through a layering method – for instance, a powder-based material (plastic, metal, ceramic or glass), fused layer by layer with a type of liquid adhesive (Baskaran et al. 2016). These models are considered very accurate replicates of both pathological and normal anatomy forms (though accuracy largely depends on the quality of the technology). Many see the value in three-dimensionally printed anatomical models for medicine, and this includes their use in neurosurgeries like cranioplasty and craniofacial repair (Vaccarezza and Papa 2015; Kelley et al. 2007; Abou-Hashem et al. 2015; Baskaran et al. 2016). Studies comparing 2D images and 3D models among students suggest that they offer more accuracy in terms of visual assessment even though the 3D models are created using 2D images (CT scans) (Kelley et al. 2007), they bypass many problems presented in surgical training of medical students (Baskaran et al. 2016), including a lack of cadavers for medical training (Lim et al. 2016), and ethical concerns of using human remains mentioned previously.

Conclusion

As a reconstructed model, it remains to be seen if 3D printer models help students understand Gage or the extent of his injuries. Curators like Dominic Hall are morally committed to ensure the skull of Gage, in its original form and as 3D replicate, is not taken up as some strange anatomy artefact, but as part of a larger, more complex story that emphasises the patient as a whole (Centor 2007). Or, in other words, he helps us recognise that Gage's skull is not simply an object, but a relational material configuration, a part of Gage as he, even in his death, shapes scientific understandings of the body, medical practice and approaches to care (Barad 2007). There is much to learn from Gage but I am doubtful that his case helps us understand how the brain functions, except to emphasise its wonderous capacity to heal.

A neurologist once explained to me, 'the only thing all neurologists know for certain is that we know very little of the brain. We cannot understand, for instance, why a big tough hockey player may sustain a mild concussion but never be able to work again, and yet a young woman with a severe traumatic brain injury is able to return to work six weeks later. There is so much that we do not know'. This comment highlights how in many ways, and no matter how advanced the technology is, neuroscientists must guess what impact the injury had on Gage. With so little reliable data and no first-hand accounts from Gage himself, what role does Gage have in medical education? Given contemporary critiques of localisation theory (Uttal 2002; Elliott 2019), and how little was really known about the changes Gage experienced after the injury, Gage's role in medical education needs to be reassessed.

Yet, Gage's story and his collection at the Warren Anatomical Museum are valued for their material power, a power that comes alive through the curated collection of objects held at the museum. While Gage's skull may not be the key to furthering neurological insight, due to the uncertainties and gaps in knowledge, Dominic Hall's curatorial labour focusing on Gage as worker, patient and sentient being lends credence to the view that medical museums have a role to play in contemporary medical education. It is Gage's *story*, the relations of the skull, of his miraculous survival of the injury and the treatments, that further our insight into how individuals survive in seemingly impossible conditions, as well as highlighting how important detailed medical records are.

References

AbouHashem, Yousef, Dayal, Manisha, Savanah, Stephane and Štrkalj, Goran (2015), 'The application of 3D printing in anatomy education', *Medical Education Online*, 20:1, p. 29847, https://doi.org/10.3402/meo.v20.29847. Accessed 11 January 2022.

Alberti, Sam (2011), 'Medical museums past, present and future', *Annals of the Royal College of Surgeons of England*, 93, pp. 56–58.

Barad, Karen (2003), 'Posthumanist performativity: Toward an understanding of how matter comes to matter', *Signs: Journal of Women in Culture and Society*, 28:3, pp. 801–31.

Baskaran, Vivek, Štrkalj, Goran, Štrkalj, Mirjana and Di Ieva, Antonio (2016), 'Current applications and future perspectives of the use of 3D printing in anatomical training and neurosurgery', *Frontiers in Neuroanatomy*, 10, p. 69.

Bennett, Jane (2010), *Vibrant Matter: A Political Ecology of Things*, Durham: Duke University Press.

Bigelow, Henry J. (1850), 'ART. I.--Dr. Harlow's case of recovery from the passage of an iron bar through the head', *The American Journal of the Medical Sciences*, 20:39, p. 10.

Centor, Robert M. (2007), 'To be a great physician, you must understand the whole story', *Medscape General Medicine*, 9:1, p. 59.

Champney, Thomas H., Hildebrandt, Sabine, Jones D. Gareth and Winkelmann, Andreas (2019), 'Bodies R US: Ethical views on the commercialization of the dead in medical education and research', *Anatomical Sciences Education* 12:3, pp. 317–25.

Coman, Jonathan, Kelly, Anne-Maree, Savulescu, Julian and Craig, Simon (2019), 'Skeletons in the closet: Towards the dignified disposal of all human bones acquired for medical education', *The BMJ*, 367: l6705, https://doi.org/10.1136/bmj.l6705. Accessed 18 May 2022.

Daehnke, Jon, and Amy Lonetree (2016), 'Repatriation in the United States: The current state of NAGPRA', *Handbook of Postcolonial Archaeology*, 3, p. 245.

Daley, Suzanne (2002), 'Exploited in life and death, South African to go home', *The New York Times*, 30 January, Section A, p. 4.

Damasio, Antonio R. (2000), 'A neural basis for sociopathy', *Archives of General Psychiatry*, 57:2, pp. 128–29.

DeBlock, Hugo (2019), 'The Africa Museum of Tervuren, Belgium: The reopening of 'the last colonial museum in the world': Issues on decolonization and repatriation', *Museum & Society*, 17:2, pp. 272–81.

Elliott, Denielle (2019), 'Neurological disturbances and time travel', *Catalyst: Feminism, Theory, Technoscience* 5:2, pp. 1–27.

Fountain, T. Kenny (2010), 'Anatomy education and the observational-embodied look', *Medicine Studies*, 2:1, pp. 49–69.

Gere, Cathy (2013), 'Curating aphasia: Pierre Paul Broca's museological science', *Interdisciplinary Science Reviews*, 38:3, pp. 200–09.

Harlow, John Martyn ([1868] 2000), 'Recovery from the passage of an iron bar through the head', *Publications of the Massachusetts Medical Society*, 2, London: Macmillan ,pp. 327–47.

Harris, Anna (2020), *A Sensory Education*, London: Routledge.

Jackson, J. B. S. (1870), *Descriptive Catalogue of the Warren Anatomical Museum*, Boston: A. Williams and Company.

Jenkins, Tiffany (2008), 'Dead bodies: The changing treatment of human remains in British museum collections and the challenge to the traditional model of the museum', *Mortality*, 13:2, pp. 105–18.

Kakaliouras, Ann M. (2012), 'An anthropology of repatriation: Contemporary physical anthropological and Native American ontologies of practice', *Current Anthropology*, 53:S5, pp. S210–21, https://www.journals.uchicago.edu/doi/pdfplus/10.1086/662331. Accessed 18 May 2022.

Kelley, Daniel, Farhoud, Mohammed, Meyerand, M. Elizabeth, Nelson, David, Ramirez, Lincoln, Dempsey, Robert, Andrew L. Alexander and Davidson, Richard (2007), 'Creating physical 3D stereolithograph models of brain and skull', *PLoS One*, 2:10, p. E1119, https://doi.org/10.1371/journal.pone.0001119. Accessed 11 January 2022.

Kwint, Marius and Wingate, Richard (2013), 'Curating the brain', *Interdisciplinary Science Reviews*, 38:3, pp. 195–99.

Lim, Kah Heng, Loo, Zhou Yaw, Goldie, Stephen, Adams, Justin and McMenamin, Paul (2016), 'Use of 3D printed models in medical education: A randomized control trial comparing 3D prints versus cadaveric materials for learning external cardiac anatomy', *Anatomical Sciences Education*, 9:3, pp. 213–21.

Lohman, Jack and Goodnow, Katherine J. (2006), *Human Remains & Museum Practice*, Oxford: Berghahn Books.

MacMillan, Malcolm (2000), 'Restoring phineas gage: A 150th retrospective', *Journal of the History of the Neurosciences*, 9:1, pp. 46–66.

MacMillan, Malcolm (2002), *An Odd Kind of Fame: Stories of Phineas Gage*, Cambridge: MIT Press.

MacMillan, Malcolm (2004), 'Inhibition and Phineas Gage: Repression and Sigmund Freud', *Neuropsychoanalysis*, 6:2, pp. 181–92.

Marreez, Yehia, Willems, Luke and Wells, Michael (2010), 'The role of medical museums in contemporary medical education,' *Anatomical Sciences Education*, 3:5, pp. 249–53.

Nott, John and Anna Harris (2020), 'Sticky models: History as friction in obstetric medicine', *Medicine Anthropology Theory*, 7:1, pp. 44–65.

Ousley, Stephen, Billeck, William and Hollinger, R. Eric (2005), 'Federal repatriation legislation and the role of physical anthropology in repatriation', *American Journal of Physical Anthropology: The Official Publication of the American Association of Physical Anthropologists*, 128:S41, pp. 2–32, https://doi.org/10.1002/ajpa.20354. Accessed 18 May 2022.

Prentice, Rachel (2005), 'The anatomy of a surgical simulation: The mutual articulation of bodies in and through the machine', *Social Studies of Science*, 35:6, pp. 837–66.

Ratiu, Peter and Talos, Ion-Florin (2004), 'The tale of Phineas Gage, digitally remastered', *The New England Journal of Medicine*, 351:23, p. 21.

Richardson, Ruth (2000), *Death, Dissection and the Destitute*, Chicago: University of Chicago Press.

Shelley, Bhaskaran (2016), 'Footprints of Phineas Gage: Historical beginnings on the origins of brain and behavior and the birth of cerebral localizationism', *Archives of Medicine and Health Sciences*, 4:2, p. 280.

Stuss, Donald and Robert Knight (2013), *Principles of Frontal Lobe Function*, 2nd ed., Oxford: Oxford University.

Uttal, William (2002), 'Précis of the new phrenology: The limits of localizing cognitive processes in the brain', *Brain & Mind*, 3:2, pp. 221–28.

Vaccarezza, Mauro and Papa, Veronica (2015), '3D printing: A valuable resource in human anatomy education', *Anatomical Science International*, 90:1, pp. 64–65.

Van Horn, John, Irimia, Andrei, Torgerson, Carinna, Chambers, Micah, Kikinis, Ron and Toga, Arthur (2012), 'Mapping connectivity damage in the case of Phineas Gage', *PloS One*, 7:5, p. e37454, https://doi.org/10.1371/journal.pone.0037454. Accessed 18 May 2022.

Wakefield, Dennis (2007), 'The future of medical museums: Threatened but not extinct', *The Medical Journal of Australia*, 187:7, pp. 380–81.

Zauld, David and Scott Rauch (2006), *The Orbitofrontal Cortex*, Oxford: Oxford University.

STETHOSCOPES

THIS THING,
A STETHOSCOPE

Claire Wendland

To use a stethoscope as a diagnostic tool, student nurses and doctors work to hear what is initially inaudible. Tuning in requires tuning out. A trainee learns to ignore the loud rustle of the stethoscope's earpieces inside her own ears, for instance, or the crackle of a paper gown intended to preserve his patient's modesty. These noises can easily drown out the subtler sounds of a heart that murmurs as circulating blood flows along unexpected pathways or encounters unexpected obstacles. If we tune out for a moment the stethoscope's function as a diagnostic tool and think about the thing itself, as an object that moves through social worlds, what subtle murmurs might become audible? What kinds of medical circulation, what pathways and obstacles, could we hear?

Stethoscopes appear in clinics and hospitals, and they feature in the publications of historians and sociologists. Through years as a medical student, a practicing physician, a patient and an anthropologist studying medical training in Malawi, I have used and noticed them. Stethoscopes served as tools for diagnosis. They were just as critical, however, as things. They circulated in gift exchanges. They marked or mitigated inequality. They were material symbols of a high-status profession, of mysterious healing practices and of a specialised way of knowing about bodies. Medical education attuned trainees to these things.

When Malawians described to me how they had come to study medicine, admiration for the stethoscope featured in some stories. In more than one instance, a student recalled not knowing what the thing was. Joe Phoya had been a sickly child. Going to the clinic was scary, but when he saw the medical staff he knew he wanted to join their ranks:

'The white attire looked so appealing to me. And they had this thing, which I never knew was a stethoscope.' Kamwachale Mandala's sister was studying to become a nurse. 'My sister was ready to go to Kamuzu College of Nursing. So, I was so interested in the stethoscopes, the thermometers!' Duncan Kasinja's grandfather had been a medical assistant. Watching his grandfather boil glass syringes and use a stethoscope was a powerful memory for Duncan. 'In a way, that influenced me to do medicine', he said. 'You know at home, you go in the village, you see this thing', and here he drew a swirl in the air with a fingertip, 'you see this stethoscope. And you think "Ah..."'

A stethoscope can be a metonym, a part standing in for a whole. During medical education and beyond it, the stethoscope can stand in for biomedicine itself, as these students' reflections indicate. Esoteric knowledge and specialist practice come together into 'this thing': a thing that can be admired or feared, loaned or borrowed, disdained or coveted; a thing that can become a commodity or a gift.

Markers of unequal power

Physically, a stethoscope connects two people: the listener in whose ears the earpieces nestle, and the person being listened to, on whose chest the stethoscope's diaphragm (or bell) rests. It makes medical discovery into a dyadic connection – which is simultaneously a separation – between a knowing subject and a known object (Lock and Nguyen 2010). The moment of that connection can be frightening. I have helped a child to put my stethoscope's earpieces in her own ears, to allow her to marvel at the sounds of my heart and then her own. Family-medicine doctors and pediatricians demonstrated this trick long ago; the idea is to try to mitigate children's fears about encounters with doctors, to put some of the power back in their hands by reversing the direction of examination. In the years since, I have taught the same technique to others. Whether children actually experience this reversal as powerful, or simply as novel, it does seem to make the examination less scary.

Children are not the only ones fearful of the connection a stethoscope creates. Medical student Anthony Boloweza had been a laboratory technician; his classmate Joe Phoya had been a surgical assistant. Each had worked in the same large Malawi hospital. In separate interviews, each described an expatriate doctor there who refused to place the stethoscope on a patient's chest himself. Both found this behavior outrageous. Joe chalked the doctor's actions up to racist squeamishness, Anthony to hauteur: 'When he went on ward rounds he would put a stethoscope in his ears and then he would request the nurse to place the diaphragm onto the patient. He was *proud*. He did not even want to touch a patient!'

Like its use, a stethoscope's possession can also mark inequality. Who owns a stethoscope, who does not, who has a hard time getting one? Students starting their third year in Malawi's medical school, about to begin examining patients on the hospital wards, often worried about how to get stethoscopes. For Andrew Kanyenda, the stethoscope stood for all the things he could not have: 'I cannot afford it. If I can't afford a simple stethoscope right now, then how am I ever going to have a complete diagnosis kit?' Students who had not yet obtained a stethoscope sometimes avoided physical-examination practice sessions rather than be shamed by their lack of gear. 'Some of us third years will skip it because we don't have what we are supposed to be using. So there we are, completely underequipped.'

Years ago, before Queen Elizabeth Central Hospital (Queens) had become an academic medical centre, I had first gone there as a visiting medical student. The flow of student visitors from other countries increased once the University of Malawi opened a College of Medicine and Queens became one of its major teaching hospitals. Students from Europe and North America circulated on its wards and in its clinics. Malawians commented on the visitors' pockets, stuffed with gear: penlights, reflex hammers, pocket emergency handbooks or (later) smartphones with emergency-handbook apps, stethoscopes. In the high-risk obstetrics clinic, Edith Koloviko – a friend and colleague – asked me to photograph her; for the picture, she borrowed my stethoscope to drape around her neck, see Figure 23.1. On a later morning in that same clinic at Queens, the head nurse remarked to an expatriate clinician who showed up bedecked with a stethoscope and other diagnostic gear, 'and now you have come here with all your ammunition'.

Symbols of authority

People whose bodies rendered them less likely to be taken seriously found that 'ammunition' to be particularly important. In Malawi, as in

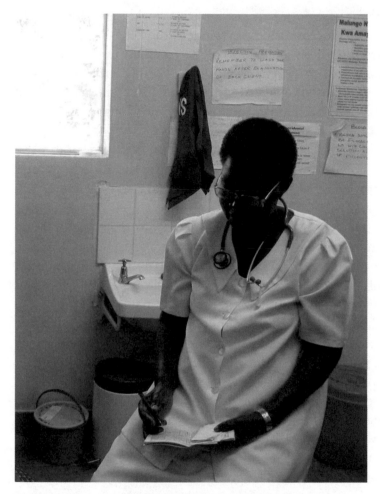

Figure 23.1: Nurse-midwife Edith Koloviko in clinic. Image courtesy of author.

the United States, women doctors sometimes chose to display stethoscopes – especially the serious-looking black or grey models – more prominently, so that they were less likely to be mistaken for nurses. A physician anthropologist working in a North American emergency room noted that the white coat, the use of lab tests, the display and use of the stethoscope, all marked the doctor as reassuringly competent and authoritative (Salhi 2016). Stethoscopes and white coats were especially powerful symbols for women physicians, who could not assume that they would be seen as authorities in the emergency room.

Stethoscopes could be mysterious and still powerful. Perhaps the mystery does not detract from the power but adds to it. Historical and ethnographic examples from many parts of the world suggest as much. In the 1930s, for instance, routine physical examinations became common sites of encounter between expatriate doctors and Tswana men aspiring to be mine-workers (Livingston 2005). Former miners remembered the stethoscope, used to auscultate recruits' chests and assess their fitness, as a mysterious mechanism to access people's interior workings. The object was unfamiliar, noted Julie Livingston (2005), but the phenomenon was not. Indigenous *dingaka* also had tools to understand the hidden interior: how those tools worked, and how the *dingaka* gained their esoteric knowledge, were secrets kept from outsiders. Of course the doctors' ways would be mysterious too.

In Pakistan, Dorothy Mull (1999) observed, informal-sector *chota doctors* used stethoscopes not to auscultate anyone's chest but as symbols of biomedical authority. The *chota doctors* were usually hospital personnel with access to pilfered drugs who set up private clinics. Lacking formal training and licensure, they built their practices instead on the indiscriminate use of antibiotics and the symbols of biomedical authority. A stethoscope placed on the top of a sick person's head could not diagnose pneumonia, but it could help to draw clientele.

A stethoscope did not have to function as an instrument of diagnosis to do as a prop. It just had to look more-or-less right. Decades ago, Arnold Wendroff (1983) encountered *nchimi* healers in northern Malawi who wore white coats, rolled herbal treatments into pill forms and used dummy stethoscopes in the course of divination. Marilyn Houlberg (2008) described Haitian *vodoun* figures who wore both fake stethoscopes and shirts bearing images of skulls, signifying their power to cure and kill.

On the cover of my book about medical training in Malawi (Wendland 2010), a stethoscope curls on the edge of a printed cloth. There too it is a prop: as the cloth symbolises Africa, the stethoscope symbolises biomedicine. The symbol resonates beyond book jacket designers. Anthony Boloweza, who spoke with me when he was just beginning medical school in Malawi's College of Medicine, knew he would feel like a real doctor 'When I go into the hospital at Queens, when I can add my knowledge to the clinical experience, when I will use a stethoscope and diagnose disease'. A faculty member in community medicine concurred: 'You should see their excitement when they reach year three – going to the hospital, you know, stethoscope around their necks.'

Objects that circulate

There is a joke about a well-loved axe: three handles and five blades, and still going strong after 50 years. My own stethoscope has accompanied me for 34 years, well over half my life, but it is a bit like the famous axe. It has been through at least six or seven sets of ear-pieces, a couple of diaphragms and at one point a refurbished plastic tube. Only the curved metal stem pieces and the metal chestpiece are from the original stethoscope, the one that arrived as an unexpected gift.

All of us got them. On the first day of class in our first year of medical school, in the autumn of 1986, each of my classmates and I found tucked in our mailboxes a box containing a dark grey stethoscope. The curved bell side of it shone dully like a steel drum. The flat plastic diaphragm had a brand name on it: Littmann Quality, it declared, with a gracefully swirling large italic L and a small TM symbol off to the side. A card in each box announced that this gift was courtesy of the Eli Lilly Company. If you looked really closely, you could see 'Lilly' engraved on the chestpiece too. I was delighted. It was free! We had been told we would need stethoscopes of our own as we learned physical examination skills, and to buy one would have taken a good seven or eight hours of my work-study job. Plus, like Anthony Boloweza twenty years later, I felt like a doctor just draping the thing around my neck, long before I knew how to listen through it.

A few – a very few – of my classmates were less excited. A handful of them had been given fancier 'cardiologist' stethoscopes as gifts from family members on being accepted to medical school. The Littman Classic that so pleased me struck them as generic, ordinary. A couple of others had ethical qualms. One of these worriers had been a sociologist and a health activist before beginning medical school. Another had been a nurse. Did we really want to start right off by accepting an expensive gift from a pharmaceutical company, they wondered? Yes we did, most of us answered, brushing off their annoying scruples. We were confident that there was no way these gifts would influence us. But for those students who were troubled, there was also no way to give the gifts back.

Sy Safransky (1985) called it a 'gift horse' in his essay on the same Lilly stethoscope, given to his wife Norma when she began medical school the year before I did. Norma's came with a brochure proudly claiming that Lilly sold more than 700 drugs in 130 countries. Malawi was one of those countries. Insulin and some key cancer medications were – and still are – among the drugs the company sold there, at high patent-protected prices that make them very difficult for most patients to access. If such a brochure accompanied our stethoscopes the next year, I do not remember it.

First-year medical students all over the United States got these stethoscopes, and many of us kept them for years. That meant there were a lot of them. If a couple of gray Littman classics were sitting on a clinic counter, how could you be sure which one was yours? Over time people personalised them. Some found snap-on nametags to clip to the metal tubes leading away from the earpieces. These nametags too were often pharmaceutical-company gifts. On the Navajo reservation in the American Southwest, where I worked for many years, several colleagues had beadwork that wrapped the Y area where the tubing converged. Some had commissioned the beadwork from a Navajo or Hopi artist; some had received it as a gift from a grateful patient or family member. Eschewing beads and nametags, I clamped a 50-cent plastic umbilical-cord clamp around mine. It is still there. In the photograph of my friend in the high-risk clinic in Malawi, the ivory-colored cord clamp of the borrowed stethoscope shows clearly against her crisp white uniform.

Some students who were troubled by their free stethoscopes ultimately gave them away to student doctors and nurses they met on journeys far away, including journeys in Malawi. Arguably, the gift stethoscopes would be more valuable in poorer places: the auscultation skills students learned so carefully in medical school were not used much in places where high-technology medical imaging was abundant, but they remained critical elsewhere. Through the alchemy of scarcity, an ethically dubious object became a welcome token of generosity. I was not one of these givers. I loaned mine, both as a diagnostic tool and as a photo prop, but never gave it away.

Not all gifts are poisonous, but some are

Gift: the word means offering or present in English, poison in German. The ambivalence of this word suits medical gifts. Second-hand medical equipment, wanted or unwanted, circulates from people and places with too much to people and places with not enough. Modest gifts salve uneasy consciences. Medical donations – ranging from valuable new equipment to expired pharmaceuticals – can testify to altruism or symbolise solidarity in the face of inequality. They can also be toxic, permitting pharmaceutical waste dumping even while garnering tax write-offs and public praise (Kamba et al. 2017).

In retrospect, I see that much of my training was sponsored by industry. The person who was chosen by faculty as best senior resident got a cheque and a walnut-and-brass plaque from the Ortho company, maker of our most commonly prescribed brand-name oral contraceptives, while the prize for best research paper came from TAP Pharmaceuticals, which made an expensive injectable medication we often used to treat endometriosis. Other prizes and goodies came from other pharmaceutical and medical-device manufacturers. No doctor or nurse ever needed to buy her own pen, their own coffee mug or his own stethoscope. Lunches for residents appeared once a month or so throughout my four years of specialty training, brought to a hospital conference room by a kindly fellow employed by Pfizer Inc. who breezed past the authorised-staff-only signs. He would talk about the special benefits of Pfizer's drug Unasyn while we helped ourselves to General Tso's chicken or green-chile enchiladas from nearby takeout places. Those 'free' lunches and his sympathetic ear for anyone's troubles surely had nothing at all to do with the exceptionally high rate of Unasyn prescriptions at our hospital.

My training programme was not unique. Those pockets stuffed with clinical ammunition? One study that asked trainees to empty their pockets found that 97 per cent of primary-care residents were carrying at least one item with a pharmaceutical manufacturer's insignia (Sigworth et al. 2001). Ninety per cent carried pocket reference books – books that guided the 'best' response for common medical problems – that were industry-sponsored giveaways. As gifts tend to do, they created a sense of obligation. The stethoscope from the Eli Lilly Company to all of the brand-new medical students of America probably delighted most of us. It also symbolised the cosy relationship between professional medicine and the commercial drug and medical-equipment industry into which we were being drawn from the very beginning.

As Carl Elliott (2010) and others have documented, commercial influence distorts what does (and does not) get researched, what does (and does not) get published, what does (and does not) get promoted or elevated into 'best clinical practice' guidelines, and what does (and does not) get prescribed. Physicians are aware that routine medical practice is shaped in all of these ways. But as the preceding two sentences' passive voice suggests, we tend to think of it as something that just happens out there somewhere. Doctors typically believe that promotional efforts and drug-company gifts affect other people's prescribing but not our own (Fickweiler et al. 2017).

The gift stethoscope can poison more directly. Carried around in a nurse's pocket, slung around a doctor's neck, hung on a wall in an intensive-care-unit cubicle, a stethoscope is an excellent *fomite*: an inanimate thing that transmits infection from one person to another, as gift blankets once carried smallpox from the immune to the vulnerable. One study showed that a third of the stethoscopes used by emergency-room doctors carried methicillin-resistant *Staphylococcus aureus*, MRSA (Merlin et al. 2009). Other researchers identified bacterial colonization in nearly all of the stethoscopes of 92 clinicians at a community hospital. Many of these bacteria – including MRSA – were potentially harmful (Schroeder et al. 2009). Similar studies conducted in other parts of the world consistently show high rates of bacterial colonisation. Besides bacteria, what else do stethoscopes carry? Viruses, including the novel coronavirus sweeping the world as I write in 2020? Fungi? Other pathogens? Probably. Beading, nametags, my cord-clamp: all of those personalising touches that clinicians add to their stethoscopes almost certainly increase the hiding places for harmful microorganisms that can be transmitted to patients. The touch of a stethoscope, like many other medical practices, can bring lethal injury (Jha et al. 2013).

Conclusion

The students who learned to love medicine by admiring the stethoscope were on to something. A stethoscope is a metonym: for the profession, the body of knowledge, the assemblage of tools and people, and the practices of care that we call biomedicine. It is very useful for its apparent purposes and for not-so-obvious ones. It attracts admiration and conveys authority – even when misused or mysterious. Its distribution is profoundly inequitable. Scarcity alters its presence, its value, and its uses. It is shaped by commercial interests. Alongside its evident benefits come concealed dangers. The student who learns to use it can inflict new harm, often unknowingly, while gaining access to new knowledge that can be healing.

Paying attention to the stethoscope's travels allows one to attune oneself to the flows and blockages of biomedical care. A stethoscope extends the reach of its user. Physicians in training think of it as a tool that can reveal evidence of dangerous biological processes. It is also an object that through its circulation extends the reach of biomedicine and provides evidence of dangerous social processes. 'You see this thing, you see this stethoscope', as Duncan Kasinja said, 'and you think, "Ah..."'

Acknowledgements

Edith Koloviko has given permission for her photo to appear here. As she prefers, I have used her real name. All other individuals' names are pseudonyms, a practice customary in anthropology and required by the ethics committees that reviewed this research.

References

Elliott, Carl (2010), *White Coat, Black Hat: Adventures on the Dark Side of Medicine*, Boston: Beacon Press.

Fickweiler, Freek, Fickweiler, Ward and Urbach, Ewuot (2017), 'Interactions between physicians and the pharmaceutical industry generally and sales representatives specifically and their association with physicians' attitudes and prescribing habits: A systematic review', *BMJ Open*, 7:e016408, http://dx.doi.org/10.1136/bmjopen-2017-016408, Accessed 18 May 2022.

Houlberg, Marilyn (2008), 'When death wears sunglasses: Negotiating life and death at the crossroads', in *Africa at Noon Symposium Series*, Madison: University of Wisconsin-Madison.

Jha, Ashish K., Larizgoitia, Itziar, Audera-Lopez, Carmen, Prasopa-Plaizier, Nittita, Waters, Hugh and Bates, David W. (2013), 'The global burden of unsafe medical care: Analytic modelling of observational studies', *BMJ Quality and Safety* 22:10, pp. 809–15.

Kamba, Pakoyo, Ireeta, Munanura, Balikuna, Sulah and Kaggwa, Bruhan (2017), 'Threats posed by stockpiles of expired pharmaceuticals in low- and middle-income countries: A Ugandan perspective', *Bulletin of the World Health Organisation*, 95, pp. 594–98.

Livingston, Julie (2005), *Debility and the Moral Imagination in Botswana*, Bloomington: Indiana University Press.

Lock, Margaret and Nguyen, Vinh-Kim (2010), *An Anthropology of Biomedicine*, Oxford: Wiley-Blackwell.

Merlin, Mark, Wong, Matthew, Pryor, Peter, Rynn, Kevin, Marques-Baptista, Andreia and Perritt, Rachael (2009), 'Prevalence of methicillin-resistant *Staphylococcus aureus* on the stethoscopes of emergency medical services providers', *Prehospital Emergency Care*, 13:1, pp. 71–74.

Mull, Dorothy (1999), 'Anthropological perspectives on childhood pneumonia in Pakistan', in R. A. Hahn (ed.), *Anthropology in Public Health: Bridging Differences in Culture and Society*, New York: Oxford University Press, pp. 84–114.

Safransky, Sy (1985), 'Gift horse', *The Sun*, 114, pp. 2–4.

Salhi, Bisan (2016), 'Beyond the doctor's white coat: Science, ritual, and healing in American biomedicine', in P. J. Brown and S. Closser (eds), *Understanding and Applying Medical Anthropology*, New York: Routledge, pp. 204–12.

Schroeder, Ariel, Schroeder, Maryellen and D'Amico, Frank (2009), 'What's growing on your stethoscope? (And what you can do about it)', *The Journal of Family Practice*, 58:8, pp. 404–09.

Sigworth, Stephen, Nettleman, Mary and Cohen, Gail (2001), 'Pharmaceutical branding of resident physicians', *JAMA: Journal of the American Medical Association*, 286:9, pp. 1024–25.

Wendland, Claire (2010), *A Heart for the Work: Journeys Through an African Medical School*, Chicago: University of Chicago Press.

Wendroff, Arnold (1983), 'Health care and social change: The case of Northeast Malawi', in J. H. Morgan (ed.), *Third World Medicine and Social Change*, Lanham: University Press of America, pp. 253–68.

TEXTILES

MATERIALITIES OF SURGERY: LEARNING THROUGH THREAD

Roger Kneebone and Fleur Oakes

Our chapter, written by a surgeon (Roger Kneebone) and a three-dimensional embroider (Fleur Oakes), builds on Oakes's three-year artistic residency in the vascular surgery unit of a large university teaching hospital in central London (St. Mary's Hospital, part of Imperial College London). It explores how a synthesis between 'artistic' and 'scientific' perspectives can bring unanticipated insights into the nature of materiality and embodied learning in the world of operative surgery. Built on a close collaboration between the authors, this account is written in the third person for the sake of narrative clarity. The chapter outlines how this unorthodox collaboration has disclosed distinct 'registers' of material awareness within the learning that happens in the operating theatre. To illustrate these different ways of experiencing surgical materiality, the chapter concludes by describing strands of work by Oakes which are opening up new educational approaches. For example, *Textile Body* (2018) and *Epiploic Cube* (2019) (see Figures 24.1–24.4) both use threads to create textile-based objects which allow learners to experience the physicality of surgical intervention without jeopardising patient safety.

Fleur and thread

Fleur trained as a fine artist and fashion designer. After graduating from art school and establishing her own fashion house, she turned to the

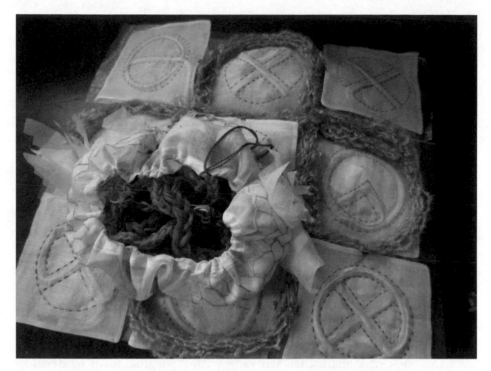

Figure 24.1: *Textile Body* detail; vascular system and gut. Image courtesy of Fleur Oakes.

world of antique textiles to explore the nature of beauty and memory. Through visits to the Victoria and Albert Museum she experienced work of the highest quality, work she learned to 'touch' through the museum glass. These visits were balanced by the scrummage of London's Brick Lane and Portobello Road, with all the decay and fragility of old garments. There Fleur learned sightless touch in the huge laundry bins of textile dealers, feeling for linen sheets amongst nylon net curtains. The two experiences fed each other. Learning about thread for Fleur was like learning the alphabet; expression and tension through line. Fleur's career then moved to making bespoke corsets, where she had to learn how to judge a tightly woven silk and gauge its breaking point. Later still she went on to learn embroidery and lacemaking. She describes how for embroidery the thread is spun clockwise, while for lacemaking it's anti-clockwise. Stitching requires you to understand many permutations – which thread to use with which needle and what fabric. You feel the vibrations of a drum tight silk on the hoop when the needle pierces it, and you hear the drag of one fibre against another. These tiny changes teach discernment. In the latest phase of her career, Fleur has become one of the UK's leading experts in stumpwork and three-dimensional embroidery. Her experience of the world as an artist is profoundly shaped by touch and colour, and all her senses come into play when she engages with her tools and materials as an expert craftsperson. There is an endless translation of line and colour into form.

Roger and thread

Roger's first career was as a general and trauma surgeon. By the time he finished his training to become a consultant, he had spent six years as a medical student and almost ten more years as a doctor. He had studied anatomy, pathology and other areas of biomedical science, and learned the techniques of operative surgery through an extended apprenticeship. He spent countless hours assisting at operations, where the ability to manage threads was just one of many skills he was expected to master. Like Fleur, he learned to manipulate threads through incessant practice – in his case, tying one-handed knots at home using lengths of string over the back of a chair, then working with a surgical team to develop his dexterity. Like Fleur, he gained these skills through constant repetition, internalising a tactile 'vocabulary' of techniques which he later drew upon almost without conscious awareness.

As a medical student, the world of surgery at first seemed alien and frightening. Yet by the time Roger had become an experienced surgeon, he felt completely at home in the operating theatre. There he focused on the patients in his care, concentrating on each one's unique problems. Much of the materiality of surgery became second nature, and it took Fleur's 'eyes of newness' several decades later to highlight the colours, textures and richness of this sensory landscape. After completing his surgical training Roger changed direction, becoming a general practitioner (family doctor) in the southwest of England and then an academic in a large university (Imperial College London). In recent years, he has explored the craft and performance of medicine (especially surgery), using simulation as a means to bring clinicians, publics and experts outside medicine together to share experiences and insights (e.g. Kneebone 2017; 2020).

Connecting through thread

In 2014, Roger was invited to stage a simulation of a surgical operation at the Art Workers' Guild in London. This remarkable organisation is made up of leading experts in over 65 fields, from textile artists (including Fleur), illustrators and potters to bookbinders, hat-makers and stone masons – though none from the world of medicine. Roger's simulation demonstrated how an expert surgical team (lead surgeon, first assistant, scrub nurse and anaesthetist) resected a segment of intestine and rejoined the ends, using a realistic silicon model. As an observer, Fleur was struck by how the surgeon and assistant used sutures to sew two segments of intestine together. She noticed similar challenges to those encountered by her own students during embroidery classes – such as preventing threads from becoming snarled, entangled or too tightly coiled. She called this 'thread management'. Fleur and Roger recognised that their perspectives were complementary. For both of them, materiality was of central importance. How they perceived that materiality was very different. What was ground for Roger was figure for Fleur, and vice versa. Where Roger saw anatomy and procedures for treating injury or disease, Fleur saw needles and threads. For Roger, threads were secondary. For Fleur, threads were prime.

Two exploratory events entitled 'Thread Management', again at the Art Workers' Guild (see Craddock 2014, 2015), invited a group of experts to explore this concept further. All the participants used thread in their practice, though in different ways. Textile artists, surgeons, puppeteers, computer modellers and a fly fisherman described their work and demonstrated their skills to one another. Consultant vascular surgeon Colin Bicknell (one of the participants) discovered common ground with Fleur around the delicacy and precision of small-scale stitching (Oakes 2020; 2021). Colin invited Fleur to become lacemaker-in-residence in his operating theatre. Her attachment continued for over three years, a role which as far as we are aware is unique.

As Fleur settled into what would become an extended residency in the operating theatre, the initial strangeness of surgery started to wear off and she became accustomed to observing quietly for hours at a time. She found that in the world of vascular surgery, as in her own workshop, the focus is on the smooth movement of curved needles through the micro-layered structure of blood vessels. Much depends on contextual awareness. In the operating theatre, it is taken for granted that an experienced surgeon would understand all the other complexities going on around his or her hands, though this may not be the case for learners. The material knowledge of muscle and fat, and an awareness of which needle to use for which anatomical structures, is as much a default setting for surgeons as Fleur's knowledge of woven fabric is to her. The heart of both worlds lies in the same place, mediated by an expert's sense of touch – but then diverges in response to surgical constraints such as the need to sew at depth, adjust to the densities of the body, and wield a curved needle in a tiny space.

In the course of this collaboration, Fleur has spent over one hundred hours observing surgical operations and keeping a record of her responses. Written by hand in brown ink on brown paper, her distinctive script interspersed with sketches, Fleur's record of her residency is unlike anything you'd expect to find in a patient's case notes or a surgeon's logbook. As an observer without medical training, Fleur responded to what she saw from her perspective as an artist and an expert in textiles. Her accounts of organs and blood vessels are descriptive, poetic and suffused with metaphor, worlds apart from the unemotional terminology of Roger's textbooks on anatomy and operative technique. Fleur responds to the physicality of what she observes and her similes are disturbingly vivid.

'Blockage [in an artery] like a dead baby mouse with a four-inch tail', she writes in her logbook. And from another operation: 'Spleen like wet bread in a wet paper bag. Removed after damage. Intestines and bowel etc. moved from side to side to access the aorta under the diaphragm – smooth silky pink. Like moving clothes in a tight packed wardrobe'. And on another occasion: 'Planes of the body, cutting across abdominal muscle and down the side of the tilted patient. Like removing a cake from a cake tin'.

As well as her responses to operative procedures, Fleur captures her experience of being amongst the team members – though always of course at one remove, as she is permitted to watch, to observe, to record, to draw and to ask questions, but never to touch. When she asks clinicians to explain what they are doing, they struggle to find appropriate words for what has become second nature. In her logbook, she describes their difficulties in articulating materiality. 'How to describe the stitches of an anastomosis into a fragile aorta'. 'Half formed sentences that are finished by gesture [...]'. Yet Fleur is also part of the team, there amongst the team members, experiencing their physicality alongside each patient's at close quarters. 'A smellscape [...]', she writes. 'Indescribable. Blood, aftershave, the sweet smell of roses, odd chemical odours, burning fat.'

Material metaphors: *Textile Body* and *Epiploic Cube*

Initially the aim of Fleur's residency was to develop training programmes for medical students and surgical trainees around 'sewing', identifying embroidery techniques that might be applicable to surgery. As the project progressed, its scope broadened, leading to a range of artistic creations which open the world of the operating theatre to wider publics by using textiles as a material metaphor for living human organs and the procedures used by surgical teams. This use of textiles provides a different mode of description from the professional lexicons of anatomy and pathology, focusing instead on the sensory landscapes of surgery and the embodied ways of knowing which it requires.

Once the residency was under way, Fleur sought ways to share her experience of surgery with colleagues outside the world of medicine. She set out to represent the physicality and team-working of the operating theatre without alienating non-clinicians by graphic descriptions of operations. These creations allow people to engage with the materiality of surgery in a way that is both authentic (presenting an experience based on surgical practice) and safe (not involving living patients). Observers can participate as well as watch.

Fleur's first piece, which she calls *Textile Body* (*TeB*), uses layers of woven, knitted and embroidered material to evoke the complex organisation of the body, see Figures 24.1–24.3. It invites people to experience how surgeons expose, separate, display, displace and restore delicate living structures, working at an intersection between hands, bodies, instruments and materials (Kneebone et al. 2019). Though not shaped like a human body, the *TeB* conveys an essence of surgical teamwork. *Epiploic Cube* (*EC*), a later creation, see Figure 24.4, is based on the well-known child's toy that can be continually transformed, bringing new surfaces into view with every rotation (Craddock 2020).

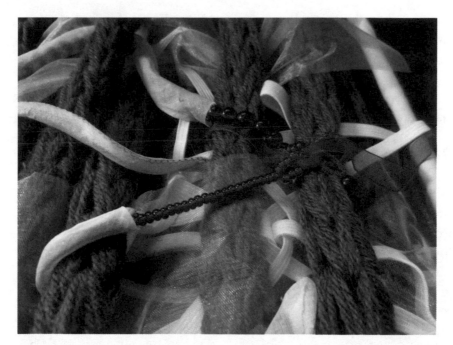

Figure 24.2: *Textile Body* detail; muscle, tendons and severed artery. Image courtesy of Fleur Oakes.

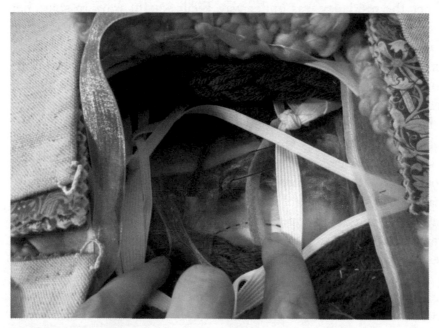

Figure 24.3: *Textile Body* detail; recreation of minimal access surgery. Image courtesy of Fleur Oakes.

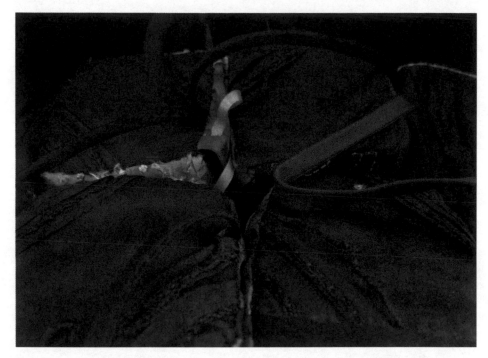

Figure 24.4: *Epiploic Cube* detail; muscular plane with arteries and fat to illustrate the visual complexity of surgery. Image courtesy of Fleur Oakes.

It further develops parallels between surgery and textile, capturing the mystery and challenge of the body's hidden spaces through a complex structure that took almost 100 hours to create. Navigating the interior landscapes of the peritoneal cavity without causing damage, for example, demands from surgeons an acute sensitivity of touch and the ability to 'listen' with their hands. Embryological convolutions within the abdomen create spaces and cul-de-sacs which surgeons like Roger had to learn to work with as they trained, recognising when anatomical structures 'give permission' to be separated and displayed. Surgeons, like artists and craftsmen, must work with the grain of their materials and not against them.

Both the *TeB* and *EC* offer parallels for surgical ways of knowing and doing, each placing an experience of surgical working into the hands of any non-medically trained person. It was important to Fleur that there should be no disturbing associations for such participants, no recognisable anatomical shapes to trigger a distracting empathy or give them the creeps. Instead, there is the language of fragile silk and robust linen. Knitting speaks for fat and elastic quivers where gut would pulse.

Layers can be gently pushed aside, with the intelligent fingertip recognising the breaking points of each material. A creak of taffeta and then the slide of one layer against another is understood as permission to rotate a structure within its safe parameters. With both these works, Fleur felt it vital to make a thing of beauty, not some whimsical shape to amuse and be passed over. The instinctive human sympathy with something well-made helps us make sense of our own selves.

Conclusion

This chapter offers insights from a surgeon–embroider collaboration around the theme of learning through thread. It shows how our unorthodox translation between modes of materiality is revealing new ways of engaging with tactile knowledge in the world of surgery and clinical medicine. By acknowledging the rich vocabulary of touch in educating, observing and engaging in surgical practice, direct contact between surgery and art can lead to a deeper understanding of the materiality on which clinical training and care depends.

At another level, the chapter can be read as a response to the multiple modes of ordering which this book explores. 'Thread' offers a physical and metaphorical framework of linkage and connection which makes sense to Fleur and Roger as practitioners. As a metaphor which is both familiar and challenging, we hope it may also prompt readers to see connections between elements of the book as a whole, whether arranged alphabetically or otherwise.

This speaks to the editors' intention to 'resist the image of biomedicine as a monolithic, singular entity', disclosing the many horizons of awareness which engagement with materiality requires. Seen as something that can bind and connect, but which can also tangle and confuse, thread speaks to the 'shifting tangle of frameworks, paradigms and practices that are hybrid, plural, multiple and readily contaminated by localised norms and alternative epistemologies' which the editors describe in their introduction.

We hope that this chapter supports the book's contention that the objects of medical reproduction resist stable classifications, meaning different things at different times and in different places. Seen through the eyes of an embroiderer and a surgeon, thread too means different things.

For us, that has been the fascination of a collaboration that crosses traditional taxonomies and challenges disciplinary distinctions.

Acknowledgements

We gratefully acknowledge the role of Dr. Paul Craddock (filmmaker and cultural historian), who has created the short videos cited in this chapter; the support and collaboration of Mr. Colin Bicknell, Consultant Vascular Surgeon and Clinical Senior Lecturer, Imperial College London and his clinical colleagues; and the support of the Royal College of Music – Imperial *Centre for Performance Science* in funding Fleur Oakes's residency. We also acknowledge the Art Workers' Guild Outreach initiative, led by Prue Cooper. Still photographs of *Textile Body* and *Epiploic Cube* by Fleur Oakes.

References

Craddock, Paul William (2014), 'Thread management short', Vimeo, https://vimeo.com/109053078. Accessed 14 November 2021.

Craddock, Paul William (2015), 'Threads', Vimeo, https://vimeo.com/123221514. Accessed 14 November 2021.

Craddock, Paul William (2020), 'Fleur's Cube', Vimeo, https://vimeo.com/382442695. Accessed 14 November 2021.

Kneebone, Roger (2017), 'Materiality and thread', *The Lancet*, 389:10066, pp. 246–47.

Kneebone, Roger (2020), *Expert: Understanding the Path to Mastery*, London: Viking Penguin.

Kneebone, Roger, Oakes, Fleur and Bicknell, Colin (2019), 'Reframing surgical simulation: The textile body as metaphor', *The Lancet*, 393:10166, pp. 22–23.

Oakes, Fleur (2020), 'Thread management', BlogSpot, http://threadmanagement.blogspot.com/search/label/Epiploic%20Cube. Accessed 12 August 2021.

Oakes, Fleur (2021), 'Thread management', BlogSpot (y) http://threadmanagement.blogspot.com/search/label/Textile%20Body. Accessed 12 August 2021.

ULTRASOUNDS

DEVELOPING ULTRASOUND: KNOWLEDGE DISSEMINATION AND TECHNOLOGICAL CHANGE, 1945–80

Jakob Lehne

The presentation of the first ultrasound picture of a foetus to family and friends has become a ritual in many contemporary societies, and patients and doctors alike see the use of ultrasound in medical settings as an innocuous routine. Yet the current ubiquity and accessibility of this technology belies its comparatively recent invention. Its rise from obscure origins to almost universal application is a fascinating example of rapid knowledge production, codification and dissemination. In this chapter, I seek to sketch how medical ultrasound developed from being the purview of a tiny group of enthusiasts, passing their knowledge on in master–pupil relationships, to being an essential part of the modern medical curriculum, with textbooks and massive online open courses (MOOC) to boot. But this (short) story of ultrasound and its development is not only about changing technologies and methods of teaching. It is also concerned with the men and women, whose lives became intertwined with and changed by a piece of technology. As I will argue, shared dedication to the development of ultrasound created a peculiar knowledge community, whose ultimate triumph – the wide dissemination of ultrasound technology – ironically rendered much of what they had created redundant.

Early Beginnings

Intellectually and materially, the Second World War laid the foundations for the 'ultrasound-boom' of the second half of the twentieth century. While the first experiments with diagnostic ultrasound were performed in competing military laboratories in the early 1940s, it was the use of similar technology (radar and sonar) on the battlefield that inspired a number of young doctors to attempt to harness its potential for medical work (Eckel 1992; Willocks and Barr 2004). The war had left them 'with a hearty respect for what electronic science can do' (Donald cited in Willocks and Barr 2004: 67), but its influence was not just intellectual. The metal scraps military action left behind – such as gun turrets – were quickly repurposed and used by early pioneers to build the first functioning ultrasound machines in the late 1940s (Goldberg et al. 1993). It is not without irony that these makeshift military research centres, using material and knowledge destined to wreak maximum damage on human bodies, should be at the origin of a most beneficial medical invention.

These beginnings, which paralleled similarly underfunded research in other medical areas – dialysis was developed under equally difficult conditions – were certainly anarchic, but within a couple of years various teams were doing research around the world (Campbell n.d.). Although working on very different projects, they helped to improve each other's ideas and constructions and slowly created an international network of knowledge about ultrasound (Kratochwil 2000). With their subject in constant flux and lacking any form of organised curriculum, younger researchers would travel to more experienced practitioners to be introduced, one-on-one, into their often-idiosyncratic methods and ideas about this new technology. Years later, Ian Donald, a Scottish ultrasound pioneer in the field of obstetrics and gynaecology, would reminisce about 'our first disciple from abroad. He was with us a month and we became great friends. I taught him all I knew and his subsequent career [...] more than vindicated the time he spent with us' (Donald 1974: 114).

Ultrasound was a complex affair and from the very beginning split into different types used for different purposes, each of them requiring in-depth knowledge of modern physics for their application. There was A-Scan – originally developed by ophthalmologists, but also used in other areas – a 1D technique with which ultrasound echoes could be plotted on a diagram. Some doctors preferred B-Scan, in which the echoes of ultrasound were translated into lighter and darker spots on a monitor and showed a static 2D image (see Figure 25.1). In cardiology meanwhile, M-Scan was the ultrasound-of-choice, able to show various aspects of the beating of the heart. All of these scanning techniques were in some way deficient. Static and unable to show clear images, they were miles away from today's technology. But the early pioneers were undaunted and, together with hand-picked engineers, racked up years of experience with unruly machines, tweaking and manipulating them to achieve better results. Knowing each aspect of the gear and being able to switch between the languages of physics and medicine was a rare trait and the circle of those who knew about contemporary ultrasound development was ever more clearly circumscribed.

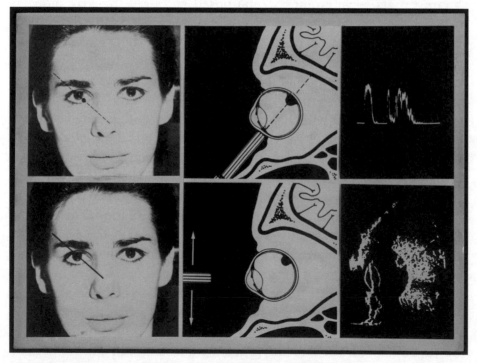

Figure 25.1: Illustrations explaining the differences between ophthalmological A-Scan and B-Scan. Archives of the Medical University of Vienna (MUW-FO-S4341-1-2).

Individual Knowledge

Among this small group of researchers, a complex vocabulary to describe what they were doing and seeing developed. The images on the monstrous and individually built machines were grainy and difficult to interpret. The classification of the appearance of different organs and masses on screen was therefore one of the most crucial aspects of the work done by these early pioneers. They were often searching for words to attribute to the shadows and white patches they were seeing, yet without formalised knowledge, they often could not help being left misunderstood. Communication among the small group of experts was difficult enough, at a time when long-distances were still a real impediment to research collaboration and journals could often not afford to print high-quality images. But to explain to colleagues from other departments that the 'white blob with a clear black comet tail in a black hole' that they were being shown 'was a gall stone' was often next to impossible (Frentzel-Beyme 2005: 368).

Along with this arcane vocabulary, early initiates often developed individual scanning techniques that were even more difficult to communicate or emulate, underscoring the individualised nature of early ultrasound knowledge. A doctor at a Glasgow hospital, for example, would describe a colleague's attempt to turn a static B-Scan ultrasound picture into a moving one and the unique technique she had perfected in order to do so. She had 'developed a system where you had a single transducer and she would make it vibrate and I remember watching her wiggle it backwards and forwards and by making it go backwards and forwards quite quickly you got the impression of real-time' (Nicholson 2003: 135). Many similar techniques to use existing machinery in alternative ways must have existed in the early decades of ultrasound. But given the continuing lack of proper textbooks, instructional videos or similar technology such individual forays remained just that. It was local knowledge about the potential of machinery, the secret of single practitioners or at best small groups, but unknown to the medical profession at large.

Yet, with the publication of a number of introductory articles in the late 1950s and 1960s, followed by several textbooks, the formalisation of ultrasound-knowledge and its presentation to the wider world had begun in earnest. These early texts demonstrated the strong understanding of physics (and obviously medicine) the early pioneers had and the in-depth of knowledge their small 'fraternity' had acquired in previous years. Trying to pack decades worth of research into a couple of pages, the authors aimed to explain everything at once and could – at times – produce slightly overwhelming material. Reminding his audience of the enormous density of this early research, a younger ultrasound-expert claimed that Ian Donald's legendary 1958 Lancet article *Investigation of Abdominal Masses by Pulsed Ultrasound* could today easily be stretched 'to about five publications' (Campbell n.d.; Donald et al. 1958). After the burst of introductory articles, followed more clearly designated and organised textbooks, which also started to appear in other languages and helped to effectively introduce ultrasound to an ever-larger audience (Kratochwil 1968).

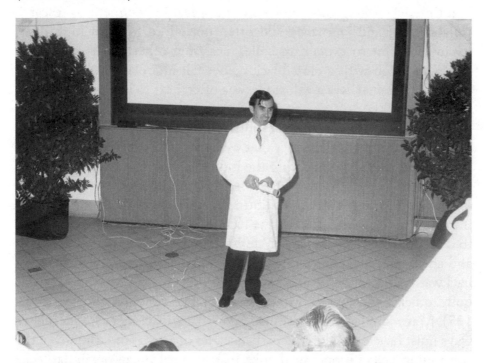

Figure 25.2: The leading Austrian ultrasound authority at the time, Alfred Kratochwil, speaks at the opening of the Ultrasound Training Center at the General Hospital in Vienna October 1970 (MUW-FO-S4362-17/29).

The Ultrasound Expansion

Partly based on these contributions, the 1970s saw an enormous change in the way knowledge about ultrasound was shared and taught; a process that uprooted the traditional structures of the ultrasound-community. While informal discussion, individual exchanges and smaller conferences had defined the life of early ultrasound-researchers, the late 1960s and early 1970s saw the introduction of large and formalised conference settings, where official communications and papers slowly replaced traditional channels of communication (World Congress on Ultrasonic Diagnostics in Medicine 1971). Simultaneously, forward-looking universities and hospitals instituted the first ultrasound training centres, formalising curricula and instituting new ways of teaching. In order to be able to teach larger classes, these centres would often employ new technology, like split-screen-videotaping and projectors, leading to a slow 'industrialisation' of ultrasound teaching (Goldberg 1974). But despite the colossal changes in some institutions, it is important to remember that this was a gradual process, with some universities and hospitals continuing to use classic master–apprentice teaching techniques until the early 1980s (Troxclair et al. 2011).

The increase of ultrasound teaching was paralleled by an expansion of research and over the next few years a number of new inventions would be made, the most important of them all being real-time-scanning (especially in obstetrics/gynaecology). The basic technology to do scanning with moving images had been around for a long time, but many pioneers had failed to see its utility, viewing the grainier images as inferior to static alternatives (Nicholson 2003). With technological developments in the early 1970s real-time-scanning was dramatically improved. The images were now much clearer and the fact that they were moving made the on-screen-identification of masses and anatomical parts much easier. For decades, highly trained experts had been exasperated by the fact that even their medical colleagues could not interpret what they were seeing. Now it seemed as if even patients could easily understand the images that they were being shown, making life easier for both sides.

Perhaps even more directly measurable was the effect the innovations in real time scanning had on hospital staff and their hierarchy. The individual scanning techniques and the complex group vocabulary, both inspired by older machines were now outdated. The result was not so much a changing of the guards, as a sudden and large-scale dissemination of knowledge and skill previously reserved for a small group. As a witness to these events remembered:

> The development of real time scanning was a great democratizing influence in obstetric scanning which was no longer confined to an elite group of experts in a few major centers. Real time scanners [...] were now widely available and many experienced practitioners of static scanning were surprised (and not a little discomfited) at how quickly their junior doctors, midwives and sonographers became experts in scanning almost overnight. (Campbell 2013: 220)

What might be termed the 'ultrasound revolution' was now complete. No longer tied to a small group of developers who shared a common set of ideas and interests, ultrasound freely developed, influencing myriad medical fields, no longer controlled by a single centre.

The early pioneers were now no longer necessary for ultrasound's success. But what could be described as their ultimate triumph had bitter side-effects. Much of the knowledge that they had produced and acquired over decades quickly became irrelevant to a new generation and the machines that they had spent years building, using only metal scraps and ingenuity, now looked like ancient history. Honorary doctorates, medals and eponymous ultrasound training centers surely reminded a younger generation of their influence, but a large part of their shared history would remain inaccessible to later followers. Today, the simplicity of ultrasound application allows it to be taught in classrooms or even online, where much of the knowledge the pioneers slowly acquired over decades is glossed over in a few slides. The time when ultrasound was a compact field, requiring simultaneous knowledge of medicine, physics and engineering, and where individual teaching was the norm, are gone forever. It is easy to understand the wistful musings of an early pioneer, looking back at 'the early days [...] when ultrasound was like a fraternity, everyone knowing everybody, each meeting being a momentous occasion' (Levi 1997: 481).

Acknowledgements

This chapter profited from previous research undertaken by the author at the Medical University of Vienna.

References

Campbell, Stuart (2013), 'A short history of sonography in obstetrics and gynaecology', *Facts, Views & Vision in Obstetrics and Gynaecology*, 5:3, pp. 213–29.

Campbell, Stuart (n.d.). 'History of ultrasound in Obstetrics and Gynecology', OBGYN.Net, http://www.obgyn.net/contraception/history-ultrasound-obstetrics-and-gynecology. Accessed 12 December 2018.

Donald, Ian (1974), 'Sonar—The story of an experiment', *Ultrasound in Medicine and Biology*, 1:2, pp. 109–17.

Donald, Ian, Macvicar, John and Brown, Tom G. (1958), 'Investigation of abdominal masses by pulsed ultrasound', *The Lancet*, 271:7032, pp. 1188–95.

Eckel, Kurt (1992), 'Die Entdeckung des ersten bildgebenden Verfahrens der Ultraschalldiagnostik durch K.-Th. Dussik vor 50 Jahren. Ein historischer Rückblick 1942–1992', *Ultraschall in Klinik und Praxis*, 7:4, pp. 299–305.

Frentzel-Beyme, Bernd (2005), 'Vom Echolot zur Farbdopplersonographie', *Der Radiologe*, 45:3, pp. 363–70.

Goldberg, Barry B. (1974), 'Use of split-screen video tapes for ultrasound training', *Journal of Clinical Ultrasound*, 2:1, pp. 17–20.

Goldberg, Barry B., Gramiak, Raymond and Freimanis, Atis K. (1993), 'Early history of diagnostic ultrasound: The role of American radiologists', *American Journal of Roentgenology*, 160:1, pp. 189–94.

Kratochwil, Alfred (1968), *Ultraschalldiagnostik in Geburtshilfe Und Gynäkologie: Lehrbuch Und Atlas*, Stuttgart: Thieme.

Kratochwil, Alfred (2000), 'Presentation of the 1999 Ian Donald Gold Medal for technical development for Carl Kretz', *Ultrasound in Obstetrics and Gynecology*, 16:1, pp. 106–07.

Levi, Salvator (1997), 'The history of ultrasound in gynecology 1950–1980', *Ultrasound in Medicine & Biology*, 23:4, pp. 481–552.

Nicholson, Deborah (2003), 'Secrets of success: The development of obstetric ultrasound in Scotland, 1963–1990', Ph.D. thesis, Glasgow: University of Glasgow.

Troxclair, Lauri, Smetherman, Dana and Bluth, Edward I. (2011), 'Shades of gray: A history of the development of diagnostic ultrasound in a large multispecialty clinic', *Ochsner Journal*, 11:2, pp. 151–55.

Willocks, James and Barr, Wallace (2004), *Ian Donald: A Memoir*, London: RCOG.

World Congress on Ultrasonic Diagnostics in Medicine (1971), *Ultrasonographia Medica: Proceedings ; 1st World Congress on Ultrasonic Diagnostics in Medicine and SIDUO III*, Vienna, Austria, 2–7 June 1969, Wien: Verlag der Wiener Medizinischen Akademie, p. 1.

WOUNDS

THE FAKE WOUND: THINKING THROUGH MATERIALS IN OSCE SIMULATIONS

Andrea Wojcik, Victor Mogre,

Anthony Amalba, Celia Yamile Rodriguez

and Francis A. Abantanga

At a medical school in Tamale, in the north of Ghana, assessment of students' clinical skills sometimes involves volunteers putting on a commercially produced fake wound (Figure 26.1). This forms part of an objective structured clinical examination (OSCE), one way to formally assess clinical skill in medicine (Elder 2018). This particular OSCE took place in 2018 at the School of Medicine and Health Sciences (SMHS) at the University for Development Studies (UDS). Here 'clinical skills' refer broadly to any skills relevant to the *practice* of medicine. Andrea Wojcik took this photograph as part of her ethnographic research on how medical students turn their bodies into diagnostic aids. Using prosthetics or replacing a volunteer with a manikin for formal assessments was exceptional, reserved for cases in which staff deemed the repetitive handling of volunteers by students inappropriate or impossible. In this case, around 140 students interacted with a 'wound' that otherwise would have required immediate treatment.

In this chapter, we draw on Wojcik's observations of the fake wound as well as on the experiences of faculty members, Victor Mogre, Anthony Amalba, Celia Yamile Rodriguez and Francis A. Abantanga in order to explore the role of materials in medical students' formal assessments. While the fake wound is visually impressive, a closer look at the clinical skills curriculum reveals that the fake wound fell short as a simulation of clinical situations for students in their first clinical year because it did not lend itself to testing students' embodied clinical judgement. We suggest the fake wound's failure is not inherent in all OSCE simulations, but rather that the materials out of which the fake wound was made did not adequately simulate the felt judgement medical practitioners often rely upon as part of their clinical judgement. This leads us to argue that thinking through the materials used in assessment simulations is one strategy that could help medical teachers assess students developing clinical judgement while accounting for practical demands and ethical considerations faced by medical education programmes.

Focusing on one prosthetic is, of course, limited in scope. The fake wound was one of several prosthetics and manikins used to train and assess medical students at the medical school, and medical educators and commercial companies across the globe experiment with materials and set-ups that enable medical educators to address the practical demands of training doctors as well as the ethical intention to minimise harm to patients who are inevitably part of the training process (Barrows 1968; Johnson 2007; Prentice 2013; Taylor 2014; Guarrasi 2015; Underman 2015; Harden 2016; Harris and Rethans 2018). With this in mind, we do not aim to criticise one assessment situation, but instead use the fake wound scenario to think about the clinical judgement teachers expect medical students to develop and the ways this is and can be assessed.

In the next section, we provide some background on OSCEs and their implementation at the SMHS, with a focus on teachers' expectation that students in their first clinical year – that is, the same cohort of students that Wojcik observed being assessed with the fake wound – started developing clinical judgement. We then show how the fake wound lent itself to assessing procedural knowledge as opposed to clinical judgement while also considering the difficulties of assessing clinical judgement at the SMHS. Finally, we consider how thinking through materials used in simulations could more adequately simulate clinical practice and therefore better assess clinical judgement.

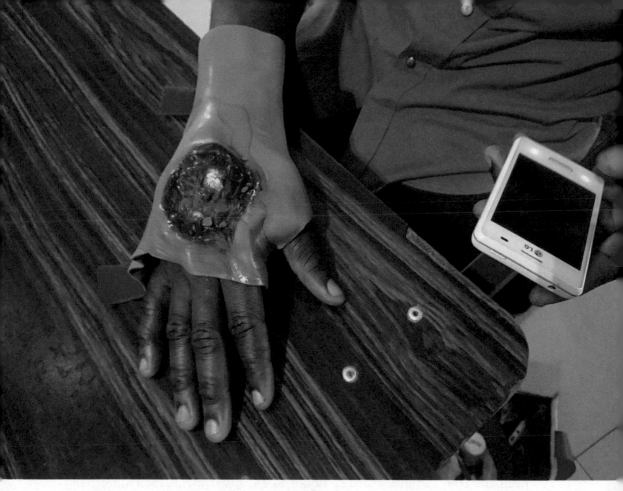

Figure 26.1: Photo of fake wound worn by a volunteer taken before a clinical skills assessment of medical students in the School of Medicine and Health Sciences at the University for Development Studies in Tamale, Ghana. Image courtesy of Andrea Wojcik.

Beyond procedure, towards judgement

In Tamale, OSCE's were held alongside written assessments as part of students' final examinations, or in the case of students finishing their final year, to determine if students would become doctors ready for licensing. Each OSCE consists of a series of simulated clinical situations often referred to as stations. At each station, students perform a task within a specified amount of time. At the SMHS, for example, the fake wound was one of twelve OSCE stations. Students had five minutes to examine the wound, report their observations and explain how to treat it. An examiner observed, questioned and graded students with the help of checklists designed by SMHS staff in the weeks before the assessment. These checklists outlined grading criteria and sometimes acceptable interventions for examiners to make during an assessment (Figure 26.2).

Examiners were students' teachers, who were also practicing doctors, and sometimes doctors from other hospitals and universities.

More advanced students would have additional OSCEs throughout the academic year. Wojcik observed two of these mid-year OSCEs for students in their first clinical year. Students in their first clinical year were in their fourth year of studying medicine, but the primary site of their education had shifted from the classrooms, lecture halls and laboratories at the SMHS campus to the Tamale Teaching Hospital (TTH). This move marked a transition from learning about bodies and pathologies in the absence of patients to interacting with patients under the supervision of healthcare professionals.

The curriculum for first-year clinical students focused on physical examination skills, which entailed looking, listening, feeling and sometimes even smelling bodies for signs of patients' conditions. While preclinical medical students at the SMHS began learning physical examination in their first-year of medical school by practicing on manikins as well as on each other, their first clinical year was when students often first began sensing many of the pathologies they had learned about in the classroom. Heart murmurs skipped through their stethoscopes. Enlarged livers pushed against their fingertips, and gangrene pinched at their noses. The transition to the clinic, therefore, marked a moment when students' bodies started acting as diagnostic tools.

To become a walking diagnostic instrument, students had to learn that physical examination was more than a series of memorised steps. Dr. Emmanuel (all the names of research participants are pseudonyms) was a clinician and teacher at the teaching hospital, and he indicated in an interview that the 'robotic' tendencies of preclinical students were no longer enough upon their arrival in the clinic; if they were not doing so before, students now had to start reasoning why they were instructed to perform a series of steps. Students moving beyond memorisation also had to improve their sensory skills. Dr. Sanne was a teacher as well as a curriculum coordinator at the medical school, and she made a distinction between touching and feeling. She explained that students 'touched' when they moved too quickly through examinations, likely missing key diagnostic information at their fingertips in their haste to execute the steps they had learned in class. This was especially true of preclinical students learning and practicing their physical examination skills on manikins whose lumps and bumps, once found, could be memorised. Feeling, however, entailed the ability to search the body for previously unidentified abnormalities. Feeling hands were more attentive to changes in, for example, tissue consistency, skin temperature and pulse rhythm.

Together, Dr. Emmanuel and Dr. Sanne pointed to an expectation that students in their first clinical year moved beyond memorising procedure and towards developing a clinical judgement distinguishing the expert from the novice. This is a clinical judgement as informed by bodily skill as it is by cognitive reasoning. In other words, clinical judgement is embodied (Prentice 2013). Dr. Sanne hinted at this with her distinction between touching and feeling, and she is not alone in her alignment of clinical judgement with bodily skills. For example, Paul Craddock (this volume) illuminates how stitching requires surgeons to assess how their stitches affect the integrity of tissue as they sew it together by feeling the pull of needle and thread. Roger Kneebone and Fleur Oakes (this volume) explain how surgeons cannot assume a surgical route through the body because the position and flexibility of various organs and tissues must be felt during surgery. Truly feeling, then, is part of how practitioners determine how to treat patients, and clinical judgement requires a 'felt judgement'.

In this section, we have described the SMHS clinical skills curriculum and identified an expectation that first-year clinical students began to develop their clinical judgement, which includes honing their ability to feel. But how to assess whether clinical students have begun developing this sensory, clinical judgement? In the next section, we return to the fake wound OSCE station to raise questions about the role of simulations in assessing what we have called felt judgement.

The pull of procedural knowledge

The following observations have been adapted from Wojcik's field-notes about the fake wound OSCE station designed as part of a mid-year OSCE for first-year clinical students.

The OSCE was well underway, with twelve stations distributed between the auditorium and the classrooms accessible via doors to either side of the stage (Figure 26.3). I (Wojcik) sat at one of the stations in the auditorium looking at two young women. One woman introduced herself as Jill, a medical student, and asked for her patient's name, to which the other woman responded, 'Selasi'. Jill then asked Selasi for permission to examine

OSCE **PBL 2: DAY 4**

STATION: MOTOR FUNCTION OF THE LOWER LIMBS (SKILLS)

INDEX NR: SMS/.../...........

EXAMINER: ....

EXAMINER SIGNATURE:

PLEASE DEMONSTRATE HOW TO EXAMINE THE MOTOR FUNCTION OF THE LOWER LIMBS

You have 5 minutes for this station.

Good luck.

	POINTS
1. Student explains the procedure and obtains consent, ensures adequate exposure *(1 point)*	
2. Inspects for wasting *(1 point)*	

3. Tests the tone of the lower limbs by at least one of the following methods:
   - Passive movement of the knee and ankle varying the speed of the movement.
   - Passive rolling of the lower limbs on the cough
   Compares right and left *(2 points)*
   2 points: good
   1 point: needs some practice
   0 points: very poor/not done	

4. Tests the strength of major muscle groups of the hip: flexion, extension, abduction and adduction comparing right and left *(2 points)*
   2 points: good technique, logical order, good communication, up-to-speed
   1 point: needs practice
   0 points: very poor/ not done	

5. Tests the strength of flexors and extensors of the knees comparing right and left *(1 point)*	
6. Tests the strength of plantar and dorsal flexors of the ankle *(1 point)*	
7. Tests the strength of the flexors and extensors of the toes, digit 1 separately. *(1 point)*	
8. Gives clear explanations to the patient throughout the examination *(1 point)*	
TOTAL (out of 10):	

NOTE:
- **IF THE TIME IS SHORT, LET THE STUDENT DEMONSTRATE THE TESTS ON ONLY ONE SIDE AFTER HAVING SHOWN AT ITEM 1 THAT (S)HE KNOWS LEFT AND RIGHT SHOULD BE COMPARED.**
- **IT IS ALLOWED TO GIVE 0.5 POINTS FOR AN ITEM**

Figure 26.2: Example OSCE grading rubric previously used for students in their second year of medical school. Courtesy of the SMHS.

the (fake) wound on the back of her hand (Figure 26.1). Upon receiving nearly inaudible approval, Jill rubbed her hands with hand sanitizer from a pump sitting on a nearby examination bed turned table. She pulled on a pair of latex gloves and moved closer to look at Selasi's hand resting on a desk. At this point, Jill's examiner, Dr. Sanne, jotted a few number '1's' in the grading checklist: Jill had adequately introduced herself and prepared for a hygienic physical examination of the wound.

The wound was an odd sight. It was a bloodless thing for a gash with the bone supposedly exposed, although there was a faint line of dried red liquid running from the edge of the wound. The dirt and pebbles contaminating it were the same rust-red colour as when Dr. Sanne had adhered them to the wound with pus-like petroleum jelly earlier that morning. The skin around the wound gleaned unnaturally in the light, and it was several shades lighter than Selasi's skin with folds at the knuckles because Selasi's wrist and hand were too slight to pull the silicone taught, even with the help of the adjustment straps.

Jill had transitioned from merely looking at the wound to feeling it through her gloved hands. Not once did Selasi feign pain or discomfort while Jill palpated the perimeter of the wound for tenderness and hardened tissue. Jill then checked for signs of infection by feeling for temperature differences between the silicone wristlet and Selasi's upper arm. Finally, Jill felt Selasi's pulse at the wrist of her 'injured' hand. When she placed her fingers close to Selasi's elbow crease on the same arm, Dr. Sanne intervened: 'I know what you are doing. It's ok. You did it. Move on.' I glanced over to Dr. Sanne and saw her awarding a point for 'testing the surrounding intravascular area', even though the comparison between the radial and brachial pulses had not been completed. The intention to compare was apparently enough.

Jill reported her findings verbally to Dr. Sanne. She commented on the size of the wound, its uncleanliness and the raised silicone edges. Signs of infection and poor intravascular health, both assessed via touch, were left out of her report because Selasi's healthy body did not exhibit them. Jill then moved deftly through her final minutes, identifying the materials and instruments she would need to stitch and bandage the wound from an overabundance of props laid out on the examination bed. These include gauze strips, gloves, hand sanitizer, tweezers, forceps, various sizes and types of sutures, bottles of local anaesthetic with and without adrenaline, syringes, and saline. When a bell rang and marked the end of five minutes, Jill moved to the next station in her exam. Dr. Sanne turned to me and said, 'Wow. Way above average. If they were all like this, I would be so happy.' I asked what Jill had done well. 'She had an answer to everything,' Dr. Sanne said. 'She knew all the instruments, and how to hold them.' The bell sounded again, marking the start of a new five minutes, and the next student introduced himself to Selasi.

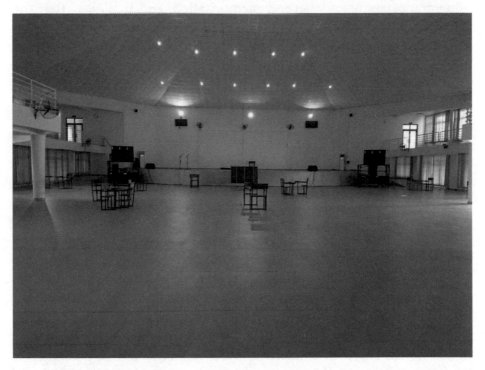

Figure 26.3: Photograph of auditorium in which part of the OSCE was held. Staff spaced out desks a semi-circle around the stage. Privacy screens, like the one in front of the stage, were placed around desks to demarcate stations. Image courtesy of Andrea Wojcik.

Wojcik had witnessed a star performance, but there is something puzzling about her observations considering teachers' desire that students at this stage in their education started developing clinical judgement. Opportunities to exercise felt judgement at the fake wound station were limited. The prosthetic, while visually impressive, partially thanks to Dr Sanne's embellishments, offered little in relation to what it feels like to examine and treat a wound. The result is that students' tactile engagement became an exercise in ticking boxes, an indication of procedural knowledge rather than a demonstration of developing dexterity.

To be clear, SMHS staff may not have intended to assess students' development of clinical judgement with the fake wound station. Indeed, many medical educators at the SMHS and elsewhere would doubtless argue that procedural knowledge is necessary and therefore deserves to be assessed, especially at the undergraduate level (see e.g. Norman et al. 1991: 125; Elder 2018: 548), but the purpose of this chapter is to think along with the expressed desire of medical educators about ways to push undergraduate students beyond memorisation, and it is clear that the fake wound assessment falls short of this goal in its inability to more thoroughly engage students' bodies. The question, then, is if and how prosthetics and other objects can be used to assess felt judgement.

The medical education literature on OSCEs indicates rather dismal prospects. Norman et al. (1991) that research suggest that checklists, like those commonly employed in OSCEs, encourage rote memorisation. A few years later, Hodges et al. (1999) similarly found that OSCE checklists emphasise procedural knowledge. More contemporary literature couches its critique in different terms: OSCEs ask students to 'show how' rather than 'do', particularly when they do not employ actual patients (van der Vleuten et al. 2010; Elder 2018). In other words, OSCEs ask students to demonstrate memorised steps, but they do not test whether students have developed the skills necessary to perform a given task. Considering this literature, Wojcik's observations of the fake wound are unsurprising, but teachers and curriculum designers wanting to move beyond memorisation are left to wonder about alternatives.

One alternative suggested in the literature is 'workplace assessment', or assessment based on students' and trainees' tasks and responsibilities in clinics and wards. This assessment focuses on students' and trainees' performance, and therefore better assesses what they can do (van der Vleuten et al. 2010; Elder 2018). SMHS relied on some workplace assessment of undergraduate students. For instance, teachers' signatures were required in individual logbooks listing topics and tasks students were expected to cover as part of their clinical education. Another option is to include more patients in OSCE assessments, but at the SMHS, these alternatives have practical and ethical limitations.

Practically, the medical school and teaching hospital in Tamale do not have the budgets for this kind of testing. Raymond Bagulo Bening's (2005) history of the UDS demonstrates that this limitation is, at least in part, a result of the historical peripherality of northern Ghana in relation to the south during colonial and post-independence developments in tertiary education. Northern Ghana has a long history of limited education and health provision, and the UDS began in the 1990s in order to address this. At the time of writing, the persistence of limited re-sources is evidenced by SHMS's high student to staff ratio. For instance, the first clinical year alone included roughly 140 students. Andrea often observed bedside teaching sessions about physical examination with fif-teen–twenty students around one patient bed. During these sessions, only a few students had the opportunity to examine a patient under their teacher's supervision. In addition to overseeing undergraduate students, the hospital teaching staff supervised graduate students completing their residencies, all while treating patients. In truth, the opportunities for teaching staff to assess undergraduate students' interactions with pa-tients were limited. Asking students to run through clinical simulations during OSCEs was one way of addressing this limitation.

Ethically, while patients were recruited and paid a modest sum to participate in clinical students' OSCEs, there were physical exami-nations and other clinical procedures that were difficult to include in OSCEs because of the physical and emotional discomfort they would or were assumed to cause patients. For example, wounds should only be stitched once, and breast, gynaecology and digital rectal examinations raised questions among staff and students about the appropriateness of subjecting patients to repeated examinations. Some medical programmes do recruit volunteers for such training, and while these programmes do much to calm students' nerves, teach about normal anatomical variation and improve the experiences of future patients (Kapsalis 1997; Under-man 2015), volunteers likely do not have pathologies, and therefore an assessment relying on them would ultimately fall into the trap of assess-ing procedure rather than felt judgement.

In the face of large numbers of students and tight budgets, educators at the SMHS walked a tightrope of encouraging students to develop bodily skills enabling felt judgement while minimising the potential harm to patients that were part of this training process. One might then suggest that relying on prosthetics and other objects in OSCE simula-tions and tending towards assessing procedural knowledge is a neces-sary trade-off – the best solution given the circumstances. We, however, would like to propose another possibility. In the next section, we con-sider how attention to the physical materials used in OSCE simulations could enable educators to work within the existing format to assess stu-dents' developing felt judgement.

Thinking through materials

In her work on the use of simulators in medical education, Ericka Johnson (2008) wrote about a manikin intended to help train students to perform gynaecology examinations. Some medical educators in Sweden did not consider the manikin a useful teaching aid because the limited range of movement of the artificial uterus did not allow trainees to feel the back of the uterus for abnormal growths during bimanual examination as the teachers were accustomed to doing as part of their medical practice. Johnson argued that this disapproval showed that simulations mimic specific practices, which may differ across the globe. Indeed, the gynaecology manikin described by Johnson appeared to be tailored to American gynaecology practice. These differences in medical practice, however slight, have important consequences for medical education. She wrote:

> Understanding that simulators are representing practice means that we must start to think about which practices are being recreated and taught to new medical practitioners, and start to ask how and why these practices are being standardized, rather than assuming that the simulator apolitically and objectively mimics an ontologically 'true' patient body. (Johnson 2008: 123)

In other words, the simulators themselves should be interrogated. It is not given that they help to teach desirable practices, but it is also not given what 'desirable' practice is. The former can only be judged in relation to the latter. We have indicated that desirable practice changes throughout students' medical education. Their first clinical year marks a moment in time when students' bodies are expected to become more capable of sensing disease. The fake wound, however, does not invite students to engage in the tactile skills necessary to treat the wound.

There are simulators better suited to assessing the ability to feel. After receiving a grant from Nuffic, the Dutch Organisation for Internationalisation in Education, to collaborate with the School of Health Professions Education at Maastricht University, the SMHS purchased such manikins (Figures 26.4–26.6): gynaecology and breast manikins that required students to identify potentially cancerous lumps with their fingers, and other manikins that required students to feel for the position of a baby inside a womb. The point, however, is not to suggest that the

SMHS, or any university, invest in more commercially produced manikins. Such manikins can be costly, and will inevitably need to be repaired or even replaced simply because of their repeated use at the hands of hundreds of students over time. For medical programmes with tight budgets, this dependency on teaching aids produced and sold in the Global North is an unsustainable drain on limited resources (Nott and Harris 2020). Furthermore, Johnson (2008) demonstrated that teaching aids produced by industry may impose a standard of practice that does not fit within the context of local medical practices (see also Nott and Harris 2020). This point is worth emphasising given an expressed need from within the African medical education community for locally relevant teaching materials (Kumoji and Nott, this volume). Rather than encouraging medical education to rely on industry for a solution, we suggest educators might turn to locally available materials to make their own simulators.

Experimentation with available materials to make teaching aids aimed at instructing sensory skills is part of medical education's past and present. Anna Harris (2019), for instance, has written about the various ways in which food has been used in medical programmes to simulate clinical situations, providing novice students the opportunity to practice sensory skills. Marijke Kruithof, a teacher at Maastricht University in the Netherlands, explained how a sponge covered with shammy cloth and mounted to a piece of wood (Figure 26.7) looks nothing like the human body, but a needle passing through these materials mimics the sensation of a needle passing through muscle to meet the resistance of skin. We are suggesting that experimenting with available materials to make 'sensorily analogous' simulators could be key to enabling OSCE examiners to assess the development of embodied clinical judgement.

Of course, even cheaply made manikins have their costs. They still require materials to be purchased, but even more so, experimentation with materials requires time to design and create. Indeed, such attention to the relationship between materials and clinical judgement could possibly benefit from a collaboration between medical schools and artists or craftspeople who are familiar with materials other than the human body. But perhaps the benefits of attention to material can outweigh the costs. A closer look at the fake wound revealed its inappropriateness for assessing felt judgement. At the same time, however, the use of prosthetics and other simulators in OSCEs are not easily dismissed due to the practical and ethical circumstances under which SMHS teachers provided medical education. Instead, what was needed was assessors' attention to the simulation in order to craft situations that could elicit the kinds of responses, techniques and affects they wanted students to develop in the clinic. Thinking through the materials used in OSCE simulations could enable teachers to better align assessments with embodied clinical judgement while also accounting for the contexts in which their programmes are situated.

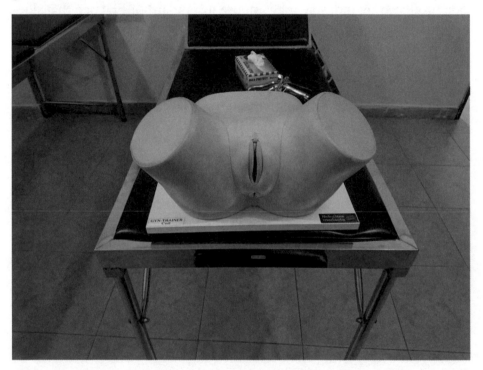

Figure 26.4: Photograph of manikin used to train and assess gynaecology examinations. Some manikins include lumps to be tactilely identified. Image courtesy of Andrea Wojcik.

Acknowledgements

This research received funding from the ERC under the European Union's Horizon 2020 research and innovation programme (Grant agreement no. 678390) and was conducted as part of the project 'Making Clinical Sense', for which Wojcik conducted seven and a half months of fieldwork at University for Development (USD) during the 2017/2018 academic year. The authors would like to thank the UDS students and staff who contributed to this research.

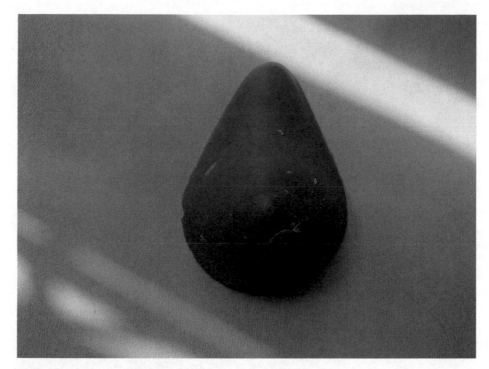

Figure 26.5: Photograph of manikin used to train students how to palpate the breast for possible tumours. Image courtesy of Andrea Wojcik.

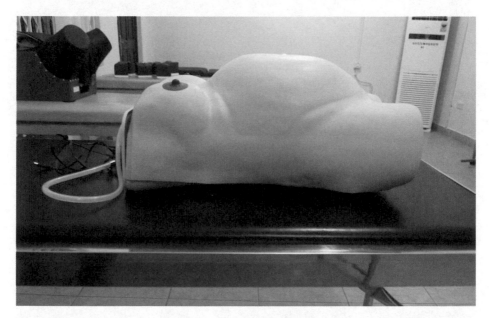

Figure 26.6: Photograph of manikins in foreground and background used to teach students how to feel for the position of the baby during pregnancy and labour. Image courtesy of Andrea Wojcik.

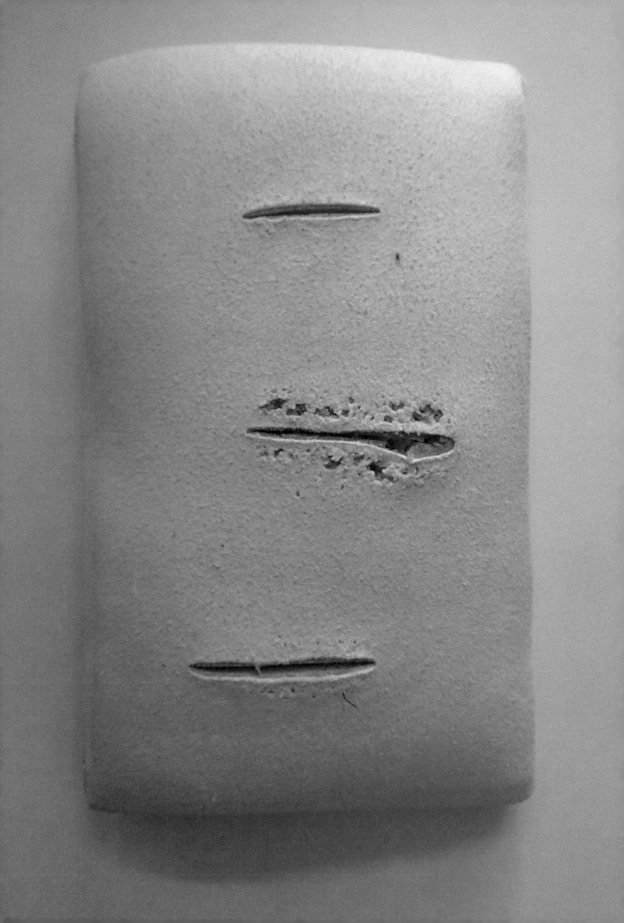

References

Barrows, Howard S. (1968), 'Simulated patients in medical teaching', *Canadian Medical Association Journal*, 98:14, pp. 674–76.

Bening, Raymond Bagulo (2005), *University for Development Studies in the History of Higher Education in Ghana*, Accra: Hish Tahawah Publications.

Elder, Andrew (2018), 'Clinical skills assessment in the twenty-first century', *Medical Clinics*, 102:3, pp. 545–58.

Guarrasi, Ivana (2015), 'Residual categories in medical simulation: The role of affect in the performance of disease', *Mind, Culture, and Activity*, 22:2, pp. 112–28.

Harden, Ronald M. (2016), 'Revisiting "Assessment of clinical competence using an objective structured clinical examination (OSCE)"', *Medical Education*, 50:4, pp. 376–79.

Harris, Anna (2019), 'The culinary art of clinical simulation', *The Gourmand*, 12, pp. 40–47.

Harris, Anna and Rethans, Jan-Joost (2018), 'Expressive instructions: Ethnographic insights into the creativity and improvisation entailed in teaching physical skills to medical students', *Perspectives on Medical Education*, 7:4, pp. 232–38.

Hodges, Brian, Regehr, Glenn, McNaughton, Nancy, Tiberius, Richard and Hanson, Mark (1999), 'OSCE checklists do not capture increasing levels of expertise', *Academic Medicine*, 74:10, pp. 1129–34.

Johnson, Ericka (2007), 'Surgical simulators and simulated surgeons: Reconstituting medical practice and practitioners in simulations', *Social Studies of Science*, 37:4, pp. 585–608.

Johnson, Ericka (2008), 'Simulating medical patients and practices: Bodies and the construction of valid medical simulators', *Body & Society*, 14:3, pp. 105–28.

Kapsalis, Terri (1997), *Public Privates: Performing Gynecology from Both Ends of the Speculum*, Durham, Duke University Press.

Norman, G. R., Van der Vleuten, C. P. M. and Graaff, E. de (1991), 'Pitfalls in the pursuit of objectivity: Issues of validity, efficiency and acceptability', *Medical Education*, 25:2, pp. 119–26.

Nott, John and Harris, Anna (2020), 'Sticky models: History as friction in obstetric education', *Medicine Anthropology Theory*, 7:1, pp. 44–65.

Prentice, Rachel (2013), *Bodies in Formation: An Ethnography of Anatomy and Surgery Education*, Durham: Duke University Press.

Taylor, Janelle S. (2014), 'The demise of the bumbler and the crock: From experience to accountability in medical education and ethnography', *American Anthropologist*, 116:3, pp. 523–34.

Underman, Kelly (2015), 'Playing doctor: Simulation in medical school as affective practice', *Social Science Medicine*, 136–37, pp. 180–88.

Van der Vleuten, C. P. M., Schuwirth, L. W. T., Scheele, F., Driessen, E. and Hodges, B. (2010), 'The assessment of professional competence: Building blocks for theory development', *Best Practice & Research Clinical Obstetrics & Gynaecology*, 24: 6, pp. 703–19.

Figure 26.7: Photograph of a simulator previously used to train medical students at Maastricht University in suturing. It is made shammy cloth over sponge mounted on a wooden board. Original inventor unknown, 2020. Image courtesy of Andrea Wojcik.

ch
ays of
eal to

X

sion of any
s he is a
and druggist
h of it in
is ordinance.

unds or

. . . .

X

LICENCE No. 2/

NATIVE PHYSICIANS LICENCE.

✠✠✠✠✠✠✠

BEKWAI DIVISION
Eastern Province, Ashanti.

✠✠✠✠✠✠✠

PRINTED BY THE SCOS PRINTING PRESS
P. O. BOX 282, KUMASI.

IN THE NATIVE COURT OF BEKWAI,
Eastern Province, Ashanti.

Licence No. 2/36

NATIVE PHYSICIANS LICENCE.
THIS IS TO CERTIFY THAT

Kobina Kusi + Kofi Boakyi
of Atobiasi

has been granted Licence to practise as Physician
within the Division of Bekwai, for twelve
months, commencing from the _12th_ day of
November 19_36_ until the
_12th_ day of _November_ 19_37_

Dated at Bekwai, the _12th_ day of _November_ 19_36_

Recommended by: Approved by:

Writer & Witness to   _Yaw Gyanti II_

mark & Signature: Bekwaihene

Ji. Asah

Registrar

ZEBRAS

ZEBRAS, NOT HORSES: ON LIMITS AND MARGINS OF BIOMEDICAL KNOWLEDGE

Candida F. Sánchez Burmester

When you hear hoofbeats, think of horses not zebras.

(Theodore E. Woodward)

The aphorism cited above was coined in the late 1940s by Theodore Woodward, a physician and educator at the School of Medicine at the University of Maryland, in Baltimore, the United States. With this phrase, he meant to advise his students not to think of an extraordinary diagnosis, the zebras, but instead to think of more common explanations, the horses. Woodward's phrase spread and is today widely known in the medical community (Levine and Bleakley 2012; Sotos 2006). Born and trained in Maryland, Woodward took for granted that domestic horses are common while zebras are 'exotic animals'. This expression echoes the contested concept of 'tropical disease'. Both presuppose a European or North American standard, which is cast against a geographically-distant 'other'. In the case of 'tropical diseases', an ethnocentric view took for granted that tropical climates were hostile and degenerative to Europeans and that indigenous physiologies and diseases encountered in European and North

Figure TE6: 'Native Physicians Licence', 1937. Produced in what is now Ghana and subsequently confiscated by the British-colonial government for contravening the Medical Practitioners and Dentists' Ordinance. Image courtesy of Public Records and Archives Administration Department (PRAAD), Accra, CSO/5/1/916.

American colonies were inherently other (Anderson 2006; Vaughan 1991). Woodward's phrase, its underlying assumption and its dissemination are representative of a broader trend in the construction and transmission of biomedical knowledge.

The biomedical framework consists of many interrelated sociotechnical systems that have developed in specific historical, political and social conditions, contributing to highly heterogeneous theories and practices. The development of these theories and practices has been strongly informed by the ideal of objectivity (see Wyatt, this volume) and a universal 'truth' about the body, in all its molecular and anatomical detail (Lock and Nguyen 2010). These ideas and practices show that biomedicine represents a paradox. On the one hand, it is temporally, spatially and culturally situated, on the other hand, it resists any such situatedness by conceptualising all human bodies as universally equivalent.

As scholarship in fields such as medical anthropology has shown, these universalising assumptions exist in the context of medical pluralism (see, for instance, Berger-González et al. 2016). Medical pluralism means that there are various interacting and contradictory ways of understanding health and disease, of practising treatment and of passing on this knowledge (see, for instance, Levin and Browner 2005; Helman 2007). Thus, the biomedical framework is only one of many approaches to medicine. Despite this multiplicity of medical knowledge systems, the biomedical narrative claims epistemic hegemony (Nogueira 2018). Based on the use of the scientific method and its epistemic authority (Shapin 2008), biomedical theories and practices are often presented as the only medical knowledge system that is valid and scientific, in turn, devaluing other medical knowledge systems as invalid or pseudoscientific, or dismissing them entirely (Nogueira 2018).

Scholars have criticised these dynamics as reinforcing colonial power relations on an epistemic level (Subramaniam et al. 2017). Alan Bleakley et al. (2008) focus particularly on medical education and discuss the dangers of the global diffusion of a unified medical curriculum that is largely based on European and North American ideas, practices and technologies. For them, a globally unified curriculum poses the risks of a '"new wave" of imperialism' (Bleakley et al. 2008: 266). To apply a key term of decolonial theory, coined by the Colombian philosopher Santiago Castro-Gómez, the danger of a globally unified curriculum and biomedical knowledge in general is the use of 'punto cero' ('point zero' or 'zero point') (2005: 40). The concept of punto cero refers to the perspective of an all-knowing subject that is observing and classifying from a neutral point of view, unaffected by a racialised body and colonial power structures. In other words, it is a perspective that hides its own particular perspective behind an abstract universalism (Grosfoguel 2007). By employing the strategy of *punto cero*, the biomedical framework pushes other knowledge systems to the margins.

Several contributions to this volume illuminate different medical knowledges that operate on the inner or outer edges of the biomedical framework, or which cross its boundaries. While one author draws particular attention to a peripheral knowledge system *within* the biomedical framework, others delineate medical epistemologies that have their roots *outside* of it. In other cases, authors discuss the interaction *between* biomedical and non-biomedical systems by focusing on specific objects that travel among them. Lastly, some authors highlight the importance of locally specific medical knowledge as a means to resist biomedicine's *punto cero*.

In her contribution, Rachel Prentice (this volume) discusses a certain type of knowledge that is based on biomedical ontology but nevertheless exists, as she mentions herself, at 'biomedicine's outer edges'. She calls this knowledge 'kinetic consciousness' and describes it as a form of understanding the physics of bodies in motion and the interdependency of different body parts. Prentice laments that the atomistic epistemology of biomedicine neglects kinetic consciousness by primarily focusing on molecular mechanisms.

In contrast to Prentice, Stacey Langwick and Mary Mosha (this volume) and Lan Li (this volume) highlight epistemic traditions rooted outside of biomedical tradition. Langwick and Mosha discuss the garden project Uzima in Tanzania, which is based on an epistemology that conceptualises the human body and well-being in close relation to its environmental surrounding. By shedding light on this garden project, they invite the reader to re-envision ideas on the biomedical body and anthropocentric medical education. Li, by contrast, discusses the materiality of Chinese medical epistemology. By analysing diverging drawings of the spleen meridian, Li demonstrates how medical illustrations give insight into ontological and cultural paradoxes; for example, how these drawings illustrate both a physical and an ephemeral ontology at the same time. They furthermore show how the bodies on which the spleen meridian is depicted represent a cultural negotiation between classical Chinese epistemology, Communist materialism and European realism.

Others have employed a different focus by shedding light on objects which travel between biomedical and non-biomedical spheres and which can change meaning in this process. For example, Claire Wendland (this volume) discusses how the stethoscope circulates between different social and geographical worlds. She describes how the stethoscope, which is often sent from companies that are headquartered in the Global North, is perceived in an educational context in Malawi. Based on ethnographic insight, Wendland suggests that the stethoscope symbolises 'the profession, the body of knowledge, the assemblage of tools and people, and the practices that we call biomedicine'. As a result of this symbolic meaning, she argues that the stethoscope also carries the epistemic authority that biomedicine is granted. While Wendland addresses the stethoscope's journey from the Global North to the Global South, other authors have focused on objects or organisms that travel the opposite direction. For instance, the historian of science Abena Dove Osseo-Asare (2014) gives insight into how various actors, including biomedical drug companies from the Global North, have worked since the 1880s to transform medicinal plants drawn from African countries into pharmaceutical drugs. Both Osseo-Asare and Wendland show how the movement of certain medical objects can mark economic and epistemic inequalities between the Global North and South.

Andrea Wojcik et al. (this volume) also address inequalities that manifest through materials used in medical contexts. They emphasise that the costs associated with purchasing and maintaining manikins and other simulation materials make them often unaffordable for educational institutions in the Global South. They therefore argue for the use of less costly, locally available resources in medical education. Wojcik et al. suggest that the consideration of local material would also encourage a shift in the conception of medical skills, from a unified set that is universally applicable to skills that are context-dependent.

In line with Wojcik et al., Robert Kumoji and John Nott (this volume) draw attention to the importance of local specificities in medical education. Through their conversation in the pathology museum at Ghana's Korle Bu Teaching Hospital, they show how the disintegration of specimens leads to a slow decay of knowledge regarding local pathologies. This material and epistemic decay stands in relation to the continuous expansion of biomedical knowledge. Kumoji and Nott argue that educative materials often carry certain practices that stem from 'imperial centres of knowledge production'. They suggest countering this epistemic force by making space for local biologies in medical education.

All these contributions provide interesting insights into different possibilities for understanding and teaching medicine. Based on their reflections on geographical and/or historical specificities, many of these authors raise questions on the universalising tendency of biomedicine and its implications for knowledge on the margins. Therefore, it can be said that they engage in what the Argentinian literary scholar Walter Mignolo calls 'epistemic disobedience' (2009: 160): they counter the *punto cero* perspective by providing diverse examples that challenge the idea of one universal form of medical knowledge. They acknowledge the existence of various medical epistemologies and highlight the importance of situated ways of producing and reproducing medical knowledge. Most importantly, they raise questions about who is constructing medical knowledge, with which materials and by which means, with what underlying assumptions and with what implications.

These chapters illustrate the value of engaging in epistemic disobedience within medical education. Based on the insights gained from them, Theodore Woodward's advice might be changed slightly. Instead of thinking of horses when hearing hoofbeats, it might sometimes be enriching to think of zebras – not in the sense of the animal, an extraordinary diagnosis, or an 'exotic' disease, but in the sense of those medical epistemologies which have been pushed to the margins.

References

Anderson, Warwick (2006), *Colonial Pathologies: American Tropical Medicine, Race, and Hygiene in the Philippines*, Durham: Duke University Press.

Berger-González, Mónica, Stauffacher, Michael, Zinsstag, Jakob, Edwards, Peter and Krütli, Pius (2016), 'Transdisciplinary research on cancer-healing systems between biomedicine and the maya of guatemala: A tool for reciprocal reflexivity in a multi-epistemological setting', *Qualitative health research*, 26:1, pp. 77–91.

Bleakley Alan, Brice, Julie and Bligh, John (2008), 'Thinking the post-colonial in medical education', *Medical Education*, 42:3, pp. 266–70.

Castro-Gómez, Santiago (2005), *La Hybris del Punto Cero: Ciencia, Raza e ilustración en la Nueva Granada (1750–1816)*, Bogotá: Editorial Pontificia Universidad Javeriana.

Grosfoguel, Ramón (2007), 'The epistemic decolonial turn: Beyond political-economy paradigms', *Cultural Studies*, 21:2–3, pp. 211–23.

Helman, Cecil G. (2007), *Culture, Health and Illness: An Introduction for Health Professionals*, 5th ed., London: Hodder Arnold.

Levin, Betty Wolder and Browner, Caroke H. (2005), 'The social production of health: Critical contributions from evolutionary, biological, and cultural Anthropology', *Social Science & Medicine*, 61:4, pp. 745–50.

Levine, David and Bleakley, Alan (2012), 'Maximising medicine through aphorisms: Maximising medicine through aphorisms', *Medical Education*, 46:2, pp. 153–62.

Lock, Margaret and Nguyen, Vinh-Kim (2010), *An Anthropology of Biomedicine*, Chichester: Wiley-Blackwell.

Mignolo, Walter D. (2009), 'Epistemic disobedience, independent thought and decolonial freedom', *Theory, Culture and Society*, 26:7–8, pp. 159–81.

Nogueira, Claudia (2018), 'Um olhar sociológico sobre o privilégio epistémico da biomedicina: desconstruindo a metanarrativa' ('A sociological view on the epistemic privilege of biomedicine: Deconstructing the metanarrative'), *Saúde E Sociedade*, 27:4, pp. 1019–32.

Osseo-Asare, Abena Dove Agyepoma (2014), *Bitter Roots: The Search for Healing Plants in Africa*, Chicago: University of Chicago Press.

Shapin, Steven (2008), 'Science and the modern world', in E. J. Hackett (ed.), *The Handbook of Science and Technology Studies*, 3rd ed., Cambridge: MIT Press, pp. 433–48.

Sotos, John G. (2006), *Zebra Cards: An Aid to Obscure Diagnoses*, Mount Vernon: Mount Vernon Book Systems.

Subramaniam, Banu, Foster, Laura, Harding, Sandra, Roy, Deboleena and TallBear, Kim (2017), 'Feminism, post-colonialism, technoscience', in U. Felt (ed.), *The Handbook of Science and Technology Studies*, 4th ed. Cambridge: MIT Press.

Vaughan, Megan (1991), *Curing Their Ills: Colonial Power and African Illness*, Stanford: Stanford University Press.

CONTRIBUTORS

Francis A. Abantanga is professor of paediatric surgery at the University for Development Studies, Tamale, Ghana. Until recently, he was also dean of the School of Medicine and Health Sciences. Between 1994 and 2015, he worked at the Kwame Nkrumah University of Science and Technology, in Kumasi, where he became professor of paediatric surgery and variously acted as vice dean of the School of Medical Sciences and head of the Department of Surgery.

Annmarie Adams is an architectural historian jointly appointed in the School of Architecture and Department of Social Studies of Medicine, McGill University. Educated at the University of California at Berkeley, her research focuses on the cultural landscapes of homes and hospitals, with special emphasis on how we embed health beliefs and gender expectations into the built environment.

Claire Aland is an anatomy lecturer at the University of Queensland. Her interests are in anatomy teaching, virtual microscopy, and online teaching and learning in anatomy and histology.

Rachel Vaden Allison is a Ph.D. candidate within the ERC-funded project 'Making Clinical Sense' at Maastricht University's Department of Society Studies. As part of this project, she conducted ethnographic fieldwork at Semmelweis University in Budapest, Hungary. Her work explores knowledge translation, with a focus on the embodied nature of anatomy training.

Anthony Amalba is an associate professor in health professions education at the University for Development Studies. He is a registered pharmacist who has worked in regulatory, hospital, academic and community settings. His research interests are in health professions education, inter-professional education, integrated curriculum development and pharmacy practice. He has worked as a consultant on problem-based learning (PBL) and community-based education and service (COBES) for universities in Benin, Burundi and Ethiopia.

Drew Danielle Belsky is a Ph.D. candidate in Science and Technology Studies at York University in Toronto. She also holds an MA from York University in interdisciplinary studies and the Diplôme National Supérieur d'Etudes Plastiques (DNSEP) in studio art from the Ecole Supérieure des Arts Décoratifs in Strasbourg, France.

Christian Bonah is a professor for the history of medical and health sciences at the University of Strasbourg. He has worked on the comparative history of medical education, medicines, human experimentation and, more recently, on the history of medical film. He is the principle investigator of the ERC-funded 'The healthy self as body capital: Individuals, market-based societies and body politics in visual twentieth century Europe'.

Paul Craddock is a cultural historian and author based in London. His debut book, *Spare Parts: A Surprising History of Transplants* (Penguin, 2021) won the Special Commendation of the Royal Society of Literature Giles St Aubyn Awards and was a *Daily Mail* Book of the Week. Paul is a Science Museum Group senior research associate, an honorary senior research associate of UCL's Division of Surgery, and a visiting lecturer at Imperial College London.

Jessica M. Dandona is a professor of art history at the Minneapolis College of Art and Design, and has received research grants from the Fulbright Association, the Boston Medical Library, the American Philosophical Society, the Huntington Library, and other institutions. Her current book project, *The Transparent Woman: Medical Visualities in Fin-de-Siècle Europe and the United States, 1880–1900*, examines the visual culture of medicine at the end of the nineteenth century.

Joël Danet is a researcher at the Department for History of Medical and Health Sciences at the University Strasbourg. He has worked in the field of visual education and documentary film history, and as a film programme curator for the documentary film association Vidéo les Beaux Jours in Strasbourg.

Denielle Elliott is an associate professor at York University in Toronto where she is the graduate programme director of the Science and Technology Studies Program. She is the author of *Reimagining Science and*

Statecraft in Postcolonial Kenya: Stories from an African Scientist (Routledge, 2019) and co-editor of *A Different Kind of Ethnography* (University of Toronto Press, 2017).

Ivana Guarrasi is a visiting assistant professor/teacher-scholar postdoctoral fellow in communication studies at Minnesota State University, Mankato. Her work brings together interdisciplinary communication studies, feminist science and technology studies, and cultural historical theories of learning in non-canonical educational settings in order to interrogate dominant medical epistemologies.

Dominic Hall is the curator of the Warren Anatomical Museum at the Center for the History of Medicine in the Countway Library of Medicine of Harvard Medical School. He has a master's in museology from the University of Washington and a master's in history from the Harvard University Extension School. Dominic is a past president of the Medical Museum Association.

Christine den Harder currently works as a teacher at the Skillslab at Maastricht University, where she has been teaching a wide array of physical examination techniques to undergraduate medical students for the past six years. Previously a general practitioner, she now also helps develop teaching materials regarding physical examination.

Anne Katrine Kleberg Hansen is a medical historian specialising in the concept of fatness in Western European medicine. She reived her Ph.D. from the University of Copenhagen (KU) and has since been a postdoctoral researcher at Max Planck Institute for the history of science, KU and a research associate at The School of Anthropology and Museum Ethnography, University at Oxford. She is currently research advisor at the Royal Danish Academy.

Anna Harris is an associate professor of anthropology and science and technology studies at Maastricht University, the Netherlands. Her work concerns issues of learning, sensing (and other bodily practices) and the contemporary/historical role of technologies in medicine. She leads the ERC-funded project 'Making Clinical Sense'.

Roger Kneebone is a professor of Surgical Education and Engagement Science, Imperial College London and a clinician and educationalist who leads the Centre for Engagement and Simulation Science at Imperial and, with the Royal College of Music, the Imperial Centre for Performance Science. His multidisciplinary research into contextualised simulation and embodied knowledge builds on his personal experience as a surgeon and a general practitioner, and his interest in domains of expertise beyond medicine.

Kaisu Koski is a cross-disciplinary artist and an associate professor of art and design at Lab4Living at Sheffield Hallam University. Her work explores empathy, human-nonhuman relationships, and climate crisis, and it involves collaboration with scientists, clinicians and engineers.

Robert Kumoji studied medicine at the Kwame Nkrumah University of Science and Technology, in Kumasi. He has recently retired from a career as a specialist pathologist for the Ghana Health Service, based at Korle Bu Teaching Hospital, in Accra.

Stacey Langwick is an associate professor in the Department of Anthropology at Cornell University. She is author of *Bodies, Politics and African Healing: The Matter of Maladies in Tanzania* (Indiana University Press, 2011) and co-editor of *Medicine, Mobility and Power in Global Africa* (Indiana University Press, 2011). In addition to collaborating with the Uzima Project, she is currently finishing a second sole-authored book entitled *Medicines That Feed Us: Plants, Healing and Sovereignty in a Toxic World*.

Jakob Lehne studied in London and Berlin and completed his Ph.D. in intellectual history at the European University Institute in 2015. He is a curator and historian at the collections of the Medical University of Vienna (Josephinum) and lectures on the history of medicine. His main interests include the historiography of medicine/science, the history of gynecology, and the public history of medicine.

Harro van Lente is a professor of science and technology studies at Maastricht University. He is one of the founders of the Sociology of Expectations, which studies how representations of the future shape current socio-technical developments. He has published more than 100 journal articles, book chapters and edited volumes on technology dynamics, innovation policy and knowledge production.

Lan A. Li is a historian of the body, focusing on medicine and health in global Johns Hopkins University. Li's work primarily centers on histories of anatomical representations of meridians and nerves with a new project on the history of numbness, drawing on approaches in postcolonial science studies, disability studies, digital and health humanities.

Mary-Louise Roy Manchadi is a Pharmacology lecturer at the University of Queensland. She is passionate about effective communication of complex concepts in a diversity of degree programmes.

Victor Mogre is an associate professor of nutrition education and training at the University for Development Studies. He has experience designing, developing and reviewing innovative curricula and teaching materials. He has expertise conducting quantitative and qualitative research into nutrition education; non-communicable disease treatment and management; and maternal and child nutrition.

Mary Vincent Mosha is a lecturer in the Community Health Department at Kilimanjaro Christian Medical University College (KCMC). She holds a M.Sc. in Nutrition for Global Health from the London School of Hygiene and Tropical Medicine and an MPH from KCMC. In addition to collaborating with the Uzima Project, she is working towards her Ph.D. in nutrition at KCMC, which examines primary school policies concerning nutrition and physical activity in Tanzania.

John Nott is an economic and medical historian, currently engaged as a research fellow on the ERC-funded project 'The epidemy: A History of epidemiological reasoning', at the University of Edinburgh. He has previously worked at the University of Ghana, the University of Leeds, and was part of the 'Making Clinical Sense' project at Maastricht University.

Fleur Oakes is a textile artist specialising in raised embroidery and lacemaking. In 2016, she became lacemaker in residence for Imperial College London, attached to the vascular surgery department.

Kirsten Ostherr is the Gladys Louise Fox professor of English and director of the Medical Humanities programme at Rice University. She is the author of *Medical Visions: Producing the Patient through Film, Television and Imaging Technologies* and *Cinematic Prophylaxis: Globalization and Contagion in the Discourse of World Health* (Oxford University Press, 2013), and editor of *Applied Media Studies* (Routledge, 2017).

Harriet Palfreyman lectures in science and health communication at the University of Manchester. Her background is in history and her research looks at the visual cultures of disease and surgery from the nineteenth century to the present day.

Rachel Prentice is an associate professor in the Department of Science & Technology Studies, Cornell University. Her work has focused on medicine, movement, the body, and animals. She is the author of *Bodies in Formation: An Ethnography of Anatomy and Surgery Education* (Duke University Press, 2013). She is currently working on the ethics, epistemics and aesthetics of humans and horses in motion.

Celia Yamile Rodriguez is the head of family medicine and primary care and is also skills coordinator at the School of Medicine and Health Sciences at the University for Development Studies in Tamale. She also works as supervising family physician for the northern cluster of Accredited Training Complexes in Ghana.

Candida Sánchez Burmester is a Ph.D. student in Science and Technology Studies at Maastricht University. Her Ph.D. is part of the ERC-funded synergy project 'NanoBubbles: How, When and Why Does Science Fail to Correct Itself?' In this project she employs ethnographic and historical methods to analyse how over-stated and erroneous claims have circulated at conferences in the field of nanobiology. Her research interests lie in scientific practices, environmentalism, and perspectives from the Global South.

Angela Saward is a research development specialist (Moving Image & Sound) at Wellcome Collection, working with the collection's extensive archive of historical medical films throughout her professional career there. She has given papers and published articles on Wellcome's unique and distinctive collections.

Nicole Shepherd is a sociologist teaching ethics and professional practice at The University of Queensland. She started her career with a science degree before moving into social science. Her scholarly interests include the interconnections between science, social science and ethics.

Belinda Swyny is an experienced lecturer of medicine at The University of Queensland. She has specialised in simulation education and clinical practice. Her scholarly pursuits lie in using creative processes to help students form clinical reasoning skills and meaning making processes.

David Theodore is Canada Research Chair in Architecture, Health, and Computation at the McGill University Peter Guo-hua Fu School of Architecture. He has co-published on the history of healthcare architecture in *Social Science & Medicine*, *Technology and Culture*, and the *Canadian Bulletin of Medical History*.

Kelly Underman is an assistant professor in the Department of Sociology and the Center for Science, Technology and Society at Drexel University.

Claire Wendland is a professor in the departments of Anthropology and Obstetrics & Gynecology at University of Wisconsin-Madison. She is the author of *A Heart for the Work: Journeys through an African Medical School* (University of Chicago Press, 2010), the first ethnography of a medical school in the Global South, and *Partial Stories: Maternal Death from Six Angles* (University of Chicago Press, 2022) .

Rebecca Whiteley is the Shreeve Fellow in the History of Medicine at the John Rylands Research Institute and Library, University of Manchester. Her work focuses on the intersections between visual culture, history of medicine and material culture. She has published in *British Art Studies* and *Social History of Medicine* and has a monograph forthcoming with University of Chicago Press on early modern illustrations of pregnancy.

Peter Winter is a sociologist of science and technology and research associate at the University of Bristol, United Kingdom. He is interested in the sociotechnical analysis of professional work, the nature of expertise and embodied practice, and challenges of developing, integrating and implementing digital technologies.

Andrea Wojcik is a Ph.D. candidate within the ERC-funded project 'Making Clinical Sense' at Maastricht University's Department of Society Studies. As part of this project, she conducted ethnographic fieldwork at the University for Development Studies in Ghana. Her work explores the role of technology in learning to touch in medical education.

Sally Wyatt is a professor of digital cultures at Maastricht University. Her research focuses on the role of digital technologies in healthcare, and on the ways digital technologies affect the production of knowledge in the humanities and the social sciences. Her book (co-authored with Anna Harris and Susan Kelly), *CyberGenetics: Health Genetics and New Media* (Routledge, 2016), was awarded the 2017 Foundation for the Sociology of Health & Illness Book Prize.

INDEX

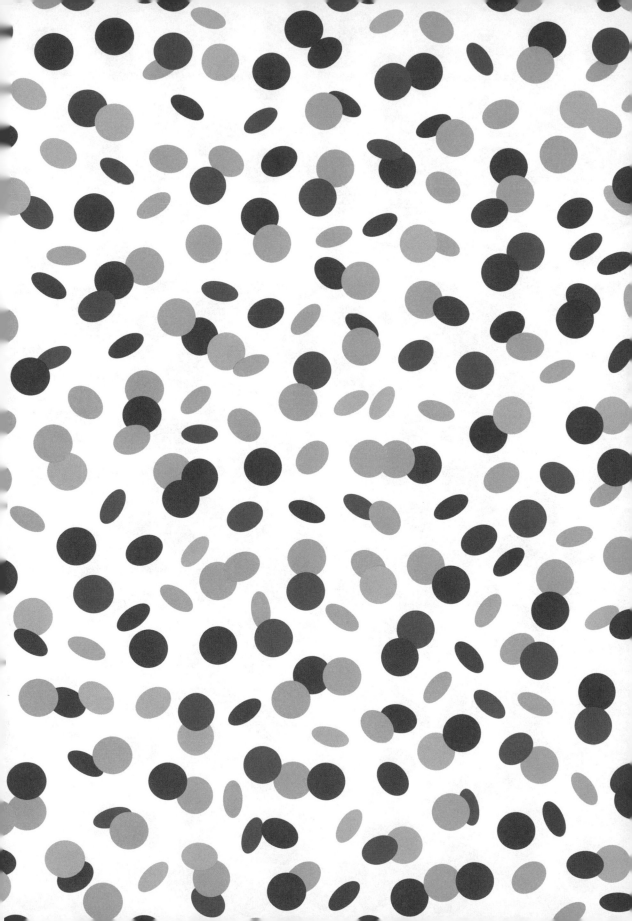

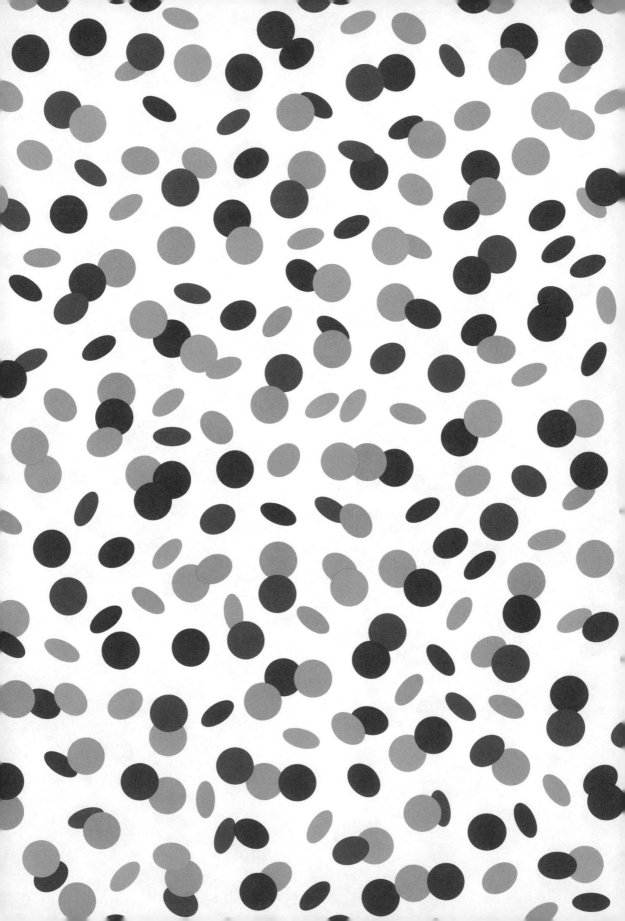

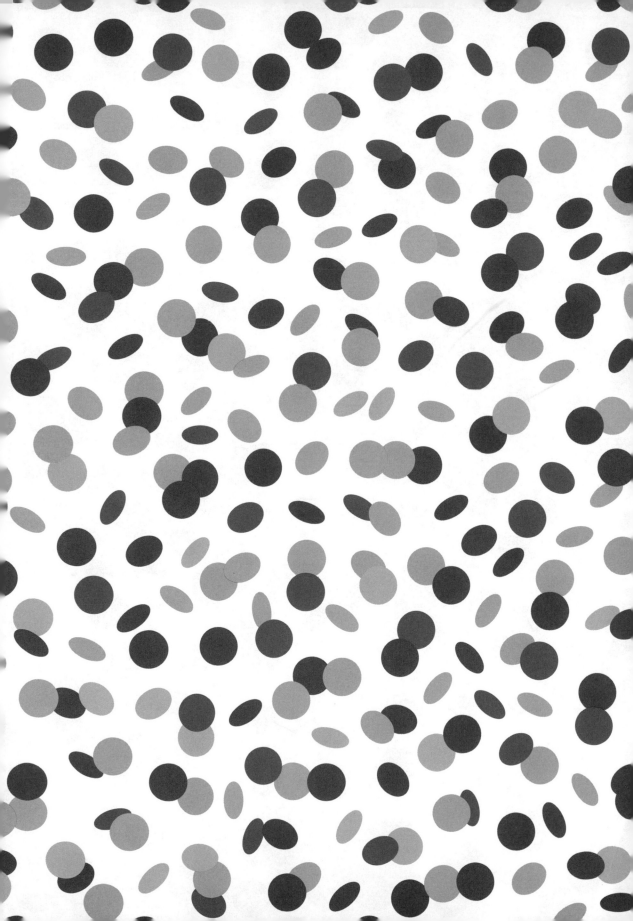

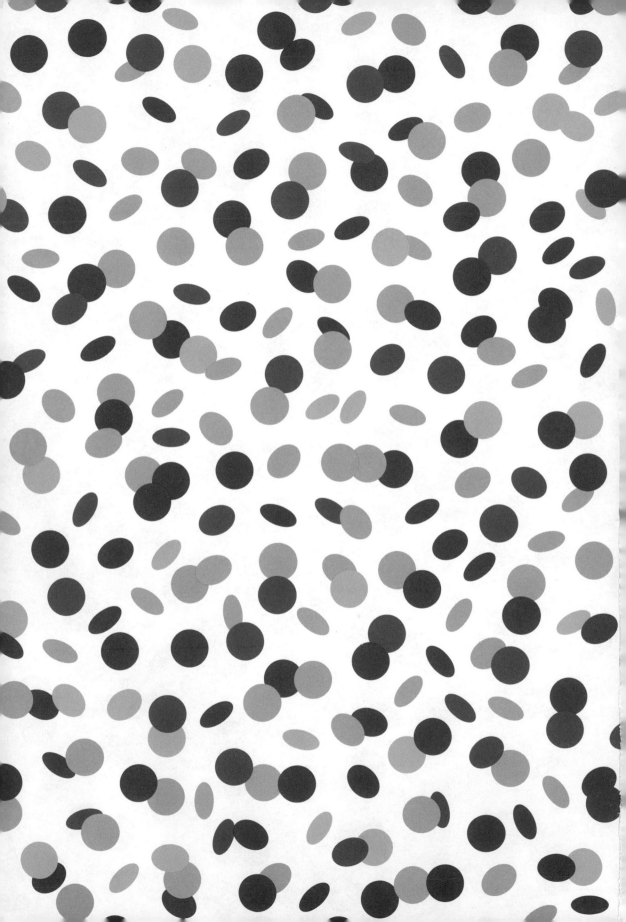